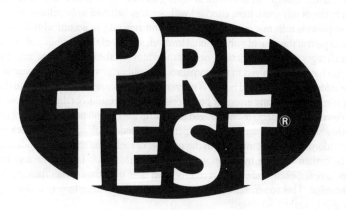

Pathology

PreTest® Self-Assessment and Review

NOTICE

Medicine is an ever-changing science. As new research and clinical experience broaden our knowledge, changes in treatment and drug therapy are required. The editor and the publisher of this work have checked with sources believed to be reliable in their efforts to provide information that is complete and generally in accord with the standards accepted at the time of publication. However, in view of the possibility of human error or changes in medical sciences, neither the editor nor the publisher nor any other party who has been involved in the preparation or publication of this work warrants that the information contained herein is in every respect accurate or complete and they are not responsible for any errors or omissions or for the results obtained from use of such information. Readers are encouraged to confirm the information contained herein with other sources. For example and in particular, readers are advised to check the product information sheet included in the package of each drug they plan to administer to be certain that the information contained in this book is accurate and that changes have not been made in the recommended dose or in the contraindications for administration. This recommendation is of particular importance in connection with new or infrequently used drugs.

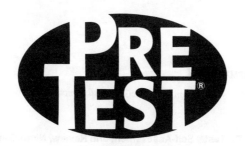

Pathology
PreTest® Self-Assessment and Review

Ninth Edition

EDITED BY
EARL J. BROWN, M.D.
Associate Professor
Department of Pathology
Quillen College of Medicine
Johnson City, Tennessee

Chief of Hematopathology
Department of Pathology
VA Medical Center
Mountain Home, Tennessee

STUDENT REVIEWERS
MARK XUEREB
St. George's University School of Medicine
Grenada, West Indies

PHILIP H. CHANG
University of Alabama School of Medicine
Birmingham, Alabama

 McGraw-Hill
Health Professions Division
PreTest® Series

NEW YORK   ST. LOUIS   SAN FRANCISCO   AUCKLAND
BOGOTÁ   CARACAS   LISBON   LONDON   MADRID
MEXICO CITY   MILAN   MONTREAL   NEW DELHI
SAN JUAN   SINGAPORE   SYDNEY   TOKYO   TORONTO

McGraw-Hill

A Division of The McGraw-Hill Companies

Pathology: PreTest® Self-Assessment and Review, Ninth Edition
International Editions 1999

3 4 5 6 7 8 9 0 KKP FC 2 0

ISBN 0-07-052686-9

The editors were John J. Dolan, Susan R. Noujaim, and Jennifer Prior.
The editing supervisor was Peter McCurdy.
The production supervisor was Helene G. Landers.
This book was set in Berkeley Book by Joanne Morbit of McGraw-Hill's Professional Book Group composition unit, Hightstown, NJ.

When ordering this title, use ISBN 0-07-116686-6

Printed in Singapore

CONTENTS

PREFACE

The study of pathology, a science so basic to clinical medicine, has been abbreviated sadly in many medical schools in recent years, and at a time when explosive growth is occurring in the science. Recent advances in immunopathology, diagnosis of bacterial and viral diseases including AIDS, and detection of infectious agents such as papillomavirus in cervical dysplasia are proceeding at a tremendous rate. The ninth edition of Pathology: PreTest® Self-Assessment and Review includes such new subject areas as predictive values in the interpretation of laboratory data, importance of cytokines, the molecular basis of genetic and other disease processes, and molecular biology techniques as these apply to lymphoproliferative disorders and other tumors.

The medical student must feel submerged at times in the flood of information—occasionally instructors may have similar feelings. This edition is not intended to cover all new knowledge in addition to including older anatomic and clinical pathology. It is, rather, a serious attempt to present important facts about many disease processes in hopes that the student will read much further in major textbooks and journals and will receive some assistance in passing medical school, licensure, or board examinations.

INTRODUCTION

Each *PreTest® Self-Assessment and Review* allows medical students to comprehensively and conveniently assess and review their knowledge of a particular basic science, in this instance Pathology. The 500 questions parallel the format and degree of difficulty of the questions found in the United States Medical Licensing Examination (USMLE) Step 1. Practicing physicians who want to hone their skills before USMLE Step 3 or recertification may find this to be a good beginning in their review process.

Each question is accompanied by an answer, a paragraph explanation, and a specific page reference to an appropriate textbook or journal article. A bibliography listing sources can be found following the last chapter of this text.

An effective way to use this PreTest is to allow yourself one minute to answer each question in a given chapter. As you proceed, indicate your answer beside each question. By following this suggestion, you approximate the time limits imposed by the Step.

After you finish going through the questions in the section, spend as much time as you need verifying your answers and carefully reading the explanations provided. Pay special attention to the explanations for the questions you answered incorrectly—but read *every* explanation. The author of this material has designed the explanations to reinforce and supplement the information tested by the questions. If you feel you need further information about the material covered, consult and study the references indicated.

The High-Yield Facts added for this edition are provided to facilitate rapid review of Pathology topics. It is anticipated that the reader will use the High-Yield Facts as a "memory jog" before proceeding through the questions.

| Laboratory Values | | |
Substance	Source	Normal
Albumin	Serum	3.2–4.5 g/dl
Alkaline phosphatase	Serum	20–130 IU/L
Bicarbonate	Plasma	21–28 mM
Bilirubin, direct (conjugated)	Serum	<0.3 mg/dL
Bilirubin, indirect (unconjugated)	Serum	0.1–1.0 mg/dL
Bilirubin, total	Serum	0.1–1.2 mg/dL
BUN	Serum	8–23 mg/dL
Calcium	Serum	9.2–11.0 mg/dl (4.6–5.5 mEq/l)
Chloride	Serum	95–103 mEq/L
Cholesterol	Serum	150–250 mg/dL
Creatinine	Serum	0.6–1.2 mg/dL
GGT (γ - glutamyltransferase)	Serum	5–40 IU/L
Glucose (fasting)	Serum	70–110 mg/dl
Insulin	Plasma	4–24 μIU/ml
Iron	Serum	60–150 μg/dL
Iron saturation	Serum	20–55%
Osmolality	Serum	280–295 mosm/L
Phosphorus	Serum	2.3–4.7 mg/dl
Potassium	Plasma	3.8–5.0 mEq/L
Protein	Serum	6.0–7.8 g/dL
Sodium	Plasma	136–142 mEq/L
T3 resin uptake	Serum	25–38 relative % uptake
Thyrotropin (TSH)	Serum	0.5–5 μIU/ml
Thyroxine, free (FT4)	Serum	0.9–2.3 ng/dL
Thyroxine, total (T4)	Serum	5.5–12.5 μg/dL
Triiodothyronine (T3)	Serum	80–200 mg/dL
Hematology		
Platelet count		150,000–450,000/μL
White cell count		4,440–11,000/μL
Lymphocyte count		1,000–4,800/μL (about 34%)
Mean corpuscular volume (MCV)		80–96 μm^3
Mean corpuscular hemoglobin (MCH)		27.5–33.2 pg
Mean corpuscular hemoglobin concentration (MCHC)		33.4–35.5%
Hemoglobin	Whole blood	Female 12–16 g/dL Male 13.5–18 g/dL

GENERAL PATHOLOGY

Questions

DIRECTIONS: Each question below contains five suggested responses. Select the **one best** response to each question.

1. A 54-year-old male develops a thrombus in his left anterior descending coronary artery. The area of myocardium supplied by this vessel is irreversibly injured. The thrombus is destroyed by the infusion of streptokinase, which is a plasminogen activator, and the injured area is reperfused. The patient, however, develops an arrhythmia and dies. An electron microscopic (EM) picture taken from the irreversibly injured myocardium reveals the presence of large, dark, irregular amorphic densities. These flocculent densities are typically found within the

a. Golgi apparatus
b. Mitochondria
c. Nucleus
d. Rough endoplasmic reticulum
e. Smooth endoplasmic reticulum

2. A 49-year-old male presents with symptoms that developed following a long weekend of binge drinking. His serum reveals a gamma-glutamyl transferase (GGT) level of 65 IU/L. A liver biopsy reveals fatty change (steatosis) of numerous hepatocytes. This patient's liver abnormality is most likely the result of

a. Decreased free fatty acid delivery to the liver
b. Decreased production of triglycerides
c. Increased mitochondrial oxidation of fatty acids
d. Increased NADH production
e. Increased release of lipoproteins

fatty change
steroid use
starvation
DM
Alcohol.

3. A 48-year-old male who has a long history of excessive drinking presents with signs of alcoholic hepatitis. Microscopic examination of a biopsy of this patient's liver reveals irregular eosinophilic hyaline inclusions within the cytoplasm of the hepatocytes. These eosinophilic inclusions are composed of

a. Immunoglobulin
b. Excess plasma proteins
c. Prekeratin intermediate filaments
d. Basement membrane material
e. Lipofuscin

4. The involution of the thymus that occurs with aging is an example of the process of programmed cell death that is best described as

a. Apoptosis
b. Pyknosis
c. Karyorrhexis
d. Karyolysis
e. Pinocytosis

5. A 49-year-old man suffers an acute myocardial infarction because of the sudden occlusion of the left anterior descending coronary artery. The areas within the ventricle of myocardial necrosis can best be described as

a. Coagulative necrosis
b. Liquefactive necrosis
c. Fat necrosis
d. Caseous necrosis
e. Fibrinoid necrosis

6. Which of the following provides an example of concomitant hyperplasia and hypertrophy?

a. Uterine growth during pregnancy
b. Left ventricular cardiac hypertrophy
c. Enlargement of skeletal muscle in athletes
d. Breast enlargement at puberty
e. Cystic hyperplasia of the endometrium

7. An adult patient presents with the sudden onset of massive diarrhea. Grossly, this individual's stool has the appearance of "rice-water" because of the presence of flecks of mucus. Cultures of this patient's stool grow *Vibrio cholera*, a curved, gram-negative rod that secretes an enterotoxin consisting of a toxic A subunit and a binding B subunit. The cholera enterotoxin causes massive diarrhea by

a. Inhibiting the conversion of Gi-GDP to Gi-GTP
b. Inhibiting the conversion of Gs-GTP to Gs-GDP
c. Stimulating the conversion of Gi-GDP to Gi-GTP
d. Stimulating the conversion of Gs-GDP to Gs-GTP
e. Stimulating the conversion of Gs-GTP to Gs-GDP

8. A patient presents with a large wound to his right forearm that is the result of a chain-saw accident. You treat his wound appropriately and follow him in your surgery clinic at routine intervals. Initially his wound is filled with granulation tissue, which is composed of proliferating fibroblasts and proliferating new blood vessels (*angiogenesis*). A growth factor that is capable of inducing all the steps necessary for angiogenesis is

a. Epidermal growth factor (EGF)
b. Transforming growth factor α (TGF-α)
c. Platelet-derived growth factor (PDGF)
d. Basic fibroblast growth factor (FGF)
e. Transforming growth factor β (TGF-β)

9. Early during the acute inflammatory process neutrophils marginate to the periphery of blood vessels. An important adhesive surface protein found on these neutrophils, but absent in patients with leukocyte adhesion deficiency type 1, is

a. E-selectin
b. L-selectin
c. Leukocyte function antigen 1 (LFA-1)
d. Intracellular adhesion molecule 1 (ICAM-1)
e. Vascular adhesion molecule 1 (VCAM-1)

10. Neutrophil movement (chemotaxis) involves the binding of certain substances to receptors (Gq) on the neutrophil membrane and the subsequent activation of phospholipase C. Plasma membrane phosphatidylinositol-4,5-biphosphate (PIP$_2$) is cleaved to form inositol-1,4,5-triphosphate (IP$_3$) and diacylglycerol (DAG). Eventually intracellular calcium ion levels are increased, which then results in the assembly of the contractile elements in the cytoplasm of leukocytes, namely actin and myosin, to cause movement. Which one of the listed components of the complement cascade is a chemotactic factor for neutrophils that is capable of activating this mechanism?

a. C3a
b. C3b
c. C5a
d. C5b
e. C5-9

11. Which one of the following substances is produced by the action of lipoxygenase on arachidonic acid, is a potent chemotactic factor for neutrophils, and causes aggregation and adhesion of leukocytes?

a. C5a
b. Prostacyclin
c. IL-8
d. Thromboxane A$_2$
e. Leukotriene B$_4$

12. A 24-year-old female presents with severe pain during menses (dysmenorrhea). To treat her symptoms you advise her to take indomethacin in the hopes that it will reduce her pain by interfering with the production of

a. Bradykinin
b. Histamine
c. Leukotrienes
d. Phospholipase A_2
e. Prostaglandin F_2

13. A very important mediator of the systemic effects of inflammation is

a. Gamma interferon (γ-IFN)
b. Beta tumor necrosis factor (β-TNF)
c. Interleukin 1 (IL-1)
d. Interleukin 2 (IL-2)
e. Interleukin 3 (IL-3)

14. The cells of the mononuclear phagocyte system originate from the

a. Spleen
b. Liver
c. Lymph node
d. Bone marrow
e. Thymus

15. Normal levels of C-reactive protein (CRP) are most often observed in

a. Acute viral illness
b. Pneumococcal pneumonia
c. Active rheumatoid arthritis
d. Active pulmonary tuberculosis
e. Acute myocardial infarction

16. A 47-year-old male presents with pain in the mid-portion of his chest. The pain is associated with eating and swallowing food. Endoscopic examination reveals an ulcerated area in the lower portion of his esophagus. Histologic sections of tissue taken from this area reveal an ulceration of the esophageal mucosa that is filled with blood, fibrin, proliferating blood vessels, and proliferating fibroblasts. Mitoses are easily found, and most of the cells have prominent nucleoli. Which one of the following correctly describes this ulcerated area?

a. Caseating granulomatous inflammation
b. Dysplastic epithelium
c. Granulation tissue
d. Squamous cell carcinoma
e. Noncaseating granulomatous inflammation

17. An exudate is the result of

a. Increased venous pressure
b. Sodium retention
c. Decreased plasma oncotic pressure
d. Increased capillary permeability
e. Lymphatic obstruction

18. "Heart failure cells" are present within the alveoli as a result of

a. Petechial hemorrhage
b. Ecchymoses
c. Purpura
d. Active hyperemia
e. Passive hyperemia

19. Procoagulant factors produced by endothelial cells include

a. Thrombomodulin
b. Prostacyclin
c. Von Willebrand factor
d. Thromboxane A_2
e. Fibrinogen

20. The action of streptokinase involves the formation of

a. Antithrombin III
b. Protein C
c. Plasmin
d. Thrombin
e. C91 inactivator

21. Which of the following conditions is most likely to predispose to thrombosis and embolism?

a. Atrial fibrillation
b. Pulmonary stenosis
c. Ventricular septal defect
d. Aortic stenosis
e. Atrial septal defect

22. A patient hospitalized for fractures of the long bones who develops mental dysfunction, increasing respiratory insufficiency, and renal failure should be suspected of having

a. Fat embolism syndrome
b. Disseminated intravascular coagulopathy
c. Myocardial infarction
d. Aortic valve disease
e. Respiratory distress syndrome

23. A 9-year-old boy suddenly develops severe testicular pain. He is taken to the emergency room where he is evaluated and immediately taken to surgery. There his left testis is found to be markedly hemorrhagic due to testicular torsion. This abnormality caused a hemorrhagic testicular infarction because of

a. Arterial occlusion
b. Septic infarction
c. The collateral blood supply of the testis
d. The dual blood supply of the testis
e. Venous occlusion

24. A 52-year-old male presents with symptoms of gastric pain after eating. While working up this patient, a 3 cm mass is found in the wall of the stomach. This mass is resected and histologic examination reveals a tumor composed of cells having elongated, spindle-shaped nuclei. The tumor does not connect to the overlying epithelium and is found only in the wall of the stomach. This tumor most likely originated from

a. Adipocytes
b. Endothelial cells
c. Glandular epithelial cells
d. Smooth muscle cells
e. Squamous epithelial cells

25. A 35-year-old male presents with the new onset of a "bulge" in his left inguinal area. After performing your physical examination, you diagnose the "bulge" to be an inguinal hernia. You refer the patient to a surgeon who repairs the hernia and sends the resected hernia sac to the pathology laboratory along with some adipose tissue, which he calls a "lipoma of the cord." The pathology resident examines the tissue grossly, microscopically, and decides that it is not a neoplastic lipoma, but instead is non-neoplastic normal adipose tissue. Which one of the following features would have been present had the lesion been a lipoma rather than normal adipose tissue?

a. Anaplasia
b. Fibrous capsule
c. Numerous mitoses
d. Prominent nucleoli
e. Uniform population of cells

26. A 45-year-old male during a routine physical examination is found to have microscopic hematuria. Further work-up finds a 4.5 cm mass in the upper pole of his right kidney. This mass is resected and reveals a tumor composed of a uniform population of cells with clear cytoplasm. Mitoses are not found. Further work-up fails to reveal the presence of any metastatic disease. Based on all of these findings, which of the following best characterizes this tumor? (Note: Assume that a low stage has a better prognosis than a high stage, and a low grade has a better prognosis than a high grade. Also assume that renal tumors composed of cells with clear cytoplasm that are larger than 2.0 cm in diameter are malignant.)

	tumor	grade	stage
a.	benign	not applicable	not applicable
b.	malignant	low	low
c.	malignant	low	high
d.	malignant	high	low
e.	malignant	high	high

Burkitts (8:14) - CMyc - IgM

CML t(9:22) bcr-abl tyrosine kinase activity

Follicular t(18:14) - bcl2

27. A 4-year-old African boy develops a rapidly enlarging mass that involves the right side of face. Biopsies of this lesion reveal a prominent "starry-sky" pattern produced by proliferating small, non-cleaved malignant lymphocytes. Based on this microscopic appearance, the diagnosis of Burkitt's lymphoma is made. This neoplasm most probably developed by which of the following mechanisms?

a. Gene amplification of erb-B
b. Point mutation of c-ras
c. Translocation of bcl-2 to the heavy chain region of chromosome 14
d. Translocation of c-abl to form the Philadelphia chromosome
e. Translocation of c-myc to the heavy chain region of chromosome 14

28. An example of a cancer suppressor gene is

a. C-abl
b. Bcr
c. C-myc
d. P53
e. Ras

29. A 35-year-old male living in a southern region of Africa presents with increasing abdominal pain and jaundice. He has worked as a farmer for many years, and sometimes his grain has become moldy. Physical examination reveals a large mass involving the right side of his liver, and a biopsy specimen from this mass confirms the diagnosis of liver cancer (hepatocellular carcinoma). The pathogenesis of this tumor involves which of the following substances?

a. Aflatoxin B_1
b. Direct acting alkylating agents
c. Vinyl chloride
d. Azo dyes
e. Beta-naphthylamine

30. A 17-year-old male presents with a lesion on his face that measures approximately 1.5 cm in greatest dimension. He has a history of numerous similar skin lesions that have occurred mainly in sun-exposed areas. This present lesion is biopsied and reveals an invasive squamous cell carcinoma. This patient most probably has one type of a group of inherited diseases associated with unstable DNA and increased incidence of carcinoma. What is the diagnosis for this patient?

a. Xeroderma pigmentosa
b. Wiskott-Aldrich syndrome
c. Familial polyposis
d. Sturge-Weber syndrome
e. Multiple endocrine neoplasia, type I (MEN I)

31. A 59-year-old male is found to have a 3.5 cm mass in the right upper lobe of his lung. A biopsy of this mass is diagnosed as a moderately differentiated squamous cell carcinoma. Work-up reveals that no bone metastases are present, but laboratory examination reveals that his serum calcium levels are 11.5 mg/dl. This patient's paraneoplastic syndrome is most likely the result of production of

a. Parathyroid hormone
b. Parathyroid hormone-related peptide
c. Calcitonin
d. Calcitonin-related peptide
e. Erythropoietin

32. An apathetic male infant in an underdeveloped country is found to have peripheral edema, a "moon" face, and an enlarged, fatty liver. Which of the following is one mechanism involved in the pathogenesis of this child's abnormalities?

a. Decreased protein intake leading to decreased lipoproteins
b. Decreased caloric intake leading to hypoalbuminemia
c. Decreased carbohydrate intake leading to hypoglycemia
d. Decreased fluid intake leading to hypernatremia
e. Decreased fat absorption leading to hypovitaminosis

33. A patient with a malabsorption syndrome who develops a deficiency of vitamin A is most likely to develop which one of the following abnormalities?

a. Acute leukemia
b. Intestinal metaplasia
c. Megaloblastic anemia
d. Night blindness
e. Soft bones

34. A significant deficiency in vitamin D might be expected to lead to

a. Hyperostosis
b. Relative excess of osteoid tissue
c. Increased absorption of calcium
d. Decreased production of bone matrix
e. Adequate serum phosphorus

35. A 70-year-old female is brought to the emergency room by her granddaughter because she has developed ecchymosis covering many areas of her body. Her granddaughter states that her grandmother lives alone at home and has not been eating well. Her diet has consisted of mainly tea and toast, as she does not eat milk, fruits, or vegetables. Your physical examination reveals small hemorrhages around hair follicles, some of these follicles having an unusual "cork-screw" appearance. You also notice swelling and hemorrhages of her gingiva. What is the most likely diagnosis?

a. Beriberi
b. Kwashiorkor
c. Pellagra
d. Rickets
e. Scurvy

36. δ-Aminolevulinic acid is excreted in increased amounts in the urine of patients with

a. Lead poisoning
b. Carcinoma of the pancreas
c. Chronic pyelonephritis
d. Vitamin C intoxication
e. Ulcerative colitis

37. An industrial foundry worker who has been chronically exposed to heavy metal vapors has developed a radiographic pattern of pulmonary "honeycombing." Which of the following heavy metals is most likely responsible?

a. Cobalt
b. Lead
c. Cadmium
d. Mercury
e. Arsenic

38. A comatose 27-year-old woman is brought to the emergency room by paramedics, and the strong odor of bitter almonds is present. The differential diagnosis must include the possibility of poisoning by

a. Ethylene glycol
b. Carbon monoxide
c. Mercury
d. Cyanide
e. Methanol

39. If a mutant gene is not expressed phenotypically in a person, this is said to represent

a. Variable expressivity
b. Reduced penetrance
c. Codominance
d. Genetic heterogeneity
e. Nondisjunction

40. A sex-linked recessive mode of inheritance exists in
a. Myotonic dystrophy
b. Limb-girdle dystrophy
c. Facioscapulohumeral dystrophy
d. Duchenne's muscular dystrophy
e. Polymyositis

41. A 23-year-old female presents with progressive bilateral loss of central vision. You obtain a detailed family history from this patient and produce the associated pedigree (dark circles or squares indicate affected individuals). Which of the following transmission patterns is most consistent with this patient's family history?

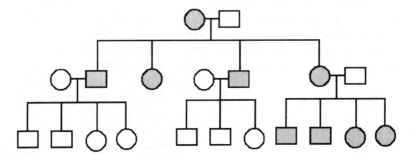

a. Autosomal recessive
b. Autosomal dominant
c. X-linked recessive
d. X-linked dominant
e. Mitochondrial

42. In tissues affected by the predominant form of Niemann-Pick disease, which of the following is found at abnormally high levels?
a. Sphingomyelin
b. Sphingomyelinase
c. Kerasin
d. Acetyl coenzyme A
e. Ganglioside

43. The abnormality most compatible with a diagnosis of von Gierke's disease is a deficiency of

a. Glucose-6-phosphatase
b. Glucose-6-phosphate dehydrogenase
c. Branching enzyme
d. Muscle phosphorylase
e. Lysosomal glucosidase

44. A 10-month-old baby is being evaluated for visual problems and motor incoordination. Examination of this child's fundus reveals a bright "cherry-red spot" at the macula. Talking to the family of this visually impaired 10-month-old infant, you find that they are Jewish and their family is from the eastern portion of Europe (Ashkenazi Jews). Based on this specific family history, which one of the following enzymes is most likely to be deficient in this infant?

a. Aryl sulfatase
b. Beta-glucocerebrosidase
c. Hexosaminidase A
d. Hexosaminidase B
e. Sphingomyelinase

45. The photomicrograph below is of the spleen from an adult patient who had marked splenomegaly. Which of the following abnormalities is most compatible with the changes seen in the spleen?

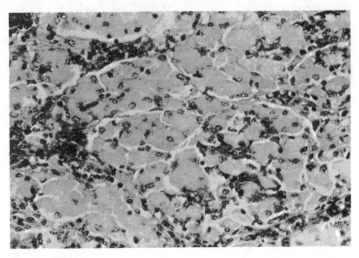

a. Glucocerebrosidase deficiency
b. Glucose-6-phosphate dehydrogenase deficiency
c. Glucuronidase deficiency
d. Lysosomal glucosidase deficiency
e. α-Galactosidase deficiency

46. The cell in the photomicrograph below was found in a bone marrow aspirate from a 25-year-old man. Such a cell is generally considered pathognomonic for

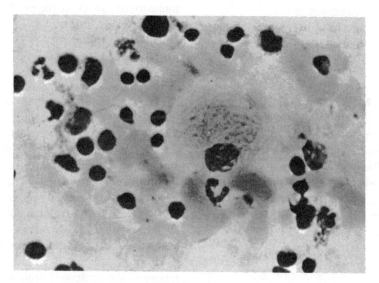

a. Niemann-Pick disease
b. Histiocytic lymphoma
c. Megaloblastic anemia
d. Gaucher's disease
e. Myelogenous leukemia

47. A 45-year-old man presents with severe pain in both knee joints. At the time of surgery, his cartilage is found to have a dark blue-black color. Further evaluation revealed that this patient's urine darkened rapidly with time. The most likely diagnosis for this abnormality is

a. Hyperphenylalaninemia
b. Tyrosinemia
c. Tyrosinase-positive oculocutaneous albinism
d. Alcaptonuria
e. Maple syrup urine disease

48. A chromosomal aberration that results in a disturbance in the normal gene balance is termed

a. Nondisjunction
b. Euploidy
c. Aneuploidy
d. Breakage
e. Variance

49. A 2-month-old girl presents with a soft, high-pitched, mewing cry and is found to have several congenital heart defects. The most likely chromosomal abnormality producing these symptoms is

a. $5p^-$
b. $11p^-$
c. $13q^-$
d. $21q^-$
e. $22q^-$

50. A young woman of average intelligence and short stature who has never menstruated is under clinical investigation for Turner's syndrome. However, a buccal smear shows some cells with one Barr body. Which of the following best explains this finding?

a. Laboratory error
b. The patient is a male
c. Classic XO pattern
d. Turner's mosaic pattern
e. Klinefelter's syndrome

51. A 15-year-old phenotypically female patient presents for workup of primary amenorrhea and is found to have an XY karyotype. The most likely diagnosis is

a. Turner's syndrome
b. Mixed gonadal dysgenesis
c. True hermaphroditism
d. Male pseudohermaphroditism
e. Female pseudohermaphroditism

52. A young boy is being evaluated for developmental delay, mild autism, and mental retardation. Physical examination reveals the boy to have large, everted ears, and a long face with a large mandible. He is also found to have macro-orchidism (large testes) and extensive work-up reveals multiple tandem repeats of the nucleotide sequence CGG in his DNA. Which one of the following is the most likely diagnosis for this patient?

a. Fragile X syndrome
b. Huntington's chorea
c. Myotonic dystrophy
d. Spinal-bulbar muscular atrophy
e. Ataxia-telangiectasia

53. An 8-year-old boy is found to have progressive corneal vascularization, deafness, notched incisors, and a flattened nose. The most likely cause of these changes is congenital infection by

a. Toxoplasma
b. Rubella
c. Cytomegalovirus
d. Herpes simplex virus
e. Treponema pallidum

54. Which one of the following abnormalities of the eye is a markedly premature infant most at risk for developing soon after birth?

a. Presbyopia
b. Pinguecula
c. Pterygium
d. Macular degeneration
e. Retrolental fibroplasia

55. A 14-month-old male infant presents with an enlarging abdominal mass. Laboratory examination reveals increased urinary levels of metanephrine and VMA (vanillylmandelic acid). A histologic section from this mass reveals a tumor composed of small primitive-appearing cells with hyperchromatic nuclei and little to no cytoplasm. Occasional focal groups of tumor cells are arranged in a ring around a central space. What is the correct diagnosis for this tumor?

a. Adrenal cortical carcinoma
b. Ganglioneuroma
c. Nephroblastoma
d. Neuroblastoma
e. Pheochromocytoma

56. Rearrangement of immunoglobulin chains is seen in

a. T lymphocytes
b. B lymphocytes
c. Macrophages
d. Langerhans' cells
e. Natural killer cells

57. If you suspect an 8-month-old infant has developed symptoms from a bacterial infection acquired after birth, you may try to find antibodies in this infant's blood that are directed against that organism. In order to know that these antibodies were not passively obtained from the mother, which one of the following antibody types would you look for in the infant's blood? (That is, what type of antibody is produced first against a bacterial infection and is also too large to have crossed the placenta?)

a. IgG
b. IgM
c. IgD
d. IgE
e. IgA

58. The cells seen in the following photomicrograph were stained by ABC technique using OKT1 (Leu-1), OKT3 (Leu-4), and OTK11 (Leu-5) cluster designation CD5, CD3, and CD2. The result indicates that the cells are of what origin?

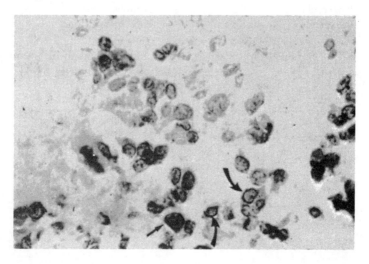

a. T lymphocytes
b. Oat cells
c. Mesothelial cells
d. EAC rosettes
e. Melanoma cells

59. Which cytokine is produced mainly by TH_1 cells and stimulates cell-mediated immunity by stimulating cytokine-driven proliferation of CD8+ cytotoxic T cells?

a. α-interferon (IFN)
b. γ-interferon
c. Interleukin 1 (IL-1)
d. IL-2
e. IL-3

60. The mixed lymphocyte reaction is used to define which one of the following?

a. HLA-A
b. HLA-DQ
c. Complement components
d. Tumor necrosis factor alpha (TNF-α)
e. Beta$_2$ microglobulin

61. In antigen recognition by cytotoxic T lymphocytes, the T-cell receptor recognizes antigens bound to

a. Class I antigens
b. Class II antigens
c. Class III antigens
d. C3b
e. Fc portion of IgG

62. There is a strong association between ankylosing spondylitis and

a. HLA-B27
b. HLA-DR3
c. HLA-DR4
d. HLA-A3
e. HLA-BW47

63. Ten minutes after being stung by a wasp, a 30-year-old male develops multiple patches of red, irregular skin lesions over his entire body. These lesions (urticaria) are pruritic, and new crops of lesions occur every day. This response is primarily the result of liberation of specific vasoactive substances by the action of

a. Activated T lymphocytes on smooth muscle cells
b. IgA on basophils and mast cells
c. IgA on lymphocytes and eosinophils
d. IgE on basophils and mast cells
e. IgE on lymphocytes and eosinophils

64. After receiving incompatible blood, a patient develops a transfusion reaction in the form of back pain, fever, shortness of breath, and hematuria. This type of immunologic reaction is classified as a

a. Systemic anaphylactic reaction
b. Systemic immune complex reaction
c. Delayed-type hypersensitivity reaction
d. Complement-mediated cytotoxicity
e. T-cell-mediated cytotoxicity

65. Delayed-type hypersensitivity reactions of the tuberculin skin test type

a. Appear within 1 or 2 h
b. Require an intact T-lymphocyte population
c. Show dermal infiltrates of granulocytes
d. Are associated uniquely with small antigens
e. Do not require previous exposure to the antigen

66. An allograft is a graft between

a. A human and an animal
b. Two individuals of different species
c. Two individuals of the same species
d. Two individuals of the same inbred strain
e. Identical twins

67. A patient with severe diabetic renal disease receives a donor cadaver kidney, following which a progressive rise in the serum creatinine occurs over a period lasting 5 months. In the photomicrograph below, what single finding is most characteristic for chronic rejection?

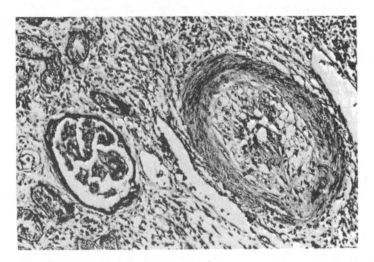

a. Damaged glomeruli
b. Interstitial fibrosis
c. Interstitial inflammation
d. Tubular atrophy
e. Vascular changes

68. A 32-year-old woman sees her physician because of "stiffness" and intolerance to cold temperatures in her fingers. Her face has a "mask-like" quality. It would be appropriate in the systems review to ask about

a. Headaches and dizziness
b. Swallowing difficulties
c. Sun hypersensitivity
d. Thyroid trouble
e. Family history

69. Which of the following conditions is most likely to be associated with cancer?

a. Systemic lupus erythematosus
b. Hypertension
c. Polymyositis
d. Autoimmune thyroiditis
e. Arteriosclerosis

70. An 87-year-old male develops worsening heart failure. Work-up reveals decreased left ventricular filling due to decreased compliance of the left ventricle. Two months later this patient dies, and post-mortem sections reveal deposits of eosinophilic, Congo red-positive material in the interstitium of his heart. When viewed under polarized light, this material displays an apple-green birefringence. What is your diagnosis?

a. Amyloidosis
b. Glycogenosis
c. Hemochromatosis
d. Sarcoidosis
e. Senile atrophy

71. A 28-year-old woman's first son died at 7 months of age due to severe combined immunodeficiency disease (SCID's). Subsequent work-up revealed a mutation in the gene for the common γ chain of the interleukin-2 receptor (IL2RG). Lymphocyte and red cell adenosine deaminase (ADA) levels were within normal limits. Work-up during her second pregnancy revealed that the fetus had the same abnormality found in her first son. Bone marrow was obtained from the 29-year-old father and was enriched with CD34+ cells (hematopoietic cell progenitors). It was then injected intraperitoneally by percutaneous, ultrasound-guided injection at 16, 17.5, and 18.5 weeks of gestation. At 11 months of life the second child was found to be clinically normal. What is the mode of inheritance of this patient's disease?

a. Autosomal dominant
b. Autosomal recessive
c. Mitochondrial
d. X-linked dominant
e. X-linked recessive

72. The most feared clinical complication of a patient with an isolated IgA deficiency is

a. Tetany
b. Anaphylaxis
c. Angioedema
d. Thrombocytopenia
e. Lymphoma

73. A 23-year-old man with full-blown AIDS is noted to be severely neutropenic. Which of the following abnormalities is most likely to be seen on further investigation?

a. Macrocytic anemia
b. Normal CD4 lymphocyte count
c. Thrombocytopenia
d. Lymphocytosis
e. Hypocellular bone marrow

74. Which of the following diseases is caused by a togavirus?

a. Epidemic keratoconjunctivitis
b. Dengue fever
c. Eastern encephalitis
d. Yellow fever
e. St. Louis encephalitis

75. A 23-year-old female presents with the recent onset of a vaginal discharge. Physical examination reveals multiple clear vesicles on her vulva and vagina. A smear of material obtained from one of these vesicles reveals several multinucleated giant cell with intranuclear inclusions and ground glass nuclei. These vesicles are most likely the result of an infection with

a. Cytomegalovirus (CMV)
b. Herpes simplex virus (HSV)
c. Human papillomavirus (HPV)
d. *Candida albicans*
e. *Trichomonas vaginalis*

76. A 19-year-old man living in New Mexico presents to a local clinic after a one-day history of fever, myalgia, chills, headache, and malaise. He complains of vomiting, diarrhea, abdominal pain, tachypnea, and a productive cough. His white cell count was elevated with an increase in the number of bands. Atypical lymphocytes were also found in the peripheral blood. He was treated with antibiotics, but the next day he developed acute respiratory failure with cardiopulmonary arrest and died. Postmortem examination of the lungs revealed intra-alveolar edema, rare hyaline membranes, and a few interstitial lymphoid aggregates. The most likely cause of this patient's illness is infection with

a. Ebola virus
b. Dengue fever virus
c. Hanta virus
d. Yellow fever virus
e. Alpha virus

77. A 6-year-old boy developed a facial rash that had the appearance of a slap to the face. The rash, which was composed of small red spots, subsequently involved the upper and lower extremities. The patient also complained of arthralgia and suddenly developed a life-threatening aplastic crisis of the bone marrow. The most likely infectious agent causing these symptoms is

a. Rhinovirus
b. Parainfluenza virus
c. Parvovirus
d. Measles virus
e. Rubella virus

78. The cells in the photomicrograph shown below are from a drop of cerebrospinal fluid. The most likely diagnosis is

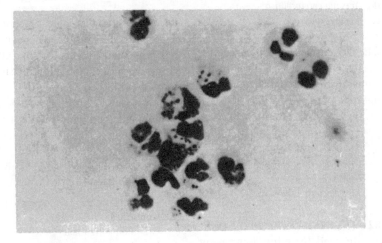

a. Subarachnoid hemorrhage
b. Viral meningitis
c. Tuberculous meningitis
d. Bacterial meningitis
e. Leukemic meningitis

79. Lobar pneumonia is caused predominantly by

a. *Klebsiella pneumoniae*
b. *Staphylococcus pyogenes*
c. *Haemophilus influenzae*
d. *Streptococcus pneumoniae*
e. *Legionella pneumophila*

80. Which of the following organisms produces signs and symptoms that mimic acute appendicitis?

a. Enteropathic *Escherichia coli*
b. *Enterobius vermicularis*
c. *Trichomonas hominis*
d. *Yersinia enterocolitica*
e. *Bacillus anthracis*

81. Organisms that can cause outbreaks around coastal areas of the United States and are characterized microscopically by a curved bacillus include

a. *Mycobacterium avium*
b. *Mycobacterium bovis*
c. *Mycobacterium marinum*
d. *Vibrio cholerae*
e. *Mycobacterium kansasii*

82. The most specific of the commonly used tests for diagnosing active syphilis is the

a. Rapid plasma reagin (RPR) test
b. *Treponema pallidum* immobilization (TPI) test
c. Fluorescent treponemal antibody-absorption (FTA-ABS) test
d. Venereal Disease Research Laboratory (VDRL) test
e. Kolmer test

83. An adult patient in the summer months suffers a rash on one of the extremities followed several weeks later by arthritis of the knee. In addition to viral and bacterial disorders and rheumatoid joint disease, which of the following should also be considered in the differential diagnosis?

a. Hemarthrosis
b. Reiter's disease
c. Lyme disease
d. Charcot's joint
e. Baker's cyst

84. A 30-year-old male presents with multiple soft, raised, beefy-red superficial ulcers in his left groin. Physical examination reveals several enlarged left inguinal lymph nodes. A histologic section from an enlarged lymph node that is stained with a silver stain reveals characteristic "Donovan bodies" within macrophages. What is the most likely diagnosis?

a. Chancroid
b. Gonorrhea
c. Granuloma inguinale
d. Lymphogranuloma venereum
e. Syphilis

85. A 35-year-old female who lives in the southeastern portion of the United States and likes to hike in the Great Smoky Mountains presents with a spotted rash that started on her extremities and spread to her trunk and face. A biopsy of one of these lesions revealed necrosis and reactive hyperplasia of blood vessels. What is the most likely causative agent of her disease?

a. Bartonella henselae
b. Bartonella quintana
c. Coxiella burnetii
d. Rickettsia prowazekii
e. Rickettsia rickettsii

86. A 21-year-old college athlete presents with a nagging cough and a 20 pound weight loss. In addition to the chronic cough and weight loss, his main symptoms consist of fever, night sweats, and chest pains. Examination of his sputum reveals the presence of rare acid-fast organisms. His symptoms are most likely due to an infection with

a. Klebsiella pneumoniae
b. Legionella pneumophila
c. Mycobacterium avium-intracellulare
d. Mycobacterium tuberculosis
e. Mycoplasma pneumonia

87. A 21-year-old HIV-positive male presents with malaise, fever, and increasing lymph nodes in his right cervical region. A microscopic section from one of the enlarged lymph nodes that is stained with an acid-fast stain reveals the presence of numerous ("too many to count") acid-fast organisms. Granulomas are not found. What organism is most likely the cause of this patient's acute illness?

a. M. avium-intracellulare
b. M. marinum
c. M. leprae
d. M. tuberculosis
e. M. kansasii

88. An adult migrant farm worker in the San Joaquin Valley of California has been hospitalized for 2 weeks with progressive lassitude, fever of unknown origin, and skin nodules on the lower extremities. A biopsy of one of the deep dermal nodules shown in the photomicrograph below reveals the presence of

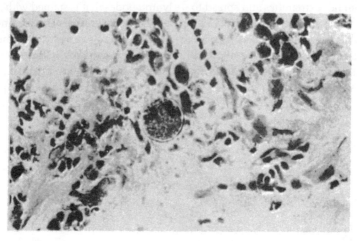

a. Russell bodies
b. Malignant lymphoma
c. Coccidioides spherule
d. Lymphomatoid granulomatosis
e. Erythema nodosum

89. Sections of tissue infected with Blastomyces would be expected to show organisms with

a. Nonbranching pseudohyphae and blastocysts
b. Acute-angle branching, septate hyphae
c. Wide-angle branching, nonseptate hyphae
d. Broad-based budding
e. Large spheres with external budding

90. Several days after exploring a new cave in eastern Kentucky, a 39-year-old female develops shortness of breath and a low-grade fever. Chest X-rays reveal several irregular areas in both upper lung fields along with enlarged hilar and mediastinal lymph nodes. A biopsy of one of these lymph nodes reveals granulomatous inflammation. Multiple small yeast surrounded by clear zones are seen within macrophages. Which one of the following organisms is most likely responsible for this individual's disease?

a. *Aspergillus* species
b. *Blastomyces dermatitidis*
c. *Candida albicans*
d. *Histoplasma capsulatum*
e. *Mucor*

91. A 38-year-old male with AIDS presents with decreasing mental status. The work-up at this time includes a spinal tap. Cerebrospinal fluid (CSF) is stained with a mucicarmine stain and India ink. The mucicarmine stain reveals numerous yeast that stain bright red. The India ink prep reveals through negative staining that these yeast have a capsule. What is your diagnosis?

a. Chromomycosis
b. Coccidiomycosis
c. Cryptococcosis
d. Cryptosporidiosis
e. Paracoccidiomycosis

92. A patient who presents to the hospital with severe headaches developed convulsions and died. At autopsy the brain grossly had a "Swiss cheese" appearance due to the presence of numerous small cysts containing milky fluid. Microscopically, a scolex with hooklets is found within one of these cysts. What is the causative agent for this disease?

a. *Taenia saginata*
b. *Taenia solium*
c. *Diphyllobothrium latum*
d. *Echinococcus granulosa*
e. *Toxocara canis*

93. The photomicrograph below of a duodenal aspiration smear shows an organism that

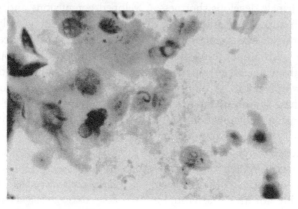

a. Is often numerous in lymph nodes
b. Infects principally the large intestine
c. Is transmitted by the genus Triatoma
d. Is the most common intestinal parasite in the U.S.
e. Is frequently identified in cervicovaginal smears

94. The photomicrograph below was prepared after a distal colonic biopsy was performed. The most likely diagnosis is

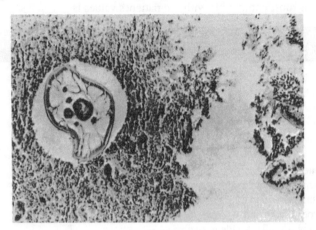

a. Clonorchiasis
b. Enterobiasis
c. Filariasis
d. Strongyloidiasis
e. Schistosomiasis

95. The enzyme activity curve labeled II, shown below, best represents the pattern for which of the following serum enzymes after an uncomplicated acute myocardial infarction?

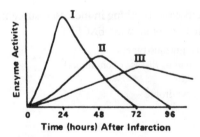

a. Aspartate aminotransferase
b. Creatine phosphokinase
c. Lactic dehydrogenase
d. Alkaline phosphatase
e. 59-Nucleotidase

96. The table below shows the normal serum values for the five isoenzymes of lactic dehydrogenase (LDH) and the values obtained for one patient. The diagnosis most compatible with the patient's values is

Isoenzyme	Normal percent activity	Patient's percent activity
LDH_1	20–35	18
LDH_2	30–40	24
LDH_3	20–30	13
LDH_4	5–15	26

a. acute hepatitis
b. Pernicious anemia
c. Pulmonary infarct
d. Myocardial infarct
e. Cerebrovascular accident

97. As visualized by the electron microscope, all the following are cell organelles EXCEPT

a. Lysosomes
b. The Golgi complex
c. The endoplasmic reticulum
d. Desmosomes
e. Microbodies

98. Defects in chemotaxis resulting in increased susceptibility to infection are associated with all the following EXCEPT

a. Diabetes mellitus, juvenile type
b. Chronic granulomatous disease of childhood
c. Chronic renal failure
d. Chédiak-Higashi syndrome
e. Thermal injury

99. The chemical mediators of inflammation listed below often proceed in a cascade after activation EXCEPT

a. Complement
b. Kinin
c. Arachidonic acid
d. Fibrinopeptides
e. Neutral proteases

100. Infectious diseases associated with a granulomatous response include all the following EXCEPT

a. Tuberculosis
b. Coccidioidomycosis
c. Schistosomiasis
d. Sarcoidosis
e. cat-scratch disease

101. Type I collagen is found in all the following EXCEPT

a. Tendon
b. Dermis
c. Cartilage
d. Fascia
e. Bone

102. Endotoxic shock is commonly caused by all the following organisms EXCEPT

a. *Pseudomonas aeruginosa*
b. *Escherichia coli*
c. *Proteus species*
d. *Corynebacterium diphtheriae*
e. *Klebsiella pneumoniae*

103. Oncogene activation has been implicated in the development of all the following malignancies EXCEPT

a. Carcinoma of the urinary bladder
b. Neuroblastoma
c. Chronic myelocytic leukemia
d. Burkitt's lymphoma
e. Retinoblastoma

104. An increased incidence of neoplasia has been observed in all the following EXCEPT

a. Primary (genetic) immunodeficient states
b. Immunosuppressed recipients of transplants
c. Acquired immunodeficiency syndrome (AIDS)
d. Therapy with radiation and radiomimetic drugs
e. Sarcoidosis

105. The incidences of all the following malignancies are higher in China or Japan when compared with those in the United States EXCEPT

a. Nasopharyngeal carcinoma
b. Liver carcinoma
c. Gastric carcinoma
d. Choriocarcinoma
e. Prostatic carcinoma

106. All the following are correct associations of special histologic stains of tumor markers with the appropriate tumors EXCEPT

a. Human chorionic gonadotropin (hCG) and trophoblastic tumors
b. Alpha-fetoprotein (AFP) and liver cell cancer
c. Prostate-specific antigen (PSA) and prostate cancer
d. Carcinoembryonic antigen (CEA) and colon cancer
e. Chloroacetate esterase (CAE) and stomach cancer

107. All the following characteristics are true of liposarcoma EXCEPT that it

a. Presents varied histology
b. Is commonly found in the retroperitoneum
c. Frequently gives rise to embolization in lymphatics
d. Is the most common soft tissue sarcoma
e. Arises very rarely in subcutaneous tissue

108. Vitamin K is required for the synthesis of all the following EXCEPT

a. Prothrombin
b. Clotting factor VII
c. Clotting factor VIII
d. Clotting factor IX
e. Clotting factor X

109. Effects of radiation exposure on tissue include all the following EXCEPT

a. Double-stranded chromosomal breaks
b. Formation of free radicals
c. Abnormal mitotic figures
d. Endothelial swelling
e. epidermal hyperplasia

110. A woman taking oral contraceptives during the reproductive years increases, even if only minimally, her risk of developing the following EXCEPT

a. Pulmonary infarction
b. Myocardial infarction
c. Vaginal adenosis
d. Venous thrombus
e. Liver cell adenoma

111. Alcohol may be the most significant cause of public health problems in the United States. All the following entities are correlated with alcohol abuse EXCEPT

a. Subdural hematoma
b. Esophageal carcinoma
c. Elevated creatine phosphokinase
d. Primary biliary cirrhosis
e. Portal vein thrombosis

112. All the following genetic disorders are autosomal recessive (AR) EXCEPT

a. Alkaptonuria
b. Familial hypercholesterolemia
c. Phenylketonuria (PKU)
d. Myeloperoxidase deficiency
e. Cystic fibrosis (CF)

113. Mechanisms responsible for Down's syndrome include all the following EXCEPT

a. Nondisjunction during first meiotic division
b. Mosaicism
c. Translocation
d. Centric fusion (Robertsonian translocation)
e. Formation of isochromosomes

114. All the following symptoms are associated with Klinefelter's syndrome EXCEPT

a. Large, soft testes
b. Gynecomastia
c. Eunuchoidism
d. Azoospermia
e. Elevated urinary gonadotropins

115. In hemolytic disease of the newborn, all the following statements are correct EXCEPT

a. Erythroblastosis fetalis develops because of prior maternal sensitization
b. Anemia and hepatosplenomegaly are characteristic
c. Anti-D immunoglobulin should be given to a sensitized mother before delivery
d. Both ABO and Rh antigens cause hemolytic disease of the newborn
e. There is transplacental transmission of maternal antibody

116. Characteristically, B lymphocytes do all the following EXCEPT

a. Constitute 10 to 15 percent of peripheral blood lymphocytes
b. Occur in lymphoid follicles and the superficial cortex of lymph nodes
c. Express surface immunoglobulins IgM and IgD
d. Express cluster differentiation antigen CD8
e. Possess complement component (C3) receptors

117. True statements concerning diagnostic specificity include all the following EXCEPT

a. Scl-70 antibody is specific for diffuse systemic sclerosis
b. Antibodies to nucleolar RNA are specific for diffuse systemic sclerosis
c. Antibodies to double-stranded DNA are specific for systemic lupus erythematosus (SLE)
d. Antibodies to antinuclear antibody (ANA) are specific for SLE
e. Anti-Sm antibodies are specific for SLE

118. Systemic lupus erythematosus (SLE), a multisystem disease of autoimmune origin, is characterized by all the following statements EXCEPT

a. Polyclonal B-cell activation is essential to the pathogenesis
b. Cardiac involvement is the most common cause of death
c. Visceral lesions are mediated by type III hypersensitivity
d. Joint involvement (arthritis) is common clinically
e. hypergammaglobulinemia is usual

119. All the following statements regarding primary Sjögren's syndrome are true EXCEPT

a. Xerostomia is a major symptom
b. Anti-SSB antibodies are major markers
c. Renal glomerular lesions are common
d. Rheumatoid factor is often present
e. There is increased frequency of HLA-DR3

120. Current knowledge concerning AIDS (acquired immunodeficiency syndrome) includes all the following EXCEPT

a. The causative agent is HIV
b. The causative agent belongs to the retrovirus group
c. T lymphocytes of the helper/inducer subset are infected
d. Cytotoxic/suppressor T cells are markedly increased
e. The incidence of non-Hodgkin's lymphomas is increased in AIDS

121. Pathogenic pneumococci typically exhibit all the following EXCEPT

a. Inhibition of growth by ethylhydrocupreine (Optochin)
b. M protein in their cell walls
c. Bile solubility
d. Positive Neufeld quellung reactions
e. Detection of capsular polysaccharides by counterimmunoelectrophoresis (CIE)

122. All the following statements about *Listeria monocytogenes* are true EXCEPT that it

a. Causes neonatal and adult meningitis
b. Causes food-borne outbreaks
c. Causes frequent epithelioid granulomas
d. Is an opportunistic agent in the immunosuppressed or pregnant
e. Is a gram-positive intracellular bacillus

123. Spirochetal infections include all the following EXCEPT

a. Bejel
b. Yaws
c. Relapsing fever
d. Weil's disease
e. Lymphogranuloma venereum

124. The organism *Mycoplasma pneumoniae* exhibits all the following characteristics EXCEPT which one?

a. It is enclosed by a membrane but lacks cell walls
b. It causes 50 percent of pneumonias in college students
c. It is often accompanied by the presence of cold agglutinins in serum
d. It is beyond resolution of light microscopy
e. It causes granuloma formation

125. Characteristic features of lepromatous leprosy include all the following EXCEPT

a. Nerve involvement
b. Numerous bacilli in histiocytes
c. Frequent polyclonal hypergammaglobulinemia
d. Association with erythema nodosum
e. Encroachment of infiltrate on basal epidermis

126. As a result of active world travel, parasitic infestations are far from being considered exotic diseases in the United States today. A pulmonary phase is part of the development of all the following helminths EXCEPT

a. *Necator americanus*
b. *Strongyloides stercoralis*
c. *Ascaris lumbricoides*
d. *Wuchereria bancrofti*
e. Toxocara

127. Parathyroid hormone, by its action on target organs, is known to cause all the following EXCEPT

a. Increased intestinal calcium absorption
b. Increased renal tubular reabsorption of calcium
c. Increased serum phosphate levels
d. Mobilization of calcium from bone
e. Decreased renal tubular reabsorption of phosphate

128. Elevated levels of serum amylase may be found in all the following conditions EXCEPT

a. Acute pancreatitis
b. Biliary tract disease
c. Mumps
d. Renal insufficiency
e. Congestive heart failure

129. Elevated levels of serum alkaline phosphatase are expected findings in each of the following conditions EXCEPT

a. Obstructive jaundice
b. Cirrhosis
c. Hepatitis
d. Polycythemia vera
e. Pregnancy (last trimester)

130. Hyperuricemia often occurs secondary to all the following disorders EXCEPT

a. Leukemias
b. Lymphomas
c. Chondrocalcinosis (pseudogout)
d. Lesch-Nyhan syndrome
e. Chronic renal disease

131. Elevated levels of serum creatine kinase (CK) are seen in all the following EXCEPT

a. Muscular dystrophy
b. Polymyositis
c. Myasthenia gravis
d. Myocardial infarction
e. Hypothyroidism

DIRECTIONS: Each group of questions below consists of lettered headings followed by a set of numbered items. For each numbered item select the **one** lettered heading with which it is **most** closely associated. Each lettered heading may be used **once, more than once, or not at all**.

Questions 132–133

Match each of the following clinical scenarios with the correct diagnosis from the following list.

a. Chédiak-Higashi syndrome
b. Chronic granulocytic leukemia
c. Chronic granulomatous disease
d. Congenital agammaglobulinemia
e. Hereditary thymic dysplasia
f. Letterer-Siwe disease
g. Leukemoid reaction
h. Wiskott-Aldrich syndrome

132. A 3-year-old boy presents with recurrent bacterial and fungal infections involving his skin and respiratory tract. Physical examination reveals the presence of oculocutaneous albinism. Examination of his peripheral blood smear reveals large granules within his neutrophils, lymphocytes, and monocytes. His total neutrophil count is found to be decreased. Further work-up reveals ineffective bactericidal capabilities of his neutrophils due to defective fusion of phagosomes with lysosomes.

133. In an evaluation of an 8-year-old boy who had had recurrent infections since the first year of life, findings included enlargement of the liver and spleen, lymph node inflammation, and a superficial dermatitis resembling eczema. Microscopic examination of a series of peripheral blood smears taken during the course of a staphylococcal infection indicated that the bactericidal capacity of the boy's neutrophils was impaired or absent.

Questions 134–135

Match each of the following clinical scenarios with the most likely substance that is deficient in each individual.

a. Biotin
b. Cyanocobalamin
c. Niacin
d. Pyridoxine
e. Riboflavin
f. Selenium
g. Thiamine

134. A 62-year-old male is brought into the emergency room by the police, who say that this patient is well-known to them. They say that he is a long-term alcoholic, but lately he has been acting very confused. Your physical examination reveals an elderly appearing male patient who is quite thin and appears emaciated. You further discover that this individual has problems with his memory, ataxia, and paralysis of his extraocular muscles. Extensive work-up reveals atrophy and small hemorrhages in the periventricular region of his brain and around the mamillary bodies.

135. A middle-aged individual presents with symptoms of diarrhea, dementia, and a dark discoloration of the skin of his neck ("necklace" dermatitis). This combination of signs and symptoms suggests the diagnosis of pellagra.

Questions 136–137

Match each of the following clinical scenarios with the correct diagnosis from the following list.

a. Chédiak-Higashi syndrome
b. Chronic granulomatous disease
c. Common variable immunodeficiency
d. DiGeorge's syndrome
e. Hodgkin's disease of nodular sclerosis subgroup
f. Pelger-Huët anomaly
g. Wiskott-Aldrich syndrome
h. X-linked agammaglobulinemia of Bruton

136. An 8-month-old male infant was admitted to the hospital because of a bacterial respiratory infection. This infant responded to appropriate antibiotic therapy, but was readmitted to the hospital several weeks later because of severe otitis media. Over the next several months, this infant was admitted to the hospital multiple times for recurrent bacterial infections. Work-up revealed extremely low serum antibody levels. This infant has no previous history of viral or fungal infections.

137. A young child presents with recurrent bacterial infections and eczema, and is found to have a platelet count of 75,000/μL. Physical examination reveals multiple enlarged lymph nodes, while an extensive work-up finds the absence of delayed-type hypersensitivity.

GENERAL PATHOLOGY

Answers

1. The answer is b. (*Cotran, 5/e, pp 4–11.*) The first effect of the interruption of blood flow (ischemia) to cells is the decrease in ATP production by aerobic cellular processes. This results in decreased oxidative phosphorylation by mitochondria and an increase in anaerobic glycolysis, which decreases intracellular pH. Decreasing ATP levels also decreases the functioning of the energy-dependent sodium pump, which results in an increased cellular influx of sodium ions and an increased efflux of potassium. The resultant net gain of intracellular ions causes isosmotic water accumulation and hydropic cellular swelling. These changes are characteristic of reversible cellular injury, but they are reversible if blood flow and oxygen supply are restored.

With prolonged ischemia, however, certain cellular events occur that are not reversible, even with restoration of oxygen supply. These cellular changes are referred to as irreversible cellular injury. This type of injury is characterized by severe damage to mitochondria (vacuole formation), extensive damage to plasma membranes and nuclei, and rupture of lysosomes. Severe damage to mitochondria is characterized by the influx of calcium ions into the mitochondria and the subsequent formation of large, flocculent densities within the mitochondria. These flocculent densities are characteristically seen in irreversibly injured myocardial cells that undergo reperfusion soon after injury. Less severe changes in mitochondria, such as mitochondrial swelling, are seen with reversible injury.

2. The answer is d. (*Cotran, 5/e, pp 25–26, 859. Chandrasoma, 3/e, pp 8–10.*) Free fatty acids are normally taken up by the liver and esterified to triglyceride, converted to cholesterol, oxidized into ketone bodies, or incorporated into phospholipids that can be excreted as very low density lipoproteins (VLDL). Abnormalities involving these normal metabolic pathways may lead to the accumulation of triglyceride within the hepatocytes. This accumulation of triglyceride is called fatty change or steatosis. Examples of abnormalities that produce hepatic steatosis include diseases that cause excess delivery of free fatty acids to the liver or diseases that cause impaired lipoprotein synthesis. Excess delivery of free fatty acids occurs in conditions that increase mobilization of adipose tissue, such as starvation, corticosteroid use, and diabetes mellitus. Impaired lipoprotein synthesis occurs with carbon tetrachloride poisoning, phosphorous poisoning, and protein malnutrition.

Alcohol can produce hepatic steatosis by several mechanisms, such as increased fatty acid synthesis, decreased triglyceride utilization, decreased fatty acid oxidation, decreased lipoprotein excretion, and increased lipolysis. Ethanol is taken up by the liver and is converted into acetaldehyde by either alcohol dehydrogenase (the major pathway), microsomal P-450 oxidase, or peroxisomal catalase. These pathways also convert NAD (nicotinamide adenine dinucleotide) to NADH. This excess production of NADH changes the normal hepatic metabolism away from catabolism of fats and toward anabolism of fats (lipid synthesis). This results in decreased mitochondrial oxidation of fatty acids and increased hepatic production of triglyceride. Ethanol also increases lipolysis and inhibits the release of lipoproteins. Increased lipolysis increases the amount of free fatty acids that reach the liver.

3. The answer is c. (*Cotran, 5/e, pp 31–32, 858.*) Hyaline is a non-specific term that is used to describe any material, inside or outside the cell, that stains a red homogenous color with the routine hematoxylin and eosin (H&E) stain. There are many different substances that have the appearance of hyaline. Alcoholic hyaline inclusions (Mallory bodies) are irregular eosinophilic hyaline inclusions that are found within the cytoplasm of hepatocytes. Mallory bodies are composed of prekeratin intermediate filaments. They are a nonspecific finding and can be found in patients with several diseases other than alcoholic hepatitis, such as Wilson's disease, and bypass operations for morbid obesity. Immunoglobulins may form intracytoplasmic or extracellular oval hyaline bodies called Russell bodies. Excess plasma proteins may form hyaline droplets in proximal renal tubular epithelial cells or hyaline membranes in the alveoli of the lungs (hyaline membrane disease). The hyaline found in the walls of arterioles of kidneys in patients with benign nephrosclerosis is composed of basement membranes and precipitated plasma proteins. Lipofuscin is an intracytoplasmic aging pigment that has a yellow-brown, finely granular appearance with H&E stains. Its appearance does not resemble hyaline material.

4. The answer is a. (*Cotran, 5/e, pp 17–21. Rubin, 2/e, pp 23–25.*) As cells die, the nuclear chromatin clumps and then aggregates along the nuclear membrane. As this clumping of chromatin continues, the nucleus becomes smaller and stains deeply basophilic (blue). This cellular process is called pyknosis. The nucleus may then break up into many clumps (karyorrhexis) or there may be decreased staining of chromatin (karyolysis). Apoptosis is a distinctive pattern of cell death that usually involves single cells. There is typically no inflammatory response. Apoptotic cells appear histologically as intensely eosinophilic (red) bodies with or without dense, fragmented nuclear material. Apoptosis is described as a programmed suicide process of cells that occurs by the stimulation of endogenous endonucleases. It is the type of cell death seen during embryonic development or hormone-induced atrophy of tissue; an example is the involution of the thymus that occurs with aging. Apoptosis may result from some bacterial toxins or viral infections, an example of which are Councilman bodies, which are found in the liver of some patients with viral hepatitis. Abnormalities of the genes involved in apoptosis may contribute to the formation of some malignancies. A different process is pinocytosis, which is the uptake of small, soluble macromolecules into the cytoplasm of phagocytic cells.

5. The answer is a. (*Cotran, 5/e, pp 5–17.*) The cause of cell injury and death may sometimes be inferred from the type of necrosis present. Coagulative necrosis, characterized by loss of the cell nucleus, acidophilic change of the cytoplasm, and preservation of the outline of the cell, is seen in sudden, severe ischemia of many organs. It is not present, however, in acute ischemic necrosis of the brain. Myocardial infarction resulting from the sudden occlusion of the coronary artery is a classic example of coagulative necrosis. In liquefactive necrosis, the dead cells are completely dissolved by hydrolytic enzymes. This type of necrosis can be seen in ischemic necrosis of the brain and in acute bacterial infections. Fat necrosis, seen with acute pancreatic necrosis, is fat cell death caused by lipases. Fibrinoid necrosis is an abnormality seen sometimes in injured blood vessels where plasma proteins abnormally accumulate within the walls of blood vessels. Caseous necrosis is a combination of coagulative and liquefactive necrosis, but the necrotic cells are not totally dissolved and remain as amorphic, coarsely granular, eosinophilic debris. This type of necrosis grossly has the appearance of clumped cheese. It is classically seen in tuberculous infections. Gangrenous necrosis of extremities is also a combination of coagulative and liquefactive necrosis. In dry gangrene the coagulative pattern is predominate, while in wet gangrene the liquefactive pattern is predominate.

6. The answer is a. (*Cotran, 5/e, pp 44–47. Rubin, 2/e, pp 7–9.*) In uterine growth during pregnancy, both cell proliferation involving the endometrial glands and muscle enlargement of the uterine wall occur. These processes offer models of both hyperplasia and hypertrophy. When both are present, DNA synthesis is markedly accelerated. Hyperplasia is an increase in the number of cells, whereas hypertrophy is an increase in cell size, as in cardiac muscle hypertrophy in response to volume overload or peripheral vascular hypertension. Enlargement of breast tissue resulting from hormonal influences is due solely to an increase in cell numbers.

7. The answer is b. (*Alberts, 3/e, pp 734–749. Cotran, 5/e, pp 37–39.*) Many extracellular substances cause intracellular actions via second messenger systems. These second messengers may bind to receptors that are located either on the surface of the cell or within the cell itself. Substances that react with intracellular receptors are lipid soluble (lipophilic) molecules that can pass through the lipid plasma membrane. Examples of these lipophilic substances include thyroid hormones, steroid hormones, and the fat soluble vitamins A and D. Once inside the cell these substances generally travel to the nucleus and bind to the hormone response element (HRE) of DNA.

Some substances that react with cell surface receptors bind to guanine-nucleotide regulatory proteins. These proteins, called G proteins, may be classified into four categories, namely Gs, Gi, Gt, and Gq. Two of these receptors, Gs and Gi, regulate the intracellular concentration of cyclic adenosine 5'- monophosphate (cAMP). In contrast, Gt regulates the intracytoplasmic levels of cyclic guanosine 5'-monophosphate (cGMP), and Gq regulates the intracytoplasmic levels of calcium ions. Gs and Gi regulate intracellular cAMP levels by their actions on adenyl cyclase, an enzyme located on the inner surface of the plasma membrane that catalyzes the formation of cAMP from ATP. The adenylate cyclase G protein complex is composed of the following components: the receptor, the catalytic enzyme (i.e., adenyl cyclase), and a coupling unit. The coupling unit consists of GTP-dependent regulatory proteins (G-proteins), which may either be stimulatory (Gs) or inhibitory (Gi). These G-proteins consist of three fragments: the α unit (either αs or αi), the β unit, and the γ unit. The a units are active only when complexed to GTP (Gαs-GTP and Gαi-GTP), and they are inactivated when GTP is converted to GDP, which forms Gαs-βγ and Gαi-βγ. To summarize, when bound to GTP and active, Gs stimulates adenyl cyclase and increases cAMP levels. (Gs can be thought of as the "on switch.") In contrast, when bound to GTP and active, Gi inhibits adenyl cyclase and decreases cAMP levels. (Gi can be thought of as the "off switch.") It is important to note that cholera toxin and pertussis toxin both act by altering this adenyl cyclase pathway. Cholera toxin inhibits the conversion of Gs-GTP to Gs-GDP. In contrast, pertussis toxin inhibits the activation of Gi-GDP to Gαi-GTP. Therefore, both cholera toxin and pertussis toxin prolong the functioning of adenyl cyclase and therefore increase intracellular cAMP, but their mechanisms are different. Cholera toxin keeps the "on switch" in the "on" position, while pertussis toxin keeps the "off switch" in the "off" position.

8. The answer is d. (*Cotran, 5/e, pp 37–41.*) Growth factors are chemicals that are associated with cell growth. For example, fibroblast growth factor (FGF) can induce the growth and proliferation of fibroblasts. Additionally one type of FGF, basic FGF, is capable of inducing all of the stages of angiogenesis, these four stages being basement membrane and extracellular matrix degradation, endothelial migration, endothelial proliferation, and finally endothelial differentiation. The epidermal growth factor family includes epidermal growth factor (EGF) and transforming growth factor-α (TGF-α). These substances can cause proliferation or many types of epithelial cells and fibroblasts. The EGF receptor is *c-erb* B_1. Platelet derived growth factor (PDGF), which is found in platelets, activated macrophages, endothelial cells, and smooth muscle cells, can cause migration and proliferation of fibroblasts, smooth muscle cells, and monocytes. TGF-β, produced by platelets, endothelial cells, T cells, and macrophages, is associated with fibrosis. In low concentrations it causes the synthesis and secretion of PDGF, but in high concentrations it is growth inhibitory due to inhibition of the expression of PDGF receptors.

9. The answer is c. (*Cotran, 5/e, pp 57–59. Rubin, 2/e, pp 49–52.*) Adhesion molecules are important in cell-to-cell interactions, such as leukocyte adhesion to endothelial cells during acute inflammation. These adhesion molecules consist of three families: integrins, selectins, and immunoglobulins. Integrins are transmembrane glycoproteins composed of alpha and beta subunits. Beta-1-integrins are found on lymphocytes, monocytes, basophils, and eosinophils, while beta-2-integrins are found on all leukocytes. The beta-2-integrins (also called CD11/CD18 molecules) consist of MO-1, leukocyte function antigen 1 (LFA-1), and gp 150,95. Activation of phagocytic cells early during inflammation increases the expression of integrins on their surface. The genetic disease leukocyte adhesion deficiency type 1 is characterized by recurrent bacterial infections and impaired leukocyte adhesion. Patients have a deficiency of the beta chains of LFA-1 and Mac-1 integrins. The selectins, in contrast, consist of E-selectin, found on endothelial cells, P-selectin, found on endothelial cells and platelets, and L-selectin, found on most leukocytes. The immunoglobulin family includes two endothelial adhesion molecules: ICAM-1 (intracellular adhesion molecule 1) and VCAM-1 (vascular adhesion molecule 1).

10. The answer is c. (*Cotran, 5/e, pp 66–67.*) The basic function of the complement system of plasma proteins is to do three things: directly lyse cells, attract leukocytes to sites of inflammation, and activate leukocytes. The main result of activation of the complement pathway is the formation of anaphylatoxins and the membrane attack complex. The anaphylatoxins, C3a, C4a, and C5a, act by causing smooth muscle contraction and increased vascular permeability. Additionally, the anaphylatoxins C3a and C5a degranulate mast cells, which causes the release of histamine. C3b is a potent opsonin, while C5a is an important chemotactic factor for leukocytes. The membrane attack complex (MAC) consists of C5b-9. MAC is inserted into the plasma membrane of cells forming transmembrane channels, which will damage cells and cause cell death.

11. The answer is e. (*Cotran, 5/e, pp 68–70, 73–74.*) Products of arachidonic acid metabolism are involved extensively in inflammation. In this pathway, arachidonic acid is broken down into leukotrienes (vasoconstrictors) and prostaglandins (vasodilators). Arachidonic acid (AA) is a polyunsaturated fatty acid that is normally found esterified in plasma membrane phospholipids. It is released by the activation of phospholipases, such as phospholipase A_2. Cyclooxygenase transforms AA into the prostaglandin endoperoxide PGG_2, which is then converted into PGH_2 and subsequently into three products: thromboxane A_2 (TxA_2), prostacyclin (PGI_2), and the more stable prostaglandins PGE_2, PGF_2, and PGD_2. Thromboxane, found in platelets, is a potent platelet aggregator and blood vessel constrictor.

In contrast, prostacyclin, which is found in the wall of blood vessels, is a potent inhibitor of platelet aggregation and is also a vasodilator. Prostaglandin E and prostacyclin probably account for most of the vasodilatation that is seen in inflammation. The prostaglandins are also involved in producing pain and fever in inflammation. In contrast to cyclooxygenase, lipoxygenase converts AA into hydroperoxyl derivatives, namely 12-HPETE in platelets and 15-HPETE in leukocytes. 5-HPETE gives rise to HETE and the leukotrienes (Lt.'s). While many substances can be chemotactic, few are known to be as potent as several of the leukotrienes. Leukotriene B_4 is a potent chemotactic agent, which also causes aggregation and adhesion of leukocytes. Additionally, the leukotrienes C_4, D_4, and E_4 cause increased vascular permeability, bronchoconstriction, and vasoconstriction. Other chemotactic factors for neutrophils include C5a and IL-8, but these substances are not formed from arachidonic acid.

12. The answer is e. (*Cotran, 5/e, pp 67–70.*) Certain drugs are important in the control of acute inflammation because they inhibit portions of the metabolic pathways involving arachidonic acid. For example, corticosteroids induce the synthesis of lipocortins, a family of proteins that are inhibitors of phospholipase A_2. They decrease the formation of arachidonic acid and its metabolites, prostaglandins and leukotrienes. Aspirin, indomethacin, and other nonsteroidal anti-inflammatory drugs (NSAID's), in contrast, inhibit cyclooxygenase and therefore inhibit the synthesis of prostaglandins and thromboxanes. The prostaglandins have several important functions. For example, prostaglandin E_2 (PGE_2), produced within the anterior hypothalamus in response to interleukin-1 secretion from leukocytes, results in fever. Therefore aspirin can be used to treat fever by inhibiting PGE_2 production. PGE_2 is also a vasodilator that can keep a ductus arteriosus open. At birth, breathing decreases pulmonary resistance and reverses the flow of blood through the ductus arteriosus. The oxygenated blood flowing from the aorta into the ductus inhibits prostaglandin production and closes the ductus arteriosus. Therefore prostaglandin E_2 can be given clinically to keep the ductus arteriosus open, while indomethacin can be used to close a patent ductus. Prostaglandin F_2 (PGF_2) causes uterine contractions, which can result in dysmenorrhea. Indomethacin can be used to treat dysmenorrhea by inhibiting the production of PGF_2.

Bradykinin is a nonapeptide that increases vascular permeability, contracts smooth muscle, dilates blood vessels, and causes pain. It is part of the kinin system and is formed from high-molecular-weight kininogen (HMWK). Histamine, a vasoactive amine that is stored in mast cells, basophils, and platelets, acts on H_1 receptors to cause dilatation of arterioles and increased vascular permeability of venules.

13. The answer is c. (*Cotran, 5/e, pp 70–71, 73–74, 84–85.*) Two of the major systemic effects of inflammation (acute-phase reactions) are fever and leukocytosis. Both of these reactions are largely under the control of the cytokines IL-1 or TNF-α (cachectin) or both. These two cytokines have many similar functions, including induction of fever, release of ACTH, leukocytosis, and other systemic acute-phase responses. IL-1 initiates fever by inducing synthesis of prostaglandin E_2(PGE_2) in the anterior hypothalamus, followed by transmission via the posterior hypothalamus, vasomotor center, and sympathetic nerves to cause skin vasoconstriction. Leukocytosis occurs initially because of rapid release of cells from the postmitotic reserve pool of the bone marrow, which is caused by IL-1 and TNF-α and associated with a "shift to the left" of immature cells. TNF-β, another cytokine, has no major role in acute-phase reactions. It takes part in T-cell cytotoxicity and its release may injure cell membranes directly in T-cell-mediated lysis.

14. The answer is d. (*Cotran, 5/e, pp 76–78. Henry, 19/e, p 607.*) There is evidence that most, if not all, macrophages originate from a committed bone marrow stem cell, which differentiates into a monoblast and then a promonocyte, which in turn matures into a monocyte in the circulating peripheral blood. When called upon, the circulating monocyte can enter into an organ or tissue bed as a tissue macrophage (previously called a histiocyte). Examples of tissue macrophages are Kupffer cells (liver), alveolar macrophages (lung), osteoclasts (bone), Langerhans cells (skin), microglial cells (central nervous system), and possibly the dendritic immunocytes of the dermis, spleen, and lymph nodes. The entire system, including the peripheral blood monocytes, constitutes the mononuclear phagocyte system.

15. The answer is a. *(Henry, 19/e, pp 248–249. Cotran, 5/e, p 84.)* C-reactive protein (CRP) elevations, as well as elevations in the erythrocyte sedimentation rate, are nonspecific markers of inflammatory conditions. The CRP rises faster and returns to normal earlier than the erythrocyte sedimentation rate in most inflammatory diseases. Most bacterial infections, rheumatoid arthritis, rheumatic fever, and diseases leading to necrosis and tissue damage will elevate the CRP. CRP elevations do not occur in most viral illnesses.

16. The answer is c. *(Cotran, 5/e, pp 85–87.)* Tissue repair occurs through the regeneration of damaged cells and the replacement of tissue by connective tissue. Tissue repair involves the formation of granulation tissue, which histologically is characterized by a combination of proliferating fibroblasts and proliferating blood vessels. Proliferating cells are cells that are rapidly dividing and usually have prominent nucleoli. This histologic feature should not be taken as a sign of dysplasia or malignancy. It is important not to confuse the term granulation tissue with the similar sounding term granuloma. The latter term refers to a special type of inflammation that is characterized by the presence of activated macrophages (epithelioid cells). One aspect of tissue repair involves wound healing, which occurs by either primary union or secondary union. Primary intention refers to healing of a clean sutured surgical incision. Healing by secondary intention differs from healing by primary intention in that it involves more initial tissue damage, more inflammatory response, takes longer to clear away debris, takes longer to granulate in, and contraction of the scar is a major factor in healing.

17. The answer is d. *(Cotran, 5/e, pp 53–57, 93–97.)* Edema is the accumulation of excess fluid in the interstitial tissue or body cavities. It may be caused by inflammation (inflammatory edema) or may be due to abnormalities involving the Starling forces acting at the capillary level (noninflammatory edema or hemodynamic edema). Inflammatory edema is caused by increased capillary permeability, which is the result of vasoactive mediators of acute inflammation. An exudate is inflammatory edema fluid resulting from increased capillary permeability. It is characterized by a high protein content, much cellular debris, and a specific gravity greater than 1.020. Pus is an inflammatory exudate having numerous leukocytes and cellular debris. In contrast, transudates result from either increased intravascular hydrostatic pressure or from decreased osmotic pressure. They are characterized by a low protein content and a specific gravity of <1.012. Noninflammatory edema is the result of abnormalities of the hemodynamic (Starling) forces acting at the level of the capillaries. Increased hydrostatic pressure may be caused by arteriolar dilatation, hypervolemia, or increased venous pressure. Hypervolemia may be caused by sodium retention seen in renal disease, and increased venous pressure can be seen in venous thrombosis, congestive heart failure, or cirrhosis. Decreased plasma oncotic pressure is caused by decreased plasma protein, the majority of which is albumin. Decreased albumin levels may be caused by loss of albumin in the urine, which occurs in the nephrotic syndrome, or by reduced synthesis, which occurs in chronic liver disease. Lymphatic obstruction may be caused by tumors, surgical resection, or infections, for example, infection with filarial worms and consequent elephantiasis.

18. The answer is e. *(Cotran, 5/e, pp 97–99.)* Hemorrhage is the leakage of blood from a blood vessel. Blood may escape into the tissue, producing a hematoma, or it may escape into spaces, producing a hemothorax, hemopericardium, or hemarthrosis. Superficial hemorrhages into the skin or mucosa are classified as petechiae (small, pinpoint capillary hemorrhages), purpura (diffuse, multiple, superficial hemorrhages), or ecchymoses (larger, confluent areas of hemorrhages). Hyperemia is an excess amount of blood within an organ. It may be caused by increased arterial supply (active hyperemia) or impaired venous drainage (passive hyperemia). Examples of active hyperemia include the increased blood flow during exercise, blushing, or inflammation. Examples of passive hyperemia, or congestion, include the changes produced by chronic heart failure. These changes include chronic passive congestion of the lung or the liver. The lung changes are characterized by intra-alveolar, hemosiderin-laden macrophages, called "heart failure cells." The congestion in the liver is characterized by centrilobular congestion, which is seen grossly as a "nutmeg" appearance of the liver.

19. The answer is c. (*Cotran, 5/e, pp 68–70, 100–103.*) The three main components of hemostasis include endothelial cells, platelets, and the coagulation system. Endothelial cells exhibit both procoagulant and anticoagulant properties. Their procoagulant activities involve activation of the extrinsic coagulation cascade by their production of tissue factor (thromboplastin) and stimulation of platelet aggregation by their production of von Willebrand's factor and platelet-activating factor. Their anticoagulant activities involve the production of prostacyclin (PGI$_2$), thrombomodulin, and plasminogen activator. The contrasting actions of the arachidonic acid metabolites prostacyclin and thromboxane A$_2$(TxA$_2$) produce a fine-tuned balance for the regulation of clotting. TxA$_2$, a product of the cyclooxygenase pathway of arachidonic acid metabolism, is synthesized in platelets and is a powerful platelet aggregator and vasoconstrictor. The prostaglandin PGI$_2$, also a product of the cyclooxygenase pathway but produced by endothelial cells, inhibits platelet aggregation and causes vasodilation. Aspirin, a cyclooxygenase inhibitor, blocks the synthesis of both TxA$_2$ and PGI$_2$ and is used in the treatment of coronary artery disease. Fibrinogen, which is produced by the liver, is cleaved by thrombin to form fibrin.

20. The answer is c. (*Henry, 19/e, pp 726–727. Cotran, 5/e, pp 103–106.*) The most important control of the coagulation cascade is the fibrinolytic system, the main component of which is plasmin. Plasminogen is converted into plasmin by either factor XII or a plasminogen activator (PA). Examples of PA's include tissue plasminogen activator (tPA), urokinase plasminogen activator, and streptokinase. Once formed, plasmin splits fibrin and also degrades both fibrinogen and coagulation factors VIII and V. Also important in the control of the coagulation cascade are plasma protease inhibitors, which include antithrombin III, protein C, and C91 inactivator. Antithrombin III in the presence of heparin inhibits thrombin, XIIa, XIa, Xa, and IXa, while protein C in the presence of heparin inhibits thrombin, XIIa, XIa, Xa, and IXa. C91 inactivator inhibits XIa, XIIa, and kallikrein. The significance of these control mechanisms is illustrated by patients with deficiencies of antithrombin III or protein C who develop recurrent thromboemboli. Thrombin acts differently in the coagulation cascade by converting fibrinogen to fibrin.

21. The answer is a. *(Cotran, 5/e, pp 105–108.)* Stasis of blood in fibrillating atria predisposes to thrombosis and embolism. Systemic embolization from left atrial thrombi may cause infarction in the brain, lower extremities, spleen, and kidneys. Endocardial mural thrombi occur as a consequence of myocardial infarction, bacterial endocarditis, or nonbacterial (marantic) endocarditis.

22. The answer is a. *(Cotran, 5/e, pp 113–114. Rubin, 2/e, pp 272–273.)* Fat embolism syndrome can supervene as a complication within 3 days following severe trauma to the long bones. However, the pathogenesis must be regarded as unknown because simple entrance of microglobular fat into the circulation as a result of damage to small vessels in marrow tissue occurs in over 90 percent of patients with trauma and bone fracture, yet the syndrome occurs in only a minority of such patients. Laboratory and clinical findings can simulate those of intravascular coagulopathy, which may be a component of fat embolism syndrome, with a major difference of split products of fibrin seen mainly in intravascular coagulopathy. Plasma levels of free fatty acids are elevated in fat embolism and may contribute to pulmonary vascular alterations. At autopsy fat material can be demonstrated in fat stains of frozen sections of lung, brain, and kidney in patients who had the syndrome.

23. The answer is e. *(Cotran, 5/e, pp 114–116, 1014–1015.)* Infarcts are localized areas of ischemic coagulative necrosis. They can be classified on the basis of their color into either red or white infarcts, or by the presence or absence of bacterial contamination into either septic or bland infarcts. White infarcts, also referred to as pale or anemic infarcts, are usually the result of arterial occlusion. They are found in solid organs such as the heart, spleen, and kidneys. Red or hemorrhagic infarcts, in contrast, may result from either arterial or venous occlusion. They occur in organs with a dual blood supply, such as the lung, or in organs with extensive collateral circulation, such as the small intestine and brain. These infarcts are hemorrhagic because there is bleeding into the necrotic area from the adjacent arteries and veins which remain patent. Hemorrhagic infarcts also occur in organs in which the venous outflow is obstructed, that is venous occlusion. Examples of this include torsion of the ovary or testis. In the latter twisting of the spermatic cord occludes the venous outflow, but the arterial inflow remains patent because these arterial blood vessels have much thicker walls. This results in venous infarction. Testicular torsion is usually the result of physical trauma in an individual with a predisposing abnormality, such as abnormal development of the gubernaculum testis.

24. The answer is d. (*Cotran, 5/e, pp 242–244. Chandrasoma, 3/e, pp 264–268.*) The names given to tumors are based on the parenchymal component of the tumor, which consists of the proliferating neoplastic cells. In general benign tumors are designated by using the suffix "-oma" attached to a name describing either the cell of origin of the tumor or the gross or microscopic appearance of the tumor. Examples of naming benign tumors based on their microscopic appearance include adenomas, which have a uniform proliferation of glandular epithelial cells, papillomas, which are tumors that form finger-like projections, fibromas, which are composed of a uniform proliferation of fibrous tissue, hemangiomas, which are formed from a uniform proliferation of endothelial cells, and lipomas, which originate from adipocytes. The suffix "-oma" is unfortunately still applied to some tumors that are not benign. Examples of this misnaming include melanomas, lymphomas, and seminomas.

Malignant tumors are generally classified as being either carcinomas or sarcomas. Carcinomas are malignant tumors of epithelial origin, while sarcomas are malignant tumors of mesenchymal tissue. Examples of malignant epithelial tumors (carcinomas) include adenocarcinomas, which consist of a disorganized mass of malignant cells that form glandular structures, and squamous cell carcinomas, which consist of a disorganized mass of malignant cells that produce keratin. Examples of malignant mesenchymal tumors include leiomyosarcomas, fibrosarcomas, and liposarcomas. One clue that a tumor developed from skeletal muscle is the presence of cross-striations. These individual cells seen histologically are called "strap cells." The wall of the stomach consists of smooth muscle, and a tumor that originates from these smooth muscle cells will consist of proliferating cells with elongated, spindle-shaped nuclei. If this tumor is benign it will be called a leiomyoma, while if it is malignant it will be called a leiomyosarcoma. This distinction is based on the number of mitoses that are present and the degree of atypia displayed by the neoplastic cells.

25. The answer is b. (*Cotran, 5/e, pp 245–252. Chandrasoma, 3/e, pp 260–264.*) Several gross and microscopic features help to differentiate benign neoplasms from malignant neoplasms. Benign neoplasms grow slowly with an expansile growth pattern that often forms a fibrous capsule. This histologic feature can also be useful in distinguishing a benign neoplastic lipoma from normal non-neoplastic adipose tissue. Benign neoplasms characteristically remain localized and do not metastasize. Histologically benign neoplastic cells tend to be uniform and well-differentiated, that is, they appear similar to their tissue of origin. This histologic feature may not distinguish between benign neoplasms and normal tissue. In contrast to benign tumors, malignant neoplasms grow rapidly in a "crab-like" pattern and are capable of metastasizing. Histologically, the malignant cells are pleomorphic because they differ from one another in size and shape. These cells have hyperchromatic nuclei and an increased nuclear to cytoplasmic ratio. Malignant cells tend to have nucleoli, and mitoses may be frequent. These two features only indicate rapidly proliferating cells and can also be seen in reactive or reparative processes. The mitoses in malignancies, however, tend to be atypical, such as tripolar mitoses. Malignant tumors are graded by their degree of differentiation into well-differentiated, moderately differentiated, and poorly differentiated malignancies. Marked pleomorphism is described as anaplasia. This histologic feature is usually seen in poorly differentiated or undifferentiated malignancies.

26. The answer is b. (*Cotran, 5/e, p 297. Chandrasoma, 3/e, pp 307–308.*) It is important to understand the difference between the grading and staging of a tumor. First of all, these terms are applied to malignant neoplasms and not to benign neoplasms. Basically, grading is done histologically, while staging is done clinically. Grading of a malignant tumor is based on the histologic degree of differentiation of the tumor cells and on the number of mitoses that are present. These histologic features are thought to be indicators of the aggressiveness of the malignant neoplasm. Cancers are generally classified as grades I through IV. Lower grades, such as grades I and II, are less aggressive and have a better prognosis, while higher grades, such as grades III and IV, are more aggressive and have a worse prognosis. In contrast to grading, the staging of cancers is based on the size of the primary lesion, the presence of lymph node metastases, and the presence of blood-borne metastases. These characteristics are determined by clinical means. One of the common staging classifications is the TNM classification. The "T" refers to the tumor size, the "N" refers to the presence of lymph node metastases, and the "M" refers to the presence of non-lymph node metastases. The location of the tumor is also important, as the TNM classification uses different staging systems depending upon the location of the primary tumor. Lower stages are smaller, localized, and have a better prognosis, while higher stages are larger, widespread, and have a worse prognosis. Staging has proved to be of greater clinical value than grading.

27. The answer is e. (*Cotran, 5/e, pp 264–265.*) There are several mechanisms by which proto-oncogenes (p-oncs) can become oncogenic (c-oncs). Normal cellular genes (proto-oncogenes) may become oncogenic by being incorporated into the viral genome (forming v-oncs), or they may by activated by other processes to form cellular oncogenes (c-oncs). These other processes include gene mutations, chromosomal translocations, and gene amplifications. Gene mutations, such as point mutations, are associated with the formation of cancers by mutant *c-ras* oncogenes. This abnormality is found in many visceral adenocarcinomas.

Chromosomal translocations are associated with the development of many types of cancers, one example of which is Burkitt's lymphoma. The most common translocation associated with Burkitt's lymphoma is t(8;14), in which the *c-myc* oncogene on chromosome 8 is brought in contact with the immunoglobulin heavy chain gene on chromosome 14. Two other examples of chromosomal translocations are the association of chronic myelocytic leukemia (CML) with t(9;22), which is the Philadelphia chromosome, and the association of follicular lymphoma with the translocation t(18;14). The former involves the proto-oncogene *c-abl*, which is rearranged in proximity to a break point cluster region (bcr) on chromosome 22. The resultant chimeric *c-abl/bcr* gene encodes a protein with tyrosine kinase activity. The t(18;14) involves the *bcl-2* oncogene on chromosome 18. Expression of the oncogene *bcl-2* is associated with the prevention of apoptosis in germinal centers. Examples of associations that involve gene amplification include *N-myc* and neuroblastoma, *c-neu* and breast cancer, and *erb-B* and breast and ovarian cancer. Gene amplification can be demonstrated by finding doublet minutes or homogenous staining regions.

28. The answer is d. (*Cotran, 5/e, pp 259–263, 265–270.*) Most proto-oncogenes are genes that encode for proteins that promote cell growth, but cancer suppressor genes encode proteins that suppress cellular proliferation. Examples of tumor suppressor genes are Rb (associated with retinoblastoma), p53, APC, NF_1, DCC, and WT_1. The p53 gene, located on chromosome 17, is the single most common target for genetic alterations in human cancers. It is found in many cases of colon, breast, and lung cancers. Mutations in the APC (adenomatous polyposis coli) gene lead to the development of tumors that may progress to adenocarcinomas of the colon, while mutations in the NF_1 (neurofibromatosis type 1) gene lead to the development of neurofibromas, some of which may progress to neurofibrosarcomas. DCC (deleted in colon carcinoma) is a tumor suppressor gene located on chromosome 18, which is related to the formation of carcinomas of the colon and stomach. Deletion of WT_1, located on chromosome 11, is associated with the development of Wilms' tumor, a childhood neoplasm of the kidney. Genes c-abl, located on chromosome 9, and bcr, located on chromosome 22, are translocated in cases of chronic myelocytic leukemia. The gene c-myc, located on chromosome 8, is translocated in cases of Burkitt's lymphoma. The c-ras oncogene is involved in the genesis of many human cancers. It is not a normal suppressor gene.

29. The answer is a. *(Cotran, 5/e, pp 283–284.)* Many chemicals are associated with an increased incidence of malignancy. These substances are called chemical carcinogens. Although there are direct acting chemical carcinogens, such as the direct acting alkylating agents that are used in chemotherapy, most organic carcinogens first require conversion to a more reactive compound. Polycyclic aromatic hydrocarbons, aromatic amines, and azo dyes must be metabolized by cytochrome P450-dependent mixed function oxidases to active metabolites. Vinyl chloride is metabolized to an epoxide and is associated with angiosarcoma of the liver, not hepatocellular carcinoma. Azo dyes, such as butter yellow and scarlet red, are metabolized to active compounds that have induced hepatocellular cancer in rats, but no human cases have been reported. Beta-naphthylamine is an exception to the general rule involving cytochrome P450, as the hydrolysis of the nontoxic conjugate occurs in the urinary bladder by the urinary enzyme glucuronidase. In the past there has been an increase in bladder cancer in workers in the aniline dye and rubber industries that have been exposed to these compounds. Aflatoxin B_1, a natural product of the fungus *Aspergillus flavus*, is metabolized to an epoxide. The fungus can grow on improperly stored peanuts and grains and is associated with the high incidence of hepatocellular carcinoma in some areas of Africa and the Far East. Hepatitis B virus is also highly associated with liver cancer in these regions.

30. The answer is a. (*Cotran, 5/e, pp 284–286, 1169–1170.*) Hereditary factors are important in the development of many types of cancers. They are particularly important in several inherited neoplasia syndromes. The autosomal recessive DNA-chromosomal instability syndromes include ataxia-telangiectasia, Bloom syndrome, Fanconi's anemia, and xeroderma pigmentosa. These disorders have in common abnormalities involving the normal repair of DNA. Patients with xeroderma pigmentosa have defective endonuclease activity, which normally repairs the pyrimidine dimers found in ultraviolet (UV) light damaged DNA. These patients have an increased incidence of skin cancers, including basal cell carcinoma, squamous cell carcinoma, and malignant melanoma. Wiskott-Aldrich syndrome, characterized by thrombocytopenia and eczema, is an immunodeficiency disease associated with an increased incidence of lymphomas and acute leukemias. Familial polyposis is characterized by the formation of numerous neoplastic adenomatous colon polyps. These individuals have a 100 percent risk of developing colorectal carcinoma unless surgery is performed. Sturge-Weber syndrome is a rare congenital disorder associated with venous angiomatous masses in the leptomeninges and ipsilateral port-wine nevi of the face. Multiple endocrine neoplasia (MEN) syndrome type I, Wermer syndrome, refers to the combination of adenomas of the pituitary, adenomas or hyperplasia of the parathyroid glands, and islet cell tumors of the pancreas.

31. The answer is b. (*Cotran, 5/e, pp 295–297. Chandrasoma, 3/e, pp 858.*) Symptoms not caused by either local or metastatic effects of tumors are called paraneoplastic syndromes. Bronchogenic carcinomas are associated with the development of many different types of paraneoplastic syndromes. These syndromes are usually associated with the secretion of certain substances by the tumor cells. For example, ectopic secretion of ACTH may produce Cushing's syndrome, while ectopic secretion of antidiuretic hormone (syndrome of inappropriate ADH secretion) may produce hyponatremia. Hypocalcemia may result from the production of calcitonin, while hypercalcemia may result from the production of parathyroid hormone-related peptide (PTHrP), which is a normal substance produced locally by many different types of tissue. PTHrP is distinct from parathyroid hormone (PTH). Therefore, patients with this type of paraneoplastic syndrome will have increased calcium levels and decreased PTH levels. As a result of decreased PTH production, all of the parathyroid glands in these patients will be atrophic. Other tumors associated with the production of PTHrP include clear cell carcinomas of the kidney, endometrial adenocarcinomas, and transitional carcinomas of the urinary bladder.

Lung cancers are also associated with multiple, migratory venous thrombosis. This migratory thrombophlebitis is called Trousseau's sign and is more classically associated with carcinoma of the pancreas. Hypertrophic osteoarthropathy is a syndrome consisting of periosteal new bone formation with or without digital clubbing and joint effusion. It is most commonly found in association with lung carcinoma, but it also occurs with other types of pulmonary disease. Erythrocytosis is associated with increased erythropoietin levels and some tumors, particularly renal cell carcinoma, hepatocellular carcinoma, and cerebellar hemangioblastoma. It is not particularly associated with bronchogenic carcinomas.

32. The answer is a. (*Damjanov, 10/e, pp 714–716. Cotran, 5/e, pp 327–328.*) Protein-calorie malnutrition in underdeveloped countries leads to a spectrum of symptoms from kwashiorkor at one end to marasmus at the other. Marasmus, caused by a lack of caloric intake (i.e., starvation), leads to generalized wasting, stunted growth, atrophy of muscles, and loss of subcutaneous fat. There is no edema or hepatic enlargement. These children are alert, not apathetic, and are ravenous. In contrast, children with kwashiorkor, which is characterized by a lack of protein despite adequate caloric intake, have peripheral edema, a "moon" face, and an enlarged, fatty liver. The peripheral edema is caused by decreased albumin and sodium retention, while the fatty liver is caused by decreased synthesis of the lipoproteins necessary for the normal mobilization of lipids from liver cells. Additionally these children have "flaky paint" areas of skin and abnormal pigmented streaks in their hair ("flag sign"). In children with marasmus, the skin is inelastic due to loss of subcutaneous fat. In either severe kwashiorkor or marasmus, thymic atrophy may result in the reduction in number and function of circulating T cells. B-cell function (i.e., immunoglobulin production) is also depressed, so that these children are highly vulnerable to infections.

33. The answer is d. (*Cotran, 5/e, pp 411–414.*) The symptoms of vitamin A deficiency result from abnormalities involving the normal functions of vitamin A. These normal functions include maintaining mucus-secreting epithelium, restoring levels of the visual pigment rhodopsin, increasing immunity to infections, and acting as an antioxidant. Deficiencies of vitamin

A will result in squamous metaplasia of mucus membranes, not intestinal metaplasia. Squamous metaplasia of the respiratory tract will lead to increased numbers of pulmonary infections due to lack of the normal protective muco-ciliary "elevator." Squamous metaplasia of the urinary tract will lead to increased numbers of urinary tract stones, while such metaplasia in sebaceous and sweat glands of dry skin causes follicular hyperkeratosis and predisposes to acne. There are numerous eye changes produced by a vitamin A deficiency. These changes include dry eyes (xerophthalmia), soft cornea (keratomalacia), and elevated white plaques of keratin debris on the conjunctiva (Bitot's spots). Because vitamin A is important in the normal function of rhodopsin, a visual pigment important for vision in dim light, a deficiency of vitamin A is associated with poor vision in dim light. This night blindness is usually the first symptom seen in patients with a vitamin A deficiency.

Rather than causing acute leukemia, vitamin A is used with good results in the treatment of a particular type of acute leukemia, namely acute promyelocytic leukemia. Megaloblastic anemia is associated with a deficiency of either vitamin B12 or folate, while a deficiency of vitamin D will lead to decreased mineralization of bones (soft bones).

34. The answer is b. (*Cotran, 5/e, pp 414–418.*) Vitamin D is essential for maintenance of normal bone remodeling in the adult; therefore, a significant deficiency in adults leads to poorly mineralized bone, or osteomalacia. Deficiency also results in decreased intestinal absorption of calcium, inadequate serum calcium and phosphorus, and, therefore, impaired mineralization of osteoid. Defective mineralization of osteoid causes formation of soft, easily deformed bones. Since there is no decreased production of osteoid matrix, a relative excess of woven bone or osteoid with wide osteoid seams results.

35. The answer is e. (*Cotran, 5/e, pp 414–418, 423–425.*) Vitamin C (ascorbic acid) is a water-soluble vitamin that is important in many body functions, such as the synthesis of collagen, osteoid, certain neurotransmitters, and carnitine. In the synthesis of collagen, vitamin C functions as a cofactor for the hydroxylation of proline and lysine and for the formation of the triple helix of tropocollagen. Patients with decreased vitamin C (scurvy) will have abnormal synthesis of connective tissue due to abnormal synthesis of collagen along with abnormal synthesis of osteoid. The former will lead to impaired wound healing. In addition, previous wounds may reopen. Because the synthesis of collagen is abnormal, the blood vessels will be fragile. This will lead to bleeding gums, tooth loss, subperiosteal hemorrhage, and petechial perifollicular skin hemorrhages. Abnormal synthesis of osteoid (unmineralized bone) will lead to decreased amounts of osteoid in the bone and increased calcification of the cartilage. Vitamin C also functions as an antioxidant and is important in neutrophil function and iron absorption in the gut. These functions will also be decreased in patients with scurvy. This syndrome is common in elderly people living on a diet deficient in milk, fruits, and vegetables.

In contrast to scurvy, which is caused by a deficiency of vitamin C, rickets is caused by a deficiency of vitamin D. Ricketts is characterized by a lack of calcium. In this abnormality the osteoblasts in bone continue to synthesize osteoid, but this material is not mineralized. This results in increased amounts of osteoid (unmineralized bone) and decreased mineralized bone. In adults this produces osteomalacia and bone pain. Histologically, the bone osteoid seams are markedly increased in thickness. In children this produces rickets, a disease that is characterized by increased osteoid at normal growth centers of bone. This produces wide epiphyses at the wrists and knees and leads to growth retardation. Beriberi is caused by a deficiency of thiamine, pellagra by a deficiency of niacin, and kwashiorkor by a deficiency of protein.

36. The answer is a. (*Cotran, 5/e, pp 390–392.*) Increased amounts of δ-aminolevulinic acid (ALA) and coproporphyrin are found in the urine of patients who have ingested lead. Lead interferes with erythropoiesis by inhibiting the activity of several enzymes, including δ-ALA synthetase and ALA dehydrase. Thus the various degrees of anemia that are usually associated with lead poisoning are likely to be mediated by interference with erythropoietic-dependent enzymes, causing a microcytic, hypochromic anemia with basophilic stippling of the erythrocytes. Additional clinical findings include abdominal colic and a wristdrop and footdrop caused by a peripheral demyelinating neuropathy.

37. The answer is c. (*Rubin, 2/e, pp 310–313.*) Heavy metal poisoning may occur via the respiratory route owing to contaminated inhalant and vapors. Such poisoning is usually industrially related, as with mercury (calomel workers), arsenic (pesticides), and lead (batteries and paints). Cadmium has been implicated in producing not only an acute form of pneumonia, but, with chronic exposure to small concentrations of cadmium vapors, diffuse interstitial pulmonary fibrosis and an increased incidence of emphysema as well. The "honeycomb" radiologic pattern is indicative of an interstitial fibrotic process and may be the result of repeated pneumonitis and bronchitis. Cadmium can also be found in tobacco smoke. Cobalt poisoning leads to myocardiopathy, mercury poisoning leads to renal tubular damage, and lead poisoning leads to liver necrosis and cerebral edema. Arsenic poisoning, in addition to carrying an increased risk of lung and skin cancer, may cause death by inhibition of respiratory enzymes and cardiac subendocardial hemorrhages complicated by gastroenteritis with shock.

38. The answer is d. (*Cotran, 5/e, p 397. Rubin, 2/e, pp 308–313.*) Many environmental chemicals are potential causes of quite serious human diseases. Cyanide causes cellular damage by binding to cytochrome oxidase and inhibiting cellular respiration. It is a component of amygdalin, which is found in the pits of several fruits, such as apricots and peaches. Cyanide poisoning is betrayed by the presence of the odor of bitter almonds. Ethylene glycol, commonly used as an antifreeze, is toxic to humans. It causes acute tubular necrosis in the kidney. Carbon monoxide replaces oxygen in hemoglobin and causes the formation of carboxyhemoglobin and anoxia. Despite the extreme cyanosis, it produces a characteristic cherry-red color to the skin. Mercury toxicity damages both the kidney (proximal tubular necrosis) and the brain. The neurologic symptoms include mental changes and a tremor. Mercury was used in the hat industry, and the symptoms of toxicity resulted in the expression "mad as a hatter." Methanol, originally called "wood alcohol," is metabolized in the body to formaldehyde and formic acid. These metabolites cause necrosis of retinal ganglion cells, which produces blindness.

39. The answer is b. (*Cotran, 5/e, pp 127–129, 152–154.*) Mendel's laws deal with single-gene mutations that may be inherited or acquired de novo, with expression of the abnormality highly variable. In autosomal dominant inheritances, if a mutant gene is unexpressed, this is called reduced penetrance and it may vary by a percentage that reflects the degree of expression. Variable expressivity refers to expression of the trait in all who harbor the mutant gene, but with different expressions of the abnormality. Nondisjunction refers to a failure of disjoining of a homologous pair of chromosomes during meiosis (may result in aneuploidy). Codominance refers to the full expression of both alleles of a gene pair. Genetic heterogeneity applies to multiple-loci mutations (each in a different location, reflecting multiple different mutations), which can result in the same or similar expressed abnormality.

40. The answer is d. (*Cotran, 5/e, pp 1285–1287.*) Classification of the muscular dystrophies is based on the mode of inheritance and clinical features. Inheritance of the Duchenne type is by an X-linked recessive trait, with the gene located on the short arm of the X chromosome, although spontaneous mutations are fairly common. Autosomal dominant inheritance characterizes both myotonic dystrophy and the facioscapulohumeral type, while limb-girdle dystrophy is autosomal recessive. In Duchenne's muscular dystrophy, males are affected and symptoms begin before the age of 4. Pelvic-girdle muscles are affected with resultant difficulty in walking, and this is followed by shoulder-girdle weakness and eventual involvement of respiratory and cardiac muscles with death from respiratory failure before age 20. Histologic changes include rounded, atrophic fibers, hypertrophied fibers, degenerative and regenerative changes in adjacent myocytes, and necrotic fibers invaded by histiocytes. Elevation of serum creatine kinase is marked.

41. The answer is e. (*Cotran, 5/e, pp 163–164, 1289–1291. Damjanov, 10/e, pp 298–299.*) Almost all genes occur on chromosomes within the nucleus. There are a few genes, however, that are located within the mitochondria. These mitochondrial genes are found on mitochondrial DNA (mtDNA). These genes are all of maternal origin because ova have mitochondria within the large amount of cytoplasm, and sperm do not. This maternal origin means that mothers transmit all of the mtDNA to both male and female offspring, but only the daughters transmit it further. No transmission occurs through males. This mtDNA contains genes that mainly code for oxidative phosphorylation enzymes, such as NADH dehydrogenase, cytochrome c oxidase, and ATP synthase. Symptoms of deficiencies of these enzymes occur in organs that require large amounts of ATP, such as the brain, muscle, liver, and kidneys. The mtDNA of these patients may be composed of either a mixture of mutant and normal DNA (heteroplasmy) or of mutant DNA entirely (homoplasmy). The severity of these diseases correlates with the amount of mutant mtDNA that is present. One disease associated with mitochondrial inheritance is Leber hereditary optic neuropathy (LHON), characterized by progressive bilateral loss of central vision, which usually occurs between 15 and 35 years of age. Other examples of mitochondrial inheritance include mitochondrial myopathies, which are characterized by the presence of abnormal size and shaped mitochondria in muscle. These abnormal mitochondria may result in the histologic appearance of the muscle as being ragged red fibers. Electron microscopy reveals the presence within large mitochondria of rectangular crystals that have a "parking-lot" appearance.

42. The answer is a. (*Cotran, 5/e, pp 142–143.*) Sphingomyelin, a lipid composed of phosphocholine and a ceramide, characteristically is found in abnormally high concentrations throughout the body tissues of patients who have any one of the forms of Niemann-Pick disease. Division of this disease into five categories is generally accepted; type A, the acute neuronopathic form, is the one that has the highest incidence. The lack of sphingomyelinase in type A is the metabolic defect that prevents the hydrolytic cleavage of sphingomyelin, which then accumulates in the brain. Patients who have the type A form usually show hepatosplenomegaly at 6 months of age, progressively lose motor functions and mental capabilities, and die during the third year of life.

43. The answer is a. (*Cotran, 5/e, pp 146–147. Rubin, 2/e, pp 240–241.*) The glycogen storage diseases are due to defective metabolism of glycogen, and at least eleven syndromes from genetic defects in the responsible enzymes have been described. Most of these glycogenoses are inherited as autosomal recessive disorders. Von Gierke's disease (type I) results from deficiency of glucose-6-phosphatase, the hepatic enzyme needed for conversion of G6P to glucose, with glycogen accumulation particularly in the enlarged liver and kidney and hypoglycemia. Diagnosis requires biopsy demonstration of excess liver glycogen plus either absent or low liver G6P activity, or a diabetic glucose tolerance curve, or hyperuricemia. Von Gierke's disease is the major hepatic or hepatorenal type of glycogenosis. Lysosomal glucosidase deficiency causes Pompe's disease (type II). Glycogen storage is widespread but most prominent in the heart (cardiomegaly). In brancher glycogenosis (type IV) there is accumulation of amylopectin or abnormal glycogen in liver, heart, skeletal muscle, and brain. The major myopathic form, McArdle's disease (type V), is due to lack of muscle phosphorylase.

Glucose-6-phosphate dehydrogenase (G6PD) deficiency may cause oxidant-induced hemolytic anemia. The gene is X-linked recessive. One variant is present in about 10 percent of African-Americans.

44. The answer is c. (*Cotran, 5/e, pp 138–144.*) One group of lysosomal storage diseases is characterized by the abnormal accumulation of sphingolipids (SL). Some types of sphingolipids are typically found within the central nervous system, and therefore abnormal accumulation of these substances will produce neurologic signs and symptoms. For example, ganglion cells within the retina, particularly at the periphery of the macula, may become swollen with excess sphingolipids. The affected area of the retina will appear pale when viewed through an ophthalmoscope. In contrast the normal color of the macula, which does not have accumulated substances, appears more red than normal. This is referred to as a cherry-red spot or a cherry-red macula. Substances that may produce this cherry-red spot include sphingomyelin, which is increased in individuals with Neiman-Pick's disease, and gangliosides, which may be increased in individuals with Tay-Sachs disease, Sandhoff's disease, or GM_1 gangliosidosis.

Autosomal recessive disorders tend to be more common in areas in which in-breeding is more common. An example of this is the increased frequency of several autosomal recessive genes in Ashkenazi Jews. "Ashkenazi" denotes an ethnic group, mostly of the Jewish faith, from Eastern Europe. People of this faith tend to marry other members of the faith. Two storage diseases that have a higher incidence in Ashkenazi Jews are Tay-Sachs disease and Type I Gaucher disease. Tay-Sachs disease is due to a deficiency of hexosaminidase A. This same enzyme is decreased in patients with Sandhoff's disease. Hexosaminidase A is composed of an α subunit and a β subunit. In contrast, hexosaminidase B is composed of two β subunits. Patients with Tay-Sachs disease have a deficiency of the α subunit. Therefore, they have a deficiency of hexosaminidase A, but not hexosaminidase B. In contrast, patients with Sandhoff's disease have a deficiency of the β subunit, and they have a deficiency of both hexosaminidase A and hexosaminidase B. In patients with Tay-Sachs disease, accumulation of GM_2 ganglioside occurs within many tissues including the heart, liver, spleen, and brain. Electron microscopy reveals cytoplasmic whorled lamellar bodies within lysosomes. There are several clinical forms of Tay-Sachs disease, but the most severe is the infantile type.

Patients develop mental retardation, seizures, motor incoordination, blindness (amaurosis), and usually die by the age of three.

Type I Gaucher's disease is due to a deficiency of β-glucocerebrosidase. Patients may have increased serum levels of acid phosphatase, an enzyme that is typically found in the prostate, erythrocytes, and platelets. Patients with Gaucher's disease have excess glucocerebrosides accumulation within phagocytic cells, not ganglion cells. Sphingomyelinase is decreased in patients with Neiman-Picks disease, while aryl-sulfatase is decreased in patients with metachromatic leukodystrophy (MLD).

45. The answer is a. (*Cotran, 5/e, pp 143–144.*) The photomicrograph in the question shows the presence of lipid-laden macrophages that have replaced much of the splenic parenchyma. The macrophages have a somewhat vacuolated cytoplasm, which is characteristic of Gaucher's disease. This is an autosomal recessive disease characterized by a reduction or a deficiency of glucocerebrosidase. Thus glucocerebroside accumulates mainly in the mononuclear phagocytic system. Three clinical types occur. The classic is type I, which occurs in adults and generally spares the central nervous system with the glucocerebrosides limited to the mononuclear phagocyte system of the spleen, liver, and bone marrow. This is mainly found in European Jewish patients and is the most common form of Gaucher's disease. Type II is the infantile form, which involves the brain and presents no detectable glucocerebrosidase activity. Death occurs at an early age. Type III may be thought of as being an intermediate between types I and II; it is found in adolescent patients and mainly involves the mononuclear phagocyte system early but will involve the brain by the third decade of life. α-Galactosidase deficiency (Fabry's disease), which is characterized by angiokeratomas of the skin, involves marked ceramide trihexosid accumulations within the endothelial and smooth muscle cells of blood vessels, ganglion cells, heart, renal tubules, and glomeruli. Glucosidase deficiency is type II glycogen storage disease, which is one of the variants of liver phosphorylase deficiency. Glucose-6-phosphate dehydrogenase deficiency results in hemolytic disease in both sexes, with the male more severely affected.

46. The answer is d. (*Cotran, 5/e, pp 140–143.*) The cell in the photomicrograph is known as Gaucher's cell, the pathognomonic histopathologic finding in Gaucher's disease, and is a histiocyte typically found in the spleen, liver, and bone marrow. The cytoplasm contains glucocerebroside in an increased concentration that is demonstrable by periodic acid-Schiff reagent staining and appears wrinkled or striated in ordinary light microscopy. Histochemical ultrastructure studies have revealed that the unique cytoplasmic wrinkles are due to the presence of many spindle-shaped bodies (Gaucher's bodies) that contain 90 percent glucocerebroside and that show increased acid phosphatase activity. A characteristic histopathologic (but not pathognomonic) finding in Niemann-Pick disease is the foam cell; this cell is found mainly in lymphoid tissues.

47. The answer is d. (*Cotran, 5/e, pp 132, 147–148, 449–450. Rubin, 2/e, pp 240–244.*) Several autosomal recessive disorders involve inborn errors of amino acid metabolism. Alkaptonuria (ochronosis) is caused by the excess accumulation of homogentisic acid. This results from a block in the metabolism of the phenylalanine-tyrosine pathway, which is caused by a deficiency of homogentisic oxidase. Excess homogentisic acid causes the urine to turn dark upon standing after a period of time. It also causes a dark coloration of the sclera, tendons, and cartilage. After years, many patients will develop a degenerative arthritis. Phenylketonuria (PKU), also called hyperphenylalaninemia, results from a deficiency of phenylalanine hydroxylase, an enzyme that oxidizes phenylalanine to tyrosine in the liver. Infants are normal at birth, but rising phenylalanine levels (hyperphenylalaninemia) results in irreversible brain damage. The excess phenylacetic acid in the urine results in a "mousy" odor. A lack of the enzyme fumarylacetoacetate hydrolase results in increased levels of tyrosine (tyrosinemia). Chronic forms of the disease are associated with cirrhosis of the liver, kidney dysfunction, and a high risk of developing hepatocellular carcinoma. Maple syrup urine disease is associated with an enzyme defect that causes the accumulation of branched-chain α-keto acid derivatives of isoleucine, leucine, and valine. Albinism refers to a group of disorders characterized by an abnormality of the synthesis of melanin. Two forms of oculocutaneous albinism are classified by the presence or absence of tyrosinase, which is the first enzyme in the conversion of tyrosine to melanin. Albinos are at a greatly increased risk for the development of squamous cell carcinomas in sun-exposed skin.

48. The answer is c. (*Cotran, 5/e, pp 152–153.*) Any deviation from the normal number of chromosomes, from their normal structure, or a combination of the two is an aberration that, if unbalanced, is termed aneuploidy. If the alterations remain balanced (balanced translocations), the condition is termed euploidy. Aneuploidy can result from the addition of a single chromosome to a pair (trisomy) or from translocations, inversions, duplications, and deletions.

49. The answer is a. (*Cotran, 5/e, p 156. Rubin, 2/e, p 220.*) Several genetic diseases are characterized by a deletion of part of an autosomal chromosome. The 5p⁻ syndrome is also called the cri du chat syndrome as affected infants characteristically have a high-pitched cry similar to that of a kitten. Additional findings in this disorder include severe mental retardation, microcephaly, and congenital heart disease. The 11p⁻ syndrome is characterized by the congenital absence of the iris (aniridia) and is often accompanied by Wilms tumor of the kidney. The 13q⁻ syndrome is associated with the loss of the Rb suppressor gene and the development of retinoblastoma. Signs and symptoms of patients with either 21q⁻ or 22q⁻ are similar to those of Down's syndrome.

50. The answer is d. (*Cotran, 5/e, pp 158–159.*) The Barr body represents a sex chromatin clump attached to the nuclear membrane that originates from an entire X chromosome and can easily be seen by using light microscopy to examine scrapings of the epithelium of the inside buccal mucosa. According to the formula $M = n - 1$, the total number of X chromatin masses equals the number of cellular X chromatin masses seen in the nucleus minus 1. Hence, normal males are $0 = 1 - 1$ (no Barr body), and normal females are $1 = 2 - 1$ (one Barr body). In classic Turner's syndrome (XO), the expected buccal smear would be $0 = 1 - 1$ (no Barr bodies seen), as in a normal male. Karyotyping is necessary when the Barr body screening test is ambiguous or inconclusive. In a young woman of short stature and average intelligence who has never menstruated, there is a strong indication that one of the forms of Turner's syndrome exists, and the presence of one Barr body indicates that the patient has XX in some percentage of cells. About 10 percent of all Turner's syndrome patients show a mosaic pattern, with some cells having XO/XX or XO/XXX patterns. In this example, the patient is likely to be XO/XX by the formula $1 = 2 - 1$. In Turner's mosaics, the likelihood of developing a seminoma or gonadoblastoma is higher than expected, and gonadectomy may be indicated.

51. The answer is d. (*Cotran, 5/e, pp 160–162, 1156–1157.*) Sexual ambiguity arises when there is disagreement between the various ways of determining sex. Genetic sex is determined by the presence or absence of a Y chromosome. Gonadal sex is based upon the histologic appearance of the gonads. Ductal sex depends on the presence of derivatives of the müllerian or wolffian ducts. Phenotypic or genital sex is based on the appearance of the external genitalia. True hermaphroditism refers to the presence of both ovarian and testicular tissue. Pseudohermaphroditism is a disagreement between the phenotypic and gonadal sex. A female pseudohermaphrodite has ovaries but external male genitalia, while a male pseudohermaphrodite has testicular tissue, resulting from an XY genital sex karyotype, but female external genitalia. Female pseudohermaphroditism results from excessive exposure to androgens during early gestation; most often this is the result of congenital adrenal hyperplasia. Male pseudohermaphroditism results from defective virilization of the male embryo, most commonly caused by complete androgen insensitivity syndrome, also called testicular feminization. Turner's syndrome, which has a 45,X0 karyotype, is characterized by a female phenotype and bilateral streak ovaries. Mixed gonadal dysgenesis consists of one well-defined testis and a contralateral streak ovary. It is a cause of ambiguous genitalia in the newborn.

52. The answer is a. (*Cotran, 5/e, pp 162–163.*) Fragile X syndrome is one of four diseases that are characterized by long repeating sequences of three nucleotides. The other diseases are Huntington disease, myotonic dystrophy, and spinal and bulbar muscular atrophy. The fragile X syndrome, which is more common in males than females, is one of the most common causes of familial mental retardation. Additional clinical features of this disorder include developmental delay, a long face with a large mandible, large everted ears, and large testicles (macro-orchidism). Examination of the DNA from patients with fragile X syndrome reveals multiple tandem repeats of the nucleotide sequence CGG on the X chromosome. Normally these repeats average up to 50 in number, but in patients with fragile X syndrome there are more than 230 repeats. This number of repeats is called a full mutation. Normal transmitting males (NTM) and carrier females have between 50 to 230 CGG repeats. This number of repeats is called a premutation. During oogenesis, but not spermatogenesis, premutations can be converted to mutations by amplification of the triplet repeats. This explains the much higher incidence of mental retardation in grandsons rather than brothers of normal transmitting males (Sherman's paradox), as the pre-mutation is amplified in females, but not in males. Since the premutation is not amplified in males, no daughters of NTM are affected. An additional finding associated with these repeat units is anticipation, which refers to the fact that the disease is worse with subsequent generations.

53. The answer is e. *(Cotran, 5/e, pp 443–444. Rubin, 2/e, pp 209–211.)* TORCH is an acronym referring to a group of microorganisms that produce similar changes during fetal or neonatal infection. The T stands for toxoplasma, the O for others, the R for rubella, the C for cytomegalovirus, and the H for herpes simplex virus. The "others" include syphilis, tuberculosis, and many other microorganisms. Manifestations of the TORCH complex include brain lesions, such as encephalitis and intracranial calcifications; ocular defects, including chorioretinitis; and cardiac abnormalities. Children born with congenital syphilis, caused by maternal infection with Treponema pallidum, initially show changes typical of the TORCH complex, but later they may develop characteristic lesions including flattening of the nose (saddle nose), notched incisors (Hutchinson's teeth), malformed molars (mulberry molars), outward bowing of the anterior tibia (saber shins), and progressive vascularization of the cornea (interstitial keratitis). The combination of deafness, interstitial keratitis, and notched incisors is referred to as Hutchinson's triad.

54. The answer is e. *(Rubin, 2/e, pp 1458, 1463, 1465, 1473.)* Retinopathy of prematurity, also called retrolental fibroplasia, is a cause of blindness in premature infants that is related to the therapeutic use of high concentrations of oxygen. The developing vessels in the retina become fibrosed, and the peripheral retina does not vascularize normally. The incidence of this complication has been markedly reduced due to close clinical monitoring of the concentration of administered oxygen. Presbyopia is an aging change resulting in loss of accommodation that affects most people at about the age of 40. Sun damage to the conjunctiva results in a yellow lesion at the limbus, a pinguecula. If the tissue encroaches on the cornea, it is called a pterygium. The macula has a large number of cones and is related to visual acuity. Degeneration of the macula occurs most often from age-related maculopathy, but it can also be caused by inherited disorders or drugs, such as chloroquine.

55. The answer is d. *(Cotran, 5/e, pp 265, 459–461.)* Neuroblastomas are malignant tumors of the adrenal medulla that occur in very young patients who present with an abdominal mass. Histologically, these tumors are composed of small cells forming Homer-Wright rosettes, which are groups of cells arranged in a ring around a central mass of pink neural filaments. Electron microscopy reveals neurosecretory granules within the cytoplasm of the tumor cells, while immunohistochemical stains are positive for neuron-specific enolase (NSE). These highly aggressive tumors are unique because some will spontaneously regress and some will de-differentiate into benign tumors, such as ganglioneuromas. Three distinct chromosomal abnormalities are associated with neuroblastomas. These abnormalities include near-terminal deletion of part of the short arm of chromosome 1 (partial monosomy 1), homogeneously staining regions (HSR) of chromosome 2, and multiple double minute chromatin bodies. The latter two are the result of amplification of the oncogene N-myc. The number of N-myc copies correlates with the aggressiveness of the tumor. De-differentiation of a neuroblastoma into a benign ganglioneuroma is associated with a marked reduction in this gene amplification. In contrast, deletion of chromosome 11 is associated with nephroblastoma (Wilm's tumor), a malignant tumor of the kidney found in young patients. This chromosome abnormality is associated with deletion of WT-1, a tumor suppressor gene.

56. The answer is b. (*Cotran, 5/e, pp 171–174.*) Some features of leukocytes are specific for certain cells of the immune system. Some of these features involve substances on the surface of these cells. B lymphocytes are the type of leukocytes that have IgM on their surface. This surface immunoglobulin participates in the binding of B cells to many different antigens. The diversity of this binding and the subsequent production of many different immunoglobulins is obtained by rearrangement of the immunoglobulin genes from their germline configuration. This rearrangement occurs only in B lymphocytes, and thus, the presence of rearranged immunoglobulin genes in a lymphoid cell indicates that the cell is a B lymphocyte. Similarly, T lymphocytes have a surface antigen-binding receptor (TCR) that consists of CD3 proteins attached to a heterodimer composed of alpha, beta, gamma, or delta polypeptide chains. Demonstration of TCR gene rearrangement is a molecular marker of T lymphocytes. Macrophages, required to process antigen to T cells, have class II HLA antigens on their surface. They are also active phagocytes and have receptors for the Fc portion of IgG and C3a. Dendritic cells, present in lymphoid tissue, and Langerhans cells, present in the epidermis, are antigen-presenting cells. They have large amounts of class II HLA antigens on their cell surfaces. Natural killer cells are identified by two cell surface molecules, CD16 and CD56.

57. The answer is b. (*Henry, 19/e, pp 913–927. Chandrasoma, 3/e, pp 59–63.*) Immunoglobulins (Ig) are the product of plasma cells, the effector cells of B lymphocyte activation. Ig's are composed of light chains and heavy chains, each of which are composed of a variable region and a constant region. The variable regions of both of these chains form the antigen-binding region of Ig, which is called the Fab portion. The portion of Ig that binds complement is called the Fc portion. Not only can the Fc portion of Ig bind to complement, but it can bind to cells that have Fc receptors. There are two types of light chains and five types of heavy chains. The two light chains are kappa, the genes of which are located on chromosome 2, and lambda, the genes of which are located on chromosome 22. The heavy chains are M, D, A, E, and G, the genes of all of these being on chromosome 14. The combination of one type of light chain with a particular heavy chain will form each of the five types of immunoglobulin.

The most abundant Ig in the serum (80 percent) is IgG. It is secreted in the second response to certain antigens, but it does not predominate early during the first response. IgG can cross the placenta, and it is the major protective immunoglobulin in the neonate. IgG can also activate complement, participate in antibody-dependent cell-mediated cytotoxicity (ADCC), neutralize toxins or viruses, and function as an opsonin. IgM, which constitutes about 5 to 10 percent of the Ig in the serum, is secreted in the first exposure to antigen (primary immune response). The monomeric form of IgM is found on the surface of some B cells, while the pentameric form is found in the serum and cannot cross the placenta. IgM is very effective at activating complement. IgD, which forms less than 1 percent of serum Ig, is found on the cell surface of some B cells and functions in the activation of these B cells. IgE, also known as reaginic antibody, is found on the plasma membrane of mast cells and basophils and participates in type I hypersensitivity reactions, such as allergies, asthma, and anaphylaxis. IgE is used to fight parasitic infections. IgA, which constitutes about 10 to 15 percent of serum Ig, exists as a monomer in the serum and a dimer in glandular secretions. IgA is synthesized by mucosal plasma cells of the GI tract, lung, and urinary tract—thus making it the immunoglobulin of "secretory immunity"—and is found in saliva, sweat, nasal secretion, and tears. It is secreted as dimer bound to a secretory piece that stabilizes the molecule against proteolysis.

58. The answer is a. *(Cotran, 5/e, pp 171–174, 635.)* With the advent of monoclonal antibodies derived from hybridomas, it is now possible to identify cells of certain specificity. These antibodies recognize epitopes of antigens found on the cell surfaces that have been used to induce immunity within the mouse. Using an immunoperoxidase technique, the OKT (Leu series) identifies T cells. In addition specific markers will identify subsets of T cells. For example, all peripheral blood T cells react with OKT1, OKT3, and OKT11 cluster designations CD5, CD3, and CD2; OKT4 (Leu-3) reacts with mature T cells; OKT4 or CD4 identifies helper T cells; and OKT8 (CD8) reacts with suppressor cells. The normal T helper/suppressor ratio in humans is about 2. These antibodies do not label cells other than those in the T-lymphocyte system. T cells as a group function in immune regulation and act in concert with B lymphocytes and macrophages. T helper cells aid the cellular immune response in reaction to antigens, while T suppressor cells help in turning the immune response off. EAC rosette cells refer to B lymphocytes that have surface receptors (C3b) that bind to sheep erythrocytes coated with IgM antibody and complement. B lymphocytes also express surface immunoglobulin.

59. The answer is d. *(Cotran, 5/e, pp 174–175. Damjanov, 10/e, pp 400–401.)* The cytokines are soluble mediators of immune reactions that are released from immune cells. Products of lymphocytes are called lymphokines, while products of monocytes or macrophages are called monokines. Two of the most important categories of cytokines are the interleukins (ILs) and the interferons (IFN's). There are two classes of IFN's, namely anti-viral IFN's (α-IFN, β-IFN, and ω-IFN) and immune IFN (γ-IFN). γ-IFN is the most potent activator of macrophages. These activated macrophages (epithelioid cells) produce granulomas. Effects of γ–IFN also include increased class I antigen expression on all somatic cells, increased class II antigen expression on antigen presenting cells (APC's), and induction of high endothelial venules.

IL-1 is produced by many types of cells, including macrophages, antigen presenting cells (APC), and other somatic cells. The functions of IL-1 include autocrine effects on the APC and paracrine effects on T cells.

Effects of IL-1 on the APC include increased expression of adhesion molecules, γ-IFN receptors, and class II antigens. Effects of IL-1 on T cells include increased IL-2 secretion and increased expression of receptors for IL-2 and γ-IFN. Other effects of IL-1 are important in acute inflammation and include stimulation of neutrophils and B cells, production of fever, and increased production of acute phase reactants.

Two of the more important cells that secrete cytokines are two subsets of T helper lymphocytes, namely TH_1 cells and TH_2 cells. TH_1 cells secrete several types of cytokines, including IL-2, γ-IFN, and lymphotoxin (β-TNF). IL-2, secreted by CD4+ TH_1 cells, has autocrine effects to increase IL-2 receptors. It also stimulates NK cells (antibody-dependent cell-mediated immunity) and CD8+ T cells (cell-mediated immunity). TH_2 cells also secrete several types of cytokines, including IL-4, IL-5, IL-6, and IL-10. IL-4 simulates TH_2 cells while at the same time it inhibits TH_1 cells. This combination inhibits cell-mediated immunity and favors humoral immunity. In addition, IL-4 regulates heavy chain class switch to IgE. The effects of IL-5 are on eosinophils. It increases their numbers and function. IL-6 is the most potent stimulator for acute phase reactant production by the liver. Additionally, it stimulates B cells, and synergistically with IL-1 it stimulates T cells. IL-10 inhibits TH_1 cells (cell-mediated immunity), NK cells, and macrophages.

IL-3, also known as multi-CSF, stimulates pluripotential stem cells. IL-7, produced by stromal cells of the thymus and bone marrow, is mitogenic for pre-B cells and thymocytes. It initiates rearrangement of TCR genes. IL-8 is produced by macrophages and other somatic cells. It is classified as a chemokine as it is a chemoattractant for neutrophils, T cells, and basophils. IL-12, produced by NK cells, B cells, and macrophages, stimulates TH_1 cells (cell-mediated immunity) and inhibits TH_2 cells (humoral immunity).

60. The answer is b. (*Cotran, 5/e, pp 175–177. Rubin, 2/e, pp 103–104.*) The genes that code for antigens that evoke tissue rejection reactions if transplanted are called histocompatibility genes. The genes that code for the strongest transplantation antigens are clustered together on chromosome 6 and are called the major histocompatibility complex (MHC), or the human leukocyte antigen (HLA) complex. The products of MHC are classified into three groups. Class I and class II genes encode for cell surface glycoproteins, while class III genes encode for components of the complement system.

Class I molecules are associated with beta$_2$ microglobulin. The loci that encode for class I antigens are HLA-A, HLA-B, and HLA-C. Class I antigens are serologically defined by using antisera (antibodies) to specific HLA antigens. Some class II antigens, e.g., HLA-DQ and HLA-DR, may also be defined serologically using antibodies. Class II DQ and DR antigens can also be defined using the mixed lymphocyte reaction, which involves mixing the patient's lymphocytes with lymphocytes of known HLA type. The patient's lymphocytes will proliferate only in response to incompatible lymphocytes. The patient's cells are assigned the DQ or DR type of the compatible lymphocytes. Some class II antigens, e.g., HLA-DP, cannot be serologically determined, and instead the primed lymphocyte assay is used. In this test, cells that have been previously typed and are primed to react with specific DP antigens are mixed with the patient's cells. The primed cells will then proliferate only in response to the patient's cells that have that specific antigen.

61. The answer is a. (*Cotran, 5/e, pp 175–177.*) CD8+ cytotoxic T lymphocytes can recognize a foreign antigen only if that antigen is complexed to self-class I antigens. In general these class I molecules bind to proteins synthesized within the cell, one example of which is the cellular production of viral antigens. The CD8 molecule of the cytotoxic T cell binds to the nonpolymorphic portion of the class I molecule, while the T-cell receptor on the surface of the T lymphocyte binds to a complex formed by the peptide fragment of the antigen and the class I antigen. In contrast, CD4+ helper T lymphocytes can recognize a foreign antigen only if that antigen is complexed to self-class II antigens. In general, class II antigens present foreign antigens that have been processed within the cell in endosomes or lysosomes, one example of which is bacteria. Macrophages and neutrophils are active phagocytes and have receptors for the Fc portion of IgG and C3b; both of these substances are important opsonins. Macrophages also ingest and present antigens to T cells in conjunction with surface class II antigens.

62. The answer is a. (*Cotran, 5/e, pp 177, 1253–1254.*) A variety of different diseases have an association with certain HLA types. The exact mechanism of this association is unknown. These diseases can be grouped into three broad categories: inflammatory diseases, such as ankylosing spondylitis, and HLA-B27; inherited errors of metabolism, such as hemochromatosis, and HLA-A3; and autoimmune diseases, which are usually associated with the DR locus. Two examples of the last are the associations of rheumatoid arthritis with DR4 and insulin-dependent diabetes with DR3/DR4. Ankylosing spondylitis is one type of spondyloarthropathy that lacks the rheumatoid factor found in rheumatoid arthritis. Other seronegative spondyloarthropathies include Reiter's syndrome, psoriatic arthritis, and enteropathic arthritis. All of these are associated with an increased incidence of HLA-B27. Ankylosing spondylitis, also known as rheumatoid spondylitis, or Marie-Strümpell disease, is a chronic inflammatory disease that primarily affects the sacroiliac joints of adult males. Reiter's syndrome is the triad of arthritis, nongonococcal urethritis, and conjunctivitis. It may be related to previous gastrointestinal or genitourinary infections.

63. The answer is d. (*Cotran, 5/e, pp 178–182.*) Hypersensitivity diseases are caused by immune mechanism. They are classified into four different categories based on the immune mechanisms that are involved. Type I hypersensitivity reactions involve IgE (reaginic) antibodies that have been bound to the surface of mast cells and basophils. These IgE antibodies are formed by a T cell dependent process. An allergen initially binds to antigen presenting cells which then activates TH_2 cells to secrete interleukin-4 (IL-4), IL-5, and IL-6. IL-5 stimulates the production of eosinophils, while IL-4 stimulates B cells to transform into plasma cells and produce IgE. This IgE then attaches to mast cells and basophils, because these cells have cell surface receptors for the Fc portion of IgE. When this "armed" mast cell or basophil is re-exposed to the allergen, the antigen bridges two IgE molecules and causes mast cells to release preformed (primary) mediators. This antigen-to-antibody binding also causes these cells to synthesize secondary mediators.

The reactions that occur as a result of the primary mediators of type I hypersensitivity are rapidly occurring since they have already been made and are present within the granules of mast cells. These substances include biogenic amines, such as histamine, chemotactic factors, enzymes, and proteoglycans. Histamine causes increased vascular permeability, vasodilatation, and bronchial smooth muscle contraction. The chemotactic factors are chemotactic for eosinophils and neutrophils. Mast cells will also produce new products (secondary mediators) by a series of reactions within the cell membrane that lead to the generation of lipid mediators and cytokines. The lipid mediators are generated from arachidonic acid. Membrane receptors bound to IgE activate phospholipase A_2, which then cleaves membrane phospholipids into arachidonic acid. Lipoxygenase produces leukotrienes, including LTB4 and the leukotrienes C_4, D_4, and E_4. These last three leukotrienes are the most potent vasoactive and spasmogenic agents known. They used to be called SRS-A (slow reactive substance of anaphylaxis). Prostaglandin D2, which is produced via the enzyme cyclooxygenase, is abundant in lung mast cells. It causes bronchospasm and increased mucus production.

Type I reactions may be either local reactions or systemic reactions. Local reactions include urticaria ("hives"), angioedema, allergic rhinitis ("hay fever"), conjunctivitis, food allergies, and allergic bronchial asthma. Systemic reactions usually follow parental administration of the antigen, such as with drug reactions (penicillin) or insect stings. The amount of antigen may be very small. Symptoms include vomiting, cramps, diarrhea, itching, wheezing, and shortness of breath, and death may occur within minutes. The main treatment is epinephrine.

64. The answer is d. (*Cotran, 5/e, pp 178–190.*) The reaction in the question is a type 2 hypersensitivity reaction that is mediated by antibodies reacting against antigens present on the surface of cells, in this case blood group antigens or irregular antigens present on the donor's red blood cells. Type 2 hypersensitivity reactions result from attachment of antibodies to changed cell surface antigens or to normal cell surface antigens. Complement-mediated cytotoxicity occurs when IgM or IgG binds to a cell surface antigen with complement activation and consequent cell membrane damage or lysis. Blood transfusion reactions and autoimmune hemolytic anemia are examples of this form. Systemic anaphylaxis is a type 1 hypersensitivity reaction in which mast cells or basophils that are bound to IgE antibodies are reexposed to an allergen, which leads to a release of vasoactive amines that causes edema and broncho- and vasoconstriction. Sudden death can occur. Systemic immune complex reactions are found in type 3 reactions and are due to circulating antibodies that form complexes upon reexposure to an antigen, such as foreign serum, which then activates complement followed by chemotaxis and aggregation of neutrophils leading to release of lysosomal enzymes and eventual necrosis of tissue and cells. Serum sickness and Arthus' reactions are examples of this. Delayed-type hypersensitivity is type 4 and is due to previously sensitized T lymphocytes, which release lymphokines upon reexposure to the antigen. This takes time—perhaps up to several days following exposure. The tuberculin reaction is the best known example of this. T-cell-mediated cytotoxicity leads to lysis of cells by cytotoxic T cells in response to tumor cells, allogenic tissue, and virus-infected cells. These cells have CD8 antigens on their surfaces.

65. The answer is b. (*Cotran, 5/e, pp 187–189.*) Delayed-hypersensitivity reactions are mediated by T lymphocytes and other mononuclear cells. The reaction requires previous exposure to antigen, frequently a large protein, and takes from 1 to 3 days to develop fully. Only true palpable induration is considered a positive reaction.

66. The answer is c. (*Damjanov, 10/e, pp 655–658.*) An allograft is also called a homograft and refers to a graft between members of the same species. An autograft is a tissue graft taken from one site and placed in a different site in the same individual. Isografts are grafts between individuals from an inbred strain of animals. A graft between individuals of two different species is a xenograft, or heterograft.

67. The answer is e. (*Cotran, 5/e, pp 190–195.*) Histocompatible antigens (HLA) are responsible for rejection of transplanted organs in humans. Organ rejection requires both humoral and cell-mediated immunologic reactions involving T cells both from the donated organ and the patient's own CD4 T helper cells and CD8 cytotoxic T cells. Hyperacute rejection occurs within minutes after transplantation and consists of neutrophils within the glomerulus and peritubular capillaries. Acute rejection occurs within days after transplantation and is marked by vasculitis and interstitial lymphocytic infiltration. Subacute rejection vasculitis occurs during the first few months after transplantation and is characterized by the proliferation of fibroblasts and macrophages in the tunica intima of arteries. In chronic rejection tubular atrophy, mononuclear interstitial infiltration, and vascular changes are encountered, with the vascular changes being characteristic and probably reflecting an end stage of arteritis. The vascular obliteration leads to interstitial fibrosis and tubular atrophy with loss of renal function. However, the histologic picture is complicated by secondary ischemic damage, and it may be difficult to discern inflammation, fibrosis, and vascular changes as cause or effect.

68. The answer is b. (*Cotran, 5/e, pp 210–213.*) The constellation of Raynaud's phenomenon, acral sclerosis, and fibrotic tightening of the muscles of facial expression should raise the specter of progressive systemic sclerosis (scleroderma), a multisystem disease that involves the cardiovascular, gastrointestinal, cutaneous, musculoskeletal, pulmonary, and renal systems through progressive interstitial fibrosis. Small arterioles in the forenamed systems show obliteration caused by intimal hyperplasia accompanied by progressive interstitial fibrosis. Evidence implicates a lymphocyte overdrive of fibroblasts to produce an excess of rather normal collagen. Eventually, myocardial fibrosis, pulmonary fibrosis, and terminal renal failure ensue. Over half of all patients have dysphagia with solid food caused by the distal esophageal narrowing in the disease.

69. The answer is c. *(Rubin, 2/e, p 140.)* Ten to twenty percent or more of cases of polymyositis are associated with underlying visceral malignancies of virtually any organ. Although the cause of this association remains unknown, it has been postulated that some cancers either produce substances that are toxic to skeletal muscle or contain antigens that are cross-reactive with skeletal muscle.

70. The answer is a. *(Cotran, 5/e, pp 231–233.)* Amyloid is a generic term that describes special properties of any protein having a tertiary structure that produces a β-pleated sheet. Amyloid stains brown with iodine ("starchlike"). Histologically the deposits always begin between or outside of cells. Eventually the amyloid deposits may strangle the cells, leading to atrophy or cell death. The histologic diagnosis of amyloid is based solely on its special staining characteristics. It stains pink with the routine hematoxylin and eosin stain, but with the Congo red stain, amyloid stains dark red and has an apple-green birefringence appearance when viewed under polarized light. There are many different types of proteins that stain as amyloid, and these proteins are associated with a wide variety of diseases. These diseases may be either systemic, such as with immune dyscrasias, reactive diseases, or hemodialysis, or they may be localized, such as with senile or endocrine disorders. Immune dyscrasias, such as multiple myeloma or B cell lymphomas, secrete amyloid light (AL) chains, while reactive systemic diseases secrete amyloid associated protein (AA). This protein is a polypeptide derived from serum amyloid-associated protein, which is produced in the liver. Systemic deposits of AA protein complicates various chronic infections and inflammatory processes, most commonly rheumatoid arthritis, other connective tissue diseases, bronchiectasis, and inflammatory bowel disease. Patients on chronic hemodialysis may develop amyloid deposits consisting of β_2-microglobulin. Patients with senile cardiac disease may develop amyloid deposits in the heart consisting of amyloid transthyretin (ATTR), while patients with senile cerebral disease, such as Alzheimer's disease, may develop amyloid deposits in the brain consisting of β_2-amyloid protein. Do not confuse β_2-amyloid protein with β_2 microglobulin, a component of the MHC class I molecule. Patients with medullary carcinoma of the thyroid, a malignancy of the calcitonin-secreting parafollicular C cells of the thyroid, characteristically have amyloid deposits of procalcitonin within the tumor. Finally, patients with type II diabetes mellitus may have amyloid deposits within pancreatic islets consisting of islet amyloid polypeptide.

71. The answer is e. (*Flake AW, N Engl J Med 335(24), pp 1806–1810, 1996. Cotran, 5/e, p 218.*) Patients with severe combined immunodeficiency disease (SCID) have defects of lymphoid stem cells involving both T-cells and B-cells. Patients have severe abnormalities of immunologic function with lymphopenia. These patients are at risk for infection with all types of infectious agents, including bacteria, mycobacteria, fungi, viruses, and parasites. Patients at birth have a skin rash, possibly due to a graft versus host reaction from maternal lymphocytes. Patients are particularly prone to chronic diarrhea, due to rotavirus and bacteria, and oral candidiasis. About 50 percent of patients with the autosomal recessive form (Swiss type) lack the enzyme adenosine deaminase (ADA) in their red cells and leukocytes. This leads to accumulation of adenosine triphosphate and deoxyadenosine triphosphate, both of which are toxic to lymphocytes. The other form of SCID's is an X-linked form due to a defect in the IL-2 receptor.

72. The answer is b. (*Cotran, 5/e, pp 217–219.*) Patients with isolated IgA deficiency, a very common immunodeficiency that affects about 1 in 600 persons in the United States, have very low levels of serum and secretory IgA. Patients commonly have recurrent sinopulmonary infections and diarrhea. These patients also have an increased incidence of respiratory tract allergy and autoimmune diseases. There is no increase in the incidence of lymphoma. Serum antibodies to IgA, however, are found in about 40 percent of these patients, who, if given blood containing normal IgA, may develop severe, possibly fatal anaphylaxis reactions. Tetany due to lack of parathyroid development is seen in patients with DiGeorge's syndrome. Angioedema, localized edema affecting the skin and mucous membranes, is seen with absence of C_1 esterase inhibitor due to the excessive generation of vasoactive C_2 kinin. Thrombocytopenia is part of the X-linked disorder Wiskott-Aldrich syndrome.

73. The answer is c. (*Cotran, 5/e, pp 219–231. Henry, 19/e, pp 708–709.*) Cytopenias occur in over 50 percent of patients with HIV infection either individually or as part of a pancytopenia. Suppression of hemopoiesis in the bone marrow as a result of mycobacterial, fungal, or protozoal infection; infiltration by lymphoma, leukemia, or Kaposi's sarcoma; and the effects of drugs (particularly zidovudine) may result in cytopenia. Anemia is seen in 80 to 85 percent of cases, usually in the pattern of anemia of chronic disease. Thrombocytopenia occurs in about 30 percent of cases and is thought to be a result of peripheral destruction of platelets, possibly by an immune mechanism. Neutropenia occurs in 40 percent of patients. Lymphopenia and a reduced ratio of CD4 to CD8 lymphocytes are characteristic of HIV infection. Atypical plasmacytoid lymphocytes are usually present in the peripheral blood smear. Examination of the bone marrow in cytopenic patients shows a normocellular or hypercellular pattern in more than 90 percent of cases.

74. The answer is c. (*Joklik, 20/e, pp 774–775. Cotran, 5/e, p 308.*) Togaviruses, a family of helical, predominantly single-stranded RNA viruses, include the genus Alphavirus (mosquito-borne), which causes eastern equine encephalitis (EEE) and western equine encephalitis (WEE). Yellow fever, dengue fever, and St. Louis encephalitis are caused by Flaviviridae; these were part of the old group B arboviruses, which used to be in the genus Flavivirus of the Togaviridae. The causative agent of epidemic hemorrhagic keratoconjunctivitis is usually the type B adenovirus, an icosahedral double-stranded DNA virus. Herpes simplex keratoconjunctivitis, although frequently recurrent, is not epidemic.

75. The answer is b. (*Cotran, 5/e, pp 340–341, 349–350. Chandrasoma, 3/e, p 805.*) The cytopathic effect of viruses is often a clue to the diagnosis of the type of infection that is present. There are several types of herpes viruses, which are relatively large, double-stranded DNA viruses. Infection by herpes simplex virus (HSV) or varicella-zoster virus (VZV) is recognized by nuclear homogenization (ground-glass nuclei), intranuclear inclusions (Cowdry type A bodies), and the formation of multinucleated cells. Herpes simplex type 2, a sexually transmitted viral disease, results in the formation of vesicles that ulcerate and cause burning, itching, and pain. These lesions will heal spontaneously, but the virus will remain dormant in the lumbar and sacral ganglia. Recurrent infections may occur, and transmission to the newborn during delivery is a feared complication that may be fatal to the infant. Shingles and chickenpox are caused by herpes zoster, which is identical to varicella.

Cytomegalovirus (CMV) causes both the nucleus and the cytoplasm of infected cells to be enlarged. Infected cells have large, purple intranuclear inclusions surrounded by a clear halo and smaller, less prominent basophilic intracytoplasmic inclusions. Adenoviruses can produce similar inclusions, but the infected cells are not enlarged. They also produce characteristic smudge cells in infected respiratory epithelial cells. Human papilloma virus (HPV) infection may produce a characteristic effect that is called koilocytosis. Histologic examination reveals enlarged squamous epithelial cells that have shrunken nuclei ("raisin-oid") within large cytoplasmic vacuoles.

Candidiasis is the most common fungal infection of the vagina, especially common in patients with diabetes or taking oral contraceptives. Candida infection causes vulvar itching and produces a white discharge. Microscopic examination of the vaginal discharge reveals yeast and pseudohyphae. *Trichomonas vaginalis*, a large, pear-shaped, flagellated protozoan, causes severe vaginal itching with dysuria. It produces a thick yellow-gray discharge.

76. The answer is c. (*Damjanov, 10/e, pp 886–887, 928–930. Duchin, N Engl J Med 330: 949–955, 1994.*) The Hantavirus genus belongs to the Bunyaviridae family and includes the causative agent of a group of diseases that occur throughout Europe and Asia and are referred to as hemorrhagic fever with renal syndrome. The characteristic features of this syndrome are hematologic abnormalities, renal involvement, and increased vascular permeability. Respiratory involvement is generally minimal in these diseases. Although several species of rodents in the United States were known to be infected with Hantavirus, no human cases had been reported until an outbreak of severe, often fatal respiratory illness occurred in the United States in May 1993 in the Four Corners area of New Mexico, Arizona, Colorado, and Utah. This illness resulted from a new member of the genus Hantavirus that caused a severe disease characterized by a prodromal fever, myalgia, pulmonary edema, and hypotension. The main distinguishing feature of this illness, which is called Hantavirus pulmonary syndrome, is noncardiogenic pulmonary edema resulting from increased permeability of the pulmonary capillaries. Laboratory features common to both Hantavirus pulmonary syndrome and hemorrhagic fever with renal syndrome include leukocytosis, atypical lymphocytes, thrombocytopenia, coagulopathy, and decreased serum protein concentrations. Abdominal pain, which can mimic an acute abdomen, may be found in both Hantavirus pulmonary syndrome and hemorrhagic fever with renal syndrome.

Dengue fever virus is a type of flavivirus, which are similar to alphaviruses. Dengue fever (breakbone fever) is initially similar to influenza but then progresses to a rash, muscle pain, joint pain, and bone pain. It can produce a potentially fatal hemorrhagic disorder. Yellow fever virus is another flavivirus that causes yellow fever. It is spread by a mosquito and produces characteristic coagulative necrosis of liver acinar zone 2 (midzonal necrosis). The necrotic hepatocytes, produced by the process of apoptosis in the absence of inflammation, result in Councilman bodies. Because of liver failure, patients become jaundiced (yellow fever) and may vomit clotted blood ("black vomit"). Another flavivirus is the cause of St. Louis encephalitis, which is spread by the Culex mosquito. Alphavirus, a type of togavirus, are similar to flaviviruses. They are the prototypical arboviruses, which are arthropod-born viruses. Clinical diseases include EEE (eastern equine encephalitis), WEE (western equine encephalitis), and VEE (Venezuelan equine encephalitis). Ebola virus is a Filoviridae that causes a severe hemorrhagic fever. Outbreaks occur in Africa and typically make the national news.

77. The answer is c. *(Joklik, 20/e, pp 1060–1063. Rubin, 2/e, pp 341–344.)* Human parvovirus may cause a serious aplastic crisis in patients with an underlying chronic hemolytic anemia. In children, infection with parvovirus produces a characteristic rash, called erythema infectiosum or fifth disease, which first appears on the face and is described as a "slapped cheek" appearance. Human parvovirus infection in adults produces a nonspecific syndrome of fever, malaise, headache, myalgia, vomiting, and a transient rash. Arthralgia is more common in adults than in children. There are many types of rhinoviruses, which are causative agents of the common cold (coryza). This infection is characterized by rhinorrhea, pharyngitis, cough, and a low-grade fever. Parainfluenza viruses, single-stranded RNA viruses that kill ciliated respiratory epithelial cells, are the most common cause of croup, which is a disease of children characterized by a barking sound on inspiration. Rubeola virus, an RNA virus, is the cause of measles. After an incubation of 10 to 21 days, measles is characterized by fever, rhinorrhea, cough, skin lesions, and mucosal lesions (Koplik spots). Rubella virus, another RNA virus, produces a mild, acute febrile illness, but if the infection occurs in the first trimester of pregnancy it can produce developmental abnormalities such as cardiac lesions, ocular abnormalities, deafness, and mental retardation.

78. The answer is d. *(Damjanov, 10/e, pp 2718–2719. Henry, 19/e, pp 1317–1318.)* In a patient who is suspected of having meningitis, microscopic examination of cerebrospinal fluid is of immediate importance. In the photomicrograph shown, all the cells are polymorphonuclear leukocytes and bacteria are visible in the cytoplasm. Neutrophils may be present in viral or tuberculous meningitis, but lymphocytes are more common. Demonstration of bacteria by Gram stain of the cerebrospinal fluid is the most valuable aid in establishing a diagnosis of early bacterial meningitis and is possible in more than 90 percent of cases.

79. The answer is d. *(Cotran, 5/e, pp 337, 696–697.)* Most cases of lobar pneumonia are caused by *Streptococcus pneumoniae* (reclassification of the pneumococcus). Streptococcal or pneumococcal pneumonia involves one or more lobes and is often seen in alcoholics or debilitated persons. Type 3 pneumococcus (*S. pneumoniae*) causes a virulent lobar pneumonia characterized by mucoid sputum, which is also seen in *Klebsiella pneumoniae*. *K. pneumoniae* (Friedländer's bacillus) usually produces a bronchopneumonia, rather than lobar pneumonia, but is clinically indistinguishable from pneumococcal lobar pneumonia. Legionella species cause a fibrinopurulent lobular pneumonia that tends to be confluent, almost appearing lobar.

80. The answer is d. *(Cotran, 5/e, pp 331, 360, 793–794.)* Yersinia (formerly called Pasteurella) is an important genus of gram-negative bacilli that causes a wide variety of human and animal disease, ranging from plague (*Y. pestis*) to acute mesenteric lymphadenitis (*Y. enterocolitica*) in older children and young adults. *Y. enterocolitica* infections also occur in the terminal ileum in young adults, causing an ileitis that produces inflammation not unlike that seen in some stages of Crohn's disease (regional enteritis). Since the organisms grow slowly on enrichment media, they may be overgrown by other coliforms at 37°C. The organisms may be isolated by means of cold enhancement at 4°C.

81. The answer is d. *(Henry, 19/e, pp 1155–1156, 1196–1200. Rubin, 2/e, pp 371–372.)* The Vibrio genus, including *V. cholerae*, is associated with gastrointestinal disease in the Far East, especially India, but is capable of inducing disease in the United States, as in pandemics occurring here around 1832 and in 1849. Along the coasts, especially the northeast and Gulf coasts of the United States, the vibrios increase in numbers in seawater and in seafood and are more likely to cause infections during the late summer and early autumn months. Patients with underlying liver disease, such as alcoholics, and those with immunosuppressive disorders are advised not to ingest raw shellfish during these months because of an increased incidence of disease with the vibrio organisms in these patients. The mycobacteria are acid-fast bacilli associated with tuberculosis and tuberculosis-like diseases; *M. avium-intracellulare* is known to be a frequent organism in AIDS. These organisms are not curved as the vibrios are.

82. The answer is c. *(Henry, 19/e, pp 1186–1187. Cotran, 5/e, p 344.)* Although the rapid plasma reagin (RPR), Kolmer, and Venereal Disease Research Laboratory (VDRL) tests are rapid and easily performed tests that can help confirm a diagnosis of active syphilis, they are associated with false positive reactions because of their low specificity for antibodies against treponemal or cardiolipin antigens. Therefore, RPR, Kolmer, and VDRL tests usually are used for screening programs. The Treponema pallidum immobilization (TPI) and the fluorescent treponemal antibody-absorption (FTA-ABS) tests have greater specificity for treponemal antigen but are technically more difficult to perform. The FTA-ABS test is generally the most sensitive and most specific procedure for diagnosis of syphilis.

83. The answer is c. *(Cotran, 5/e, pp 361–362, 1253, 1260.)* A localized skin rash in the summertime followed within a period of weeks by arthritis, especially involving less than three joints, should arouse suspicion of Lyme disease. This disorder was first described in the mid-1970s in Connecticut when small clusters of cases of children suffering from an illness resembling juvenile rheumatoid arthritis were first noted. The disease has now been shown to be caused by a spirochete, *Borrelia burgdorferi*, through the bite of a tick belonging to the genus *Ixodes*. The spirochete-infested ticks reside in wooded areas where there are deer and small rodents. The deer act as a wintering-over reservoir for the ticks. In the spring the tick larval stage emerges and evolves into a nymph, which is infective for humans if they are bitten. Adult ticks are also capable of transmitting the spirochete as well during questing. The bite is followed by a rash called erythema chronicum migrans, which may resolve spontaneously. However, many patients have a transient phase of spirochetemia, which may allow the spread of the spirochete to the meninges, heart, and synovial tissue. Originally thought to be confined to New England, Lyme disease has now been shown to be present in Europe and Australia as well. The spirochetes are sensitive to penicillin, erythromycin, and tetracycline. Reiter's disease does not present with a spreading rash, and a Baker's cyst produces swelling in the popliteal fossa behind the knee rather than joint effusions anteriorly.

84. The answer is c. (*Chandrasoma, 3/e, pp 799–806.*) Granuloma inguinale is a rare, sexually transmitted disease that is caused by *Calymmatobacterium donovani*, a small, encapsulated gram-negative bacillus. Infection results in a chronic disease that is characterized by superficial ulcers of the genital region. Regional lymph node involvement produces large nodular masses that develop extensive scarring. Specialized culture media is available, but its use is not practical. Serologic tests are also not useful. Instead, histologic examination is used to demonstrate Donovan bodies, which are organisms within the cytoplasm of macrophages. They are seen best with silver stains or Giemsa's stain. Chancroid is an acute venereal disease that is characterized by painful genital ulcers with lymphadenopathy. It is caused by *Hemophilus ducreyi*, a small, gram-negative bacillus. Gram stains of the suppurative lesions or cultures on specialized media may be used to make the diagnosis. Serologic tests are not useful. *Neisseria gonorrhea*, a gram-negative diplococcus, causes gonorrhea, an acute suppurative infection of the genital tract. In males it produces a purulent discharge (urethritis) and dysuria. In women, it may be asymptomatic (50 percent), or it may produce infection of the cervix with a vaginal discharge, dysuria, and abdominal pain. Ascending infections in women can lead to salpingitis, tubo-ovarian abscess, and pelvic inflammatory disease (PID). Fitz-Hugh-Curtis syndrome refers to perihepatitis infection. In newborns, infection acquired during birth can produce a purulent conjunctivitis (ophthalmia neonatorum). This disease has been prevented due to prophylactic therapy to newborn infants. A Gram-stain of the urethral or cervical exudate may reveal the intra-cytoplasmic gram-negative diplococci, or the exudate can be cultured on special media. Serologic tests are not useful. Characteristically, *N. gonorrhea* produces acid from glucose, but not maltose or lactose. The spirochete *Treponema pallidum*, the causative agent of syphilis, has not been grown on any culture media; therefore, other means are available to aid in the diagnosis of syphilis. Dark-field or immunofluorescence examination may be used to detect organisms in the genital ulcers of primary syphilis. Antibodies to cardiolipin, a substance in beef heart that is similar to a lipoid released by *T. pallidum*, are used to screen for syphilis. This is the basis of both the VDRL and the RPR (rapid plasma reagin) tests; however, these screening tests are not totally specific. Chlamydia are obligate intracellular parasites that form elementary bodies and reticulate bodies. The former are small, extracellular, and infectious, while the latter are intracellular forms and are noninfectious. Three chlamydia species are *C. psittaci, C. pneumoniae,* and *C. trachomatis.* The last causes several human diseases including trachoma, inclusion conjunctivitis, nongonococcal urethritis, and lymphogranuloma venereum. Specialized culture media and direct examination procedures are available to aid in the diagnosis of these diseases. The regional lymph nodes in patients with lymphogranuloma venereum have a characteristic histologic appearance characterized by necrotizing granulomas forming stellate areas of necrosis. Trachoma is the leading cause of blindness in underdeveloped countries. It is a chronic infection of the conjunctiva that eventually scars the conjunctiva and cornea. Lymphogranuloma venereum (LGV) is a sexually transmitted disease that is characterized by the formation of a genital ulcer with local necrotizing lymphadenitis. The skin test for LGV is the Frei test, which consists of intradermal injection of LGV antigen. Finally, *C. psittaci* is the causative agent of psittacosis (parrot fever). It produces a severe pulmonary disease and should be suspected in patients with a history of bird contact, such as pet shop workers or parrot owners.

85. The answer is e. (*Cotran, 5/e, pp 358–360. Damjanov, 10/e, pp 866–878.*) Rickettsia are obligate intracellular parasites that infect endothelial cells and produce symptoms as a result of vasculitis and microthrombi formation. Serologic tests for rickettsia include complement fixation tests and the Weil-Felix agglutination reaction. The basis for the latter test is the fact that the sera of infected patients can agglutinate strains of proteus vulgaris. There are numerous types of rickettsia that produce many different diseases. Examples include Rocky Mountain Spotted Fever (RMSF, caused by *R. rickettsii*), epidemic typhus (caused by *R. prowazekii* and spread by the human body louse pediculus humanus), endemic typhus (caused by *R. typhi* and spread by lice), scrub typhus (caused by *R. tsutsugamushi* and spread by mites), ehrlichiosis, and Q fever (caused by *Coxiella burnetii* and spread not by vectors but by inhalation of aerosols). RMSF is found not only in the Rocky Mountains, but also the southeast and south-central United States. The vector in the Rocky Mountains is the wood tick (*Dermacentor andersoni*), while in the southeast it is the dog tick (*Dermacentor variabilis*) and in the south-central United States, the Lone Star tick. The animal reservoir for RMSF are wild rodents and dogs. The rash of RMSF characteristically begins peripherally and spreads centrally to the trunk and face. The pathology involves infection of blood vessels producing thrombosis. Intracellular bacilli form parallel rows in an end-to-end arrangement ("flotilla at anchor facing the wind"). Patients also develop muscle pain and high fever.

Bartonella infections are also characterized by proliferations of blood vessels. Examples of Bartonella include *Bartonella quintana*, *Bartonella henselae*, and *Bartonella bacilliformis*, the causative agent of Oroya fever. *Bartonella quintana* is spread by the human body louse and is the causative agent of trench fever (seen in the trenches of WWI) and bacillary angiomatosis. This latter term refers to a lesion seen in patients with AIDS consisting of a lobular proliferation of capillaries with abundant leukocytoclastic debris. Finally, *Bartonella henselae* is the causative agent of cat-scratch fever. Histologically this disease is characterized by the formation of stellate microabscesses with necrotizing granulomas.

86. The answer is d. (*Cotran, 5/e, pp 324–327, 694–698, 700–703.*) Tuberculosis (TB) is caused by infection with *Mycobacterium tuberculosis*. Mycobacteriaceae are slow growing aerobic rods, with cell walls rich in glycolipids, true waxes, and long chain fatty acids called mycolic acids. The lipid rich mycolic acid containing cell wall is responsible for the unique staining properties of the Mycobacteria, namely their impermeability to most basic dyes and their resistance to acid decolorization (acid-fast staining). Infection with *M. tuberculosis* occurs either as a primary infection or a secondary reactivation or reinfection. The initial infection of primary tuberculosis, the Ghon complex, consists of a subpleural lesion near the fissure between the upper and lower lobes and enlarged caseous lymph nodes that drain the pulmonary lesion. The histologic lesions of TB reveal caseating granulomas with Langerhans giant cells. Although primary pulmonary tuberculosis is usually asymptomatic, systemic and localizing symptoms can occur. These symptoms include malaise, anorexia, weight loss, fever, night sweats, cough and hemoptysis. The pulmonary lesion of secondary tuberculosis is usually located in the apex of one of both lungs. Progressive pulmonary tuberculosis may result in cavitary fibrocaseous tuberculosis, miliary tuberculosis, or tuberculous bronchopneumonia. Miliary tuberculosis consists of multiple small yellow-white lesions scattered throughout the entire lung. These lesions are the result of erosion of a granulomatous lesion into a blood vessel with subsequent lymphohematogenous dissemination. While TB is often asymptomatic, the resultant hypersensitivity reaction is a marker for infection in those individuals without clinically apparent disease. The TB skin test is called the Mantoux Test and is characterized by the intradermal injection of PPD (purified protein derivative). An area of 1/2 cm or more in diameter of induration at 48 hours is a positive result. The diagnosis of TB depends upon the clinical picture and chest X-ray. Acid-fast stains of sputum are followed with culture, not only to identify the species of mycobacteria but to determine the pattern of antibiotic sensitivity. Treatment is with isoniazid (INH) combined with other antibiotics.

Klebsiella pneumoniae is a cause of bacterial pneumonia in debilitated and malnourished individuals, such as chronic alcoholics. Patients develop a thick, gelatinous sputum production. This bacterial infection has a greater mortality than pneumococcal pneumonia. Legionnaires' disease is a form of bronchopneumonia that is caused by the gram-negative bacillus, Legionella pneumophila. This organism is almost ubiquitous in water and is spread by inhalation of contaminated airborne droplets. Infection results in a patchy bronchopneumonia, and microscopically the alveolar spaces are filled with an inflammatory exudate of neutrophils and macrophages. There may be multiple, small areas of necrosis and abscess. Organisms cannot be visualized by routine stains, so instead a Dieterle silver stain is used.

87. The answer is a. (Cotran, 5/e, pp 326–327. Damjanov, 10/e, pp 850–854.) There are several types of mycobacteria that are not M. tuberculosis. These organisms are called atypical mycobacteria, or mycobacteria other than tuberculosis (MOTT). They are separated into different classes (Runyon classes) based on several culture characteristics, such as pigment production, colony morphology, and rate of growth. Examples of MOTT include *M. avium-intracellulare*, *M. marinum*, and *M. leprae*, which is the causative agent of leprosy. *M. avium-intracellulare* is an important cause of infection in patients with AIDS. Histologic sections in these immunosuppressed patients do not reveal granulomas because the cellular immune reactions of these patients are defective. Instead numerous organisms can be seen with special stains. *M. marinum* inhabits marine organisms and grows in water. It can cause superficial disease, skin and subcutaneous disease, and can be obtained from infected aquariums or swimming pools.

88. The answer is c. (*Cotran, 5/e, pp 328–329.*) In the approximate center of the photomicrograph is the classic, refractile, double-walled spherule of the deep fungus *Coccidioides immitis*, which is several times the diameter of the largest inflammatory cell nearby. Coccidioidomycosis is endemic in California, Arizona, New Mexico, and parts of Nevada, Utah, and Texas, where it resides in the arid soils and is contracted by direct inhalation of airborne dust. If inhaled, it produces a primary pulmonary infection that is usually benign and self-limiting in immunologically competent persons, often with several days of fever and upper respiratory flu-like symptoms. However, certain ethnic groups, such as some blacks, Asians, and Filipinos, are at risk of developing a potentially lethal disseminated form of the disease that can involve the central nervous system. If the large, double-walled spherule containing numerous endospores can be demonstrated outside the lungs (e.g., in a skin biopsy), this is evidence of dissemination. Antibodies of high titers are detectable by means of complement fixation studies in patients undergoing spontaneous recovery. Amphotericin B is usually reserved for treating high-risk and disseminated infection. The cultured mycelia of the organism on Sabouraud's agar present a hazard for laboratory workers.

89. The answer is d. (*Cotran, 5/e, p 310. Rubin, 2/e, pp 408–419.*) The deep fungal infections produce characteristic morphologic features in tissue sections. The two basic morphologic types of fungi are yeasts, which are oval cells that reproduce by budding, and molds, which are filamentous colonies consisting of branched tubules called hyphae. Some yeasts produce buds that do not detach. Instead they form long structures that resemble hyphae and are called pseudohyphae. This is characteristic of Candida species. Blastomyces is a larger, double contoured yeast that is characterized by broad-based budding. Aspergillus is characterized by septate hyphae with acute-angle branching of the filamentous colonies and occasional fruiting bodies. Irregular, broad, nonseptate hyphae with wide-angle branching is seen with mucormycosis (zygomycosis). Large spheres with external budding, referred to as a "ship's wheel," are seen with Paracoccidioides, while large spheres with endospores are seen with coccidiomyces infection.

90. The answer is d. (*Cotran, 5/e, pp 310, 327–328, 354–357. Rubin, 2/e, pp 408–418.*) *Histoplasma capsulatum*, a dimorphic fungus, causes one of the three major fungal infections in the United States that may result in systemic infection (Blastomyces and Coccidioides are the other two). Although it commonly produces asymptomatic primary disease, it can result in granulomatous inflammation, especially granulomatous lung disease. Multiple small, yeast surrounded by clear zones may be found within the cytoplasm of macrophages. The source for histoplasma is soil contaminated by the excreta of birds (starlings and chickens) and bats. The typical location for individuals to develop histoplasmosis is the Ohio and Mississippi Valley areas. Aspergillus species produce several clinical disease states, including allergic aspergillosis, systemic aspergillosis, and aspergilloma. Typically Aspergillus is seen in tissue as acute-angle branching septate hyphae; however, they may form fruiting bodies in cavities, such as within cystic cavities of the lungs. There they may form a large mass called a fungus ball or aspergilloma. Blastomycosis is a chronic granulomatosis disease caused by a dimorphic fungus, *Blastomyces dermatitidis*. In tissues this fungus is seen as a thick walled yeast having broad based budding. Without the budding, Blastomyces may be mistaken as cryptococcus. The infection, also known as Gilchrist's disease, is seen in individuals living in the Ohio and Mississippi Valley areas and is usually confined to the lungs. Candida species, which frequently cause human infections, grow as yeast, elongated chains of yeast without hyphae (pseudohyphae), or septate hyphae. Mucocutaneous candidal infections can produce white plaques called thrush. Mucormycosis (zygomycosis) is a disease caused by "bread-mold fungi," such as Rhizopus, Mucor, and Absidia species. These infections typically occur in neutropenic patients or diabetics. One form of the disease, typically found in diabetics, is called rhinocerebral mucormycosis and is characterized by facial pain, headache, changing mental status, and a blood-tinged nasal discharge. Tissue sections will reveal characteristic broad, non-septate, right angle branching hyphae.

91. The answer is c. (*Cotran, 5/e, pp 310, 355. Rubin, 2/e, pp 408–418.*) Cryptococcosis is caused by *Cryptococcus neoformans*, an encapsulated yeast (not dimorphic) that infects the central nervous system, primarily in immunocompromised patients. The soil-dwelling yeast is inhaled, but lung involvement tends to be mild in individuals that are not immunodeficient. Diagnosis of cryptococcal meningitis is achieved by finding encapsulated yeasts in CSF preparations. The capsule can be seen with a mucicarmine stain, or it can be negatively stained using India ink. The CSF and serum should also be tested for cryptococcal antigen by the latex cryptococcal agglutination test (LCAT), which is positive in more than 90 percent of cases. Cryptococcal meningitis varies from a chronic inflammatory and granulomatous infection to a noninflammatory meningitis with numerous yeasts massed, sometimes forming cystic "soap bubble" lesions in the brain. Do not confuse cryptococcus with cryptosporidium. *Cryptosporidium parvum* is a protozoan parasite that may cause a transient diarrhea in immunocompetent individuals or a chronic diarrhea in patients with AIDS (cryptosporidiosis). Histologically, sporozoites may be found attached to the surface of intestinal epithelial cells. They are best seen with an acid-fast stain. Chromomycosis is a chronic infection of the skin that is produced by an organism that appears as a brown thick-walled sphere ("copper penny") in tissue sections. Coccidiomycosis is a mycotic infection caused by inhalation of the arthrospores of the dimorphic fungus *Coccidioides immitis*. Within the lung the spores enlarge to from large spherules (sporangia) that become filled with many small endospores. The cyst will rupture, releasing the endospores. Unruptured spherules incite a granulomatous reaction, while the endospores cause a neutrophilic response. Paracoccidiomycosis (South American blastomycosis) is a chronic granulomatous infection caused by *Paracoccidioides brasiliensis*, a dimorphic fungus seen in tissues as a large central organism having peripheral oval budding. This histologic appearance is described as being similar to a mariner's wheel.

92. The answer is b. (*Cotran, 5/e, pp 364–365. Rubin, 2/e, pp 442, 449–452.*) Intestinal tapeworm (cestode) infections result from eating improperly prepared meat. *Taenia saginata* is acquired from ingesting contaminated beef, *Taenia solium* is acquired from contaminated pork, and *Diphyllobothrium latum* is obtained from contaminated fish. The life cycles of these tapeworms involve larval stages in animals and worm stages in humans. If the contaminated meat contains the larval forms of these organisms, then they may develop into an adult worm in the intestines of infected humans. These individuals generally remain asymptomatic, except that *D. latum* may cause a vitamin B12 deficiency. A very different disease will result from humans eating the eggs of *T. solium*, which may be found in human feces. In this case, the eggs hatch in larva, which then penetrate the gut wall and disseminate via the blood stream to lodge in different organs. There they encyst and differentiate into cysticerci. Multiple cysticerci in the brain produce a "Swiss cheese" appearance grossly, and microscopically a scolex (the head of the worm) is found with hooklets. This disease is called cysticercosis. Another cestode, *Echinococcus granulosa*, is the cause of hydatid disease in humans. Individuals become infected by eating the tapeworm eggs. Patients are usually sheep herders who get the eggs from their dogs. Larvae released from the eggs disseminate most often to the liver (75 percent), but they may also travel to the lungs or skeletal muscle. They form large, slowly growing, unilocular cysts that contain multiple scolices. *Toxocara* species, such as *Toxocara canis* and *Toxocara cati*, are one cause of visceral larval migrans. This disease is characterized by infection of visceral organs by helminthic larvae. The typical patient is a young child who develops hypereosinophilia and hypergammaglobulinemia. Ocular manifestations of toxocariasis are common, especially the loss of vision in one eye in a child. Note that this disease is different from cutaneous larva migrans, which is caused by the larval forms of the hookworms and *Strongyloides stercoralis*.

93. The answer is d. *(Damjanov, 10/e, pp 987–988.)* *Giardia lamblia*, a flagellate protozoan, is the most common cause of outbreaks of waterborne diarrheal disease in the U.S. and is seen frequently in Rocky Mountain areas. Ingestion of cysts from contaminated water results in trophozoites in duodenum and jejunum. Identification of the trophozoite stage is done by duodenal aspiration or small-bowel biopsy and of the cyst stage (intermittent) by examination of stool. The trophozoite may appear as a pear-shaped, binucleate organism ("two eyes"). Giardiasis may cause malabsorption but is often asymptomatic. Duodenal aspiration, immunofluorescence, and ELISA testing for Giardia antigens are diagnostic and therapy with metronidazole or quinacrine is effective. Lymph nodes often contain numerous parasites in trypanosomiasis and leishmaniasis. Triatoma is the vector of Chagas' disease (American trypanosomiasis). *Trichomonas vaginalis* is identified in cervicovaginal smears.

94. The answer is b. *(Damjanov, 10/e, pp 1013–1018.)* In the photomicrograph, a cross section of an Enterobius adult worm is shown. Apparent morphologic features of this nematode include the bilateral crests, the meromyarial type of musculature, and the noncellular cuticle with spines. *Enterobius vermicularis*, the agent responsible for the helminthic infection most common in the United States, usually produces pruritus ani as the outstanding and most disturbing symptom of enterobiasis (pinworm infection). Enterobius worms often attach themselves to the fecal mucosa and contiguous regions, but the usual host sites for schistosomiasis, clonorchiasis, and filariasis are the veins of the large intestine, the bile ducts, and the lymphatics, respectively. Elephantiasis is a characteristic feature in filariasis, and infection by *Strongyloides stercoralis* usually produces hyperemia and edema of the mucosa of the small intestine.

95. The answer is a. (*Henry, 19/e, pp 279–285. Cotran, 5/e, p 537.*) The levels of serum aspartate aminotransferase (AST), which is also called serum glutamic-oxaloacetic transaminase (SGOT) (curve II), become elevated within 12 h after nearly all acute myocardial infarctions; they generally reach a peak level within 48 h and return to normal within 4 to 5 days. After myocardial infarctions, creatine phosphokinase levels (curve I) rise and fall more rapidly than do SGOT levels. Lactic dehydrogenase levels (curve III) also become elevated within 1 day after infarctions, but they remain elevated for about 10 days. Alkaline phosphatase and 59-nucleotidase levels, normal during infarctions, usually show marked increases in patients who have obstructive jaundice.

96. The answer is a. (*Henry, 19/e, pp 281–284.*) The patient described probably has hepatitis, according to the values given for the five isoenzymes of lactic dehydrogenase (LDH). Liver cells contain higher proportions of LDH_4 and LDH_5 than do myocardium or red blood cells, both of which contain greater relative amounts of LDH_1 and LDH_2. Lung tissue is high in LDH_3, and brain tissue contains only small amounts of LDH_5. During the LDH increase following a myocardial infarction, levels of LDH_1 are usually higher than those of LDH_2. This pattern is called a "flipped" LDH.

97. The answer is d. (*Damjanov, 10/e, pp 123–133.*) The cytoplasmic matrix contains numerous organelles with highly specialized functions. Whereas mitochondria are the "power" units of the cell involved with the Krebs cycle and anaerobic metabolism, the endoplasmic reticulum is a complex network of rodlike tubules containing ribosomes and is involved in protein synthesis (rough endoplasmic reticulum). Lysosomes are round bodies containing enzymes involved in inflammation. These include the sulfatases, desoxyribonucleases, hydrolases, and acid phosphatases. The Golgi apparatus (complex) is made up of tiny vesicles, membranes, and vacuoles and is also involved in protein synthesis, as it receives the synthesized proteins from the endoplasmic reticulum. The Golgi complex appears to collect, segregate, and export protein. Microbodies are membrane-bound spheres that contain catalase and oxidases. Epithelial cells, especially surface-lining cells, are held together by connections referred to as intercellular junctions. Desmosomes (squamous cells), tight junctions (zonula occludens), and gap junctions (nexuses) are examples of such membrane connectors.

98. The answer is b. (*Cotran, 5/e, p 64. Rubin, 2/e, pp 60, 1031–1032.*) The enzymatic defect that exists in chronic granulomatous disease of childhood does not impair chemotaxis or the cell's ability to engulf bacteria but rather involves a failure to produce hydrogen peroxide after engulfment. Chemotactic defects resulting in inhibition of the capacity of leukocytes to infiltrate an area of infection or injury may be due to intracellular defects, as found in Chédiak-Higashi syndrome, in other genetic defects, and in diabetes mellitus. Chronic renal failure and cirrhosis may be associated with factors in the circulation that impair chemotaxis. Thermal injuries are also associated with acquired defects in leukocyte chemotaxis.

99. The answer is e. (*Cotran, 5/e, pp 21–22, 66–70.*) Lysosomes contain many substances involved in inflammation including alkaline and acid phosphatase, collagenases, lysozymes, lactoferrin, myeloperoxidase, cationic proteins, and acid proteases. Of these, the neutral proteases (elastase, collagenase, cathepsin G) function in stages of inflammatory confinement and wound healing by degrading tissue matrix like collagen, fibrin, cartilage, elastin, and basement membranes. The other mediators cascade as follows: complement cascade starts classically by an antigen-antibody complex or alternately by nonimmunologic stimuli. C5a leads to chemotaxis while the complement complex C5b-9 leads to cell lysis. The kinins are activated by Hageman factor (XIIA), via prekallikrein, into bradykinin. The fibrinopeptides of the clotting system can also be activated by Hageman factor or by extrinsic tissue thromboplastin to result in a polymerized fibrin clot. The important cascades of arachidonic acid metabolites (cyclooxygenase, lipoxygenase), leading to functioning vasodilators (prostaglandins) and membrane permeability factors (leukotrienes), are the most complex of all, beginning with the actions of phospholipase.

100. The answer is d. (*Cotran, 5/e, pp 80–82.*) Granulomatous inflammation is characterized by the presence of granulomas, consisting of 1- to 2-mm foci of modified macrophages (epithelioid cells) surrounded by mononuclear cells, mainly lymphocytes. It is a chronic inflammation initiated by a variety of infectious and noninfectious agents. Indigestible organisms or particles, or T-cell-mediated immunity to the inciting agent, or both, appear essential for formation of granulomas. Although tuberculosis is the classic infectious granulomatous disease, several other infectious disorders are characterized by formation of granulomas, including deep fungal infections (coccidioidomycosis and histoplasmosis), schistosomiasis, syphilis, brucellosis, lymphogranuloma venereum, and cat-scratch disease. In sarcoidosis, a disease of unknown cause, the granulomas are noncaseating, which may assist in histologic differentiation from tuberculosis. No organisms are found in lesions of sarcoidosis.

101. The answer is c. (*Cotran, 5/e, pp 87–89, 132–133. Rubin, 2/e, pp 70–74, 226–227.*) Type I collagen is found in skin, tendon, bone, dentin, and fascia; type II collagen is found only in cartilage; type III collagen (reticulin) appears in skin, blood vessels, uterus, and embryonic dermis. Type IV collagen, a component of basement laminae of epithelial and endothelial cells, does not have the typical 67-nm banding of types I, II, and III. Synthesis of collagen includes lysine oxidation, resulting in alpha-chain cross-linkages with structural stability of collagen. Decreased formation of cross-linkages in collagen and elastin occurs in Marfan's syndrome, an autosomal dominant disorder of connective tissues, with skeletal abnormalities including arachnodactyly, lens subluxation, and cystic medionecrosis of aorta with aneurysm and sometimes rupture.

102. The answer is d. (*Cotran, 5/e, pp 117–119.*) Septic shock is caused by the gram-negative, endotoxin-producing aerobic rods mentioned in the question. It results from pooling of blood in the peripheral circulation. A common cause of sepsis in burn wounds is *Pseudomonas aeruginosa.* The major target in severe shock is the kidneys, which suffer acute ischemic tubular necrosis, affecting proximal and distal nephrons in septic shock. Gram-negative endotoxic shock has a 70 percent mortality.

103. The answer is e. *(Cotran, 5/e, pp 259–270. Rubin, 2/e, pp 173–183.)* Proto-oncogenes are genes that code for proteins involved in normal growth and development. These normal cellular genes may become oncogenic by being incorporated into a viral genome by a process called retroviral transduction, which forms viral oncogenes (v-oncs). They can also be activated by other processes, such as mutations, that form cellular oncogenes (c-oncs). These oncogenes, which are associated with certain malignancies, can be classified into different classes based on various postulated mechanisms of cellular activation. The *c-abl* oncogene, which is associated with chronic myeloid leukemia, acts through a tyrosine-like kinase, which is a protein involved in signal transduction. The *ras* family of oncogenes, associated with neuroblastoma and urinary bladder cancer, code for a protein, p21, which is similar to GTP-binding proteins (G proteins). The product of some oncogenes, such as *c-myc*, which is associated with Burkitt's lymphoma, are found only in the nucleus and are classified as nuclear regulatory proteins. Some genes, rather than being associated with the formation of cancer, are associated with the suppression of cancer. A classic example of these "anti-oncogenes" involves the formation of retinoblastoma. Both normal alleles, the "anti-oncogenes," which are located at the retinoblastoma (Rb) locus on chromosome 13, must be inactivated for the development of retinoblastoma. This is the basis of the famous "two-hit" hypothesis developed by Knudson. There is also a higher incidence of other cancers in these patients, especially osteogenic sarcoma.

104. The answer is e. *(Cotran, 5/e, pp 215–219, 228–231, 283–286, 293, 712–714.)* Immunodeficiency states often predispose to the development of neoplasia. The primary immunodeficiencies most clearly associated with an increased incidence of malignancy are common variable immunodeficiency, severe combined immunodeficiency, Wiskott-Aldrich syndrome, and ataxia-telangiectasia (in which defective repair of DNA may also play a role). The neoplasms in these genetic immunodeficiencies are predominantly non-Hodgkin's lymphomas, often immunoblastic, and often extranodal. Secondary immunodeficiency states occur in patients immunosuppressed for organ transplantation and tumors that develop are mainly high-grade, non-Hodgkin's lymphomas, frequently extranodal, especially in the CNS.

Transplant patients also show an increased incidence of Kaposi's sarcoma, and a slight increase of squamous cell carcinoma in skin and oral tissues has been reported. The significant increase in neoplasia due to irradiation and radiomimetic drugs—primarily an increase in acute nonlymphoid leukemia—appears to be largely independent of immunosuppression. AIDS, a major devastating example of secondary immunodeficiency, was first recognized in 1981 through the increased incidence of Kaposi's sarcoma in young homosexual men. Subsequent studies established a considerable increase of high-grade, non-Hodgkin's lymphomas in patients infected with human immunodeficiency virus (HIV). Such lymphomas include small noncleaved cell, immunoblastic, and diffuse large cell lymphomas. There also may be an increase in Hodgkin's disease of aggressive type in HIV infection. Sarcoidosis is not associated with an increased incidence of malignancy.

105. The answer is e. (*Cotran, 5/e, pp 253–254. Rubin, 2/e, pp 192–197.*) There are marked differences in the incidence of various types of cancer in different parts of the world. Nasopharyngeal carcinoma, associated with the Epstein-Barr virus, is rare in most parts of the world, except for parts of the Far East, especially China. Liver cancer is associated with both hepatitis B infection and high levels of aflatoxin B_1. It is endemic in large parts of Africa and Asia. The highest rates for gastric carcinoma are found in Japan. Trophoblastic diseases, including choriocarcinoma, have high rates of disease in the Pacific rim areas of Asia. In contrast, Asian populations have a very low incidence of prostate cancer. American blacks have a high incidence, while the rate in American and European whites is in between.

106. The answer is e. (*Henry, 19/e, pp 483–490, 677–679. Cotran, 5/e, pp 300–301.*) Tumor markers are a diverse group of biochemical substances associated with the presence of some tumors and include hormones, oncofetal antigens, isozymes, proteins, mucins, and glycoproteins. Human chorionic gonadotropin (hCG) is a hormone associated with trophoblastic tumors, especially choriocarcinoma. Alpha-fetoprotein (AFP) is a glycoprotein synthesized by the yolk sac and the fetal liver and is associated with yolk sac tumors of the testes and liver cell carcinomas. Prostate-specific antigen (PSA) and prostatic acid phosphatase (PAP) are associated with cancer of the prostate. Carcinoembryonic antigen (CEA) is a glycoprotein associated with many cancers including adenocarcinomas of the colon, pancreas, lung, stomach, and breast. It may also be increased in some benign disorders. Chloroacetate esterase (CAE) (not to be confused with CEA) is a histochemical stain used in the differentiation of acute leukemias.

107. The answer is c. (*Cotran, 5/e, pp 1262–1263.*) Liposarcomas are the most common soft tissue sarcoma of adults, arise deeply in the thigh or retroperitoneum, and are liable to metastasize by embolization in blood vessels (nonmyxoid types). Histology is varied—well-differentiated, myxoid, round cell, or pleomorphic—depending on tumor type. Myxoid liposarcoma is the most common variant. The pleomorphic type is undifferentiated and easily confused with other poorly differentiated mesenchymal sarcomas. The clinical picture is also varied. Well-differentiated and myxoid types are locally invasive and recurrent, if they are not completely excised, but they are rarely metastatic. Round-cell and pleomorphic types are often aggressive with widespread metastases, local recurrence, and poor 5-year survival.

108. The answer is c. (*Lee, 9/e, pp 570–572. Henry, 19/e, pp 740–741.*) Vitamin K is not required for the biosynthesis of coagulation factor VIII, which has an uncertain participation as a trace protein in the intrinsic coagulation pathway and is also known as the antihemophilic factor. Vitamin K, although its biochemical mode of action remains unclear, is required for the biosynthesis and maintenance of normal concentrations of coagulation factors II (prothrombin), VII, IX, and X.

109. The answer is e. (*Cotran, 5/e, pp 402–408.*) Ionizing radiation, which is used in clinical diagnosis and therapy, induces changes in many different organ systems of the body. Its effects may be direct or indirect. Direct effects on target tissues produce single- or double-stranded chromosomal breaks in DNA. Indirect effects result in the formation of free radicals. Radiation also causes bizarre nuclear morphology along with abnormal mitotic figures. Changes induced in blood vessels include swelling and vacuolation of endothelial cells along with secondary thromboses and hemorrhages. The skin shows epidermal atrophy, not hyperplasia, and hyalinization and fibrosis of the dermis. There is atrophy of skin appendages and dilatation of the blood vessels. Effects on the blood include lymphopenia and granulocytopenia. Sterility is an effect on the gonads in both males and females, and the gastrointestinal tract is frequently damaged, leading to nausea and vomiting.

110. The answer is c. (_Cotran, 5/e, pp 385–387, 1044–1045._) Despite current controversy, most researchers agree that women taking oral contraceptives are at risk, however small, of developing myocardial infarction, especially if the woman is a cigarette smoker, and vascular thrombi that may lead to strokes and pulmonary embolism and infarction. Also very minimal in terms of numbers of cases are hepatic adenomas, which have been recorded in patients taking oral estrogens over a protracted period of time. Conflicting evidence is found concerning the risk of developing endometrial carcinoma. Some researchers have shown a definite risk of developing uterine cancer, but not all series have demonstrated a positive correlation. The same problem exists in estimation of the risk of developing breast cancer. Vaginal adenosis develops not in the women taking estrogens themselves, but rather in the female offspring of mothers who received diethylstilbestrol (DES) while pregnant. Some of these daughters have also developed clear cell carcinoma of the cervix, an adenocarcinoma that carries a rather poor prognosis. DES binds to cell nuclear DNA and hence may act as a cocarcinogen rather than as a mere promoter.

111. The answer is d. (_Cotran, 5/e, pp 388–390, 868–869._) The seemingly innumerable deleterious effects of alcohol abuse are recognized as constituting a major public health problem even in non-Western locations, such as Africa and Asia. The effects may be socioeconomic (divorce, absenteeism, and high insurance rates due to automobile accidents), political, moral, or organic. Indeed, it is difficult to think of an organ or organ system that does not develop a physical dysfunction, either reversible or irreversible, in response to excessive intake of ethanol. Subdural hematomas are commonly seen in alcoholics. Portal vein thrombosis is rarely seen in the absence of nutritional or Laënnec's cirrhosis. Levels of the muscle and cardiac enzyme creatine phosphokinase may be elevated in states of alcoholic myocardiosis, cardiomyopathy, alcoholic rhabdomyolysis, or trauma to skeletal muscles while the patient is in an alcoholic toxic state. Primary biliary cirrhosis occurs predominantly in middle-aged women and its etiology is unknown, although marked immunologic factors have been described, as well as marked copper deposition in the liver with normal serum ceruloplasmin.

112. The answer is b. (_Cotran, 5/e, pp 28, 63–64, 135–137, 449–454. Rubin, 2/e, pp 230–234, 240–244._) Familial hypercholesterolemia (FH) is a common autosomal dominant (AD) disorder caused by mutation in the low-density lipoprotein (LDL) receptor gene located on chromosome 19. These gene mutations impair LDL transport and catabolism, with accumulation of LDL cholesterol in plasma. Elevated cholesterol levels result in skin xanthomas, early atherosclerosis, and increased risk of myocardial infarction. There is absent or deficient LDL receptor activity in homozygotes and one-half normal receptor activity in heterozygotes. CF is a fairly common AR disorder in whites (1:2500). Exocrine glands produce viscous mucus and sweat with high sodium and chloride concentration. The mutant gene product is unknown but the CF gene is localized on the long arm of chromosome 7. CF is manifest clinically only in homozygotes; parents are asymptomatic heterozygous carriers of the trait. PKU is an AR disorder of amino acid metabolism due to mutation in the gene coding for phenylalanine hydroxylase. Chromosome location is 12 and six different mutations are known. Myeloperoxidase deficiency has a frequency of 1:2000; slow bacterial killing is the major problem. Alkaptonuria is rare, the mutant gene product is homogentisic acid oxidase, and abnormal pigmentation of connective tissue (ochronosis) will result.

113. The answer is e. (*Cotran, 5/e, pp 152–156. Rubin, 2/e, pp 216–220.*) Nondisjunction is the failure of paired chromosomes or chromatids to separate during anaphase, either during mitosis or meiosis. Nondisjunction during the first meiotic division is responsible for trisomy 21 in about 93 percent of patients with Down's syndrome. Nondisjunction during mitosis of a somatic cell early during embryogenesis results in mosaicism in about 2 percent of patients with Down's syndrome. Translocation of an extra long arm of chromosome 21 causes about 5 percent of Down's syndrome cases. An important type of translocation, the Robertsonian translocation (centric fusion), involves two nonhomologous acrocentric chromosomes with the resultant formation of one large metacentric chromosome and one small chromosomal fragment, which is usually lost. Carriers of this type of translocation may produce children with Down's syndrome. Isochromosomes result from abnormal division of the centromere in a transverse plane. They are important in the pathogenesis of Turner's syndrome, not Down's syndrome.

114. The answer is a. (*Damjanov, 10/e, p 252. Cotran, 5/e, pp 159–160.*) The findings of small, firm testes, eunuchoidism, gynecomastia, and mental retardation constitute the classic manifestations of Klinefelter's syndrome, a type of hypogonadism. The seminiferous tubules may be sclerosed and hyalinized. Urinary levels of gonadotropin are usually elevated; the elevation is thought to result from the absence of controlling testicular hormones, not from pituitary dysfunction.

115. The answer is c. (_Cotran, 5/e, pp 446–449._) Hemolytic disease of the newborn is characterized by anemia, jaundice, tissue edema, and hepatosplenomegaly. The transmission of maternal antibody (transplacental transmission) causes the disease because of incompatibility between maternal and fetal blood types. ABO incompatibilities occur often but are not severe; however, both ABO and Rh antigens may cause the disease. There are many Rh antigens that do not cause disease, but Rh D is the usual antigen that causes mild to very severe disease, except in the first pregnancy. The frequency increases with repeat pregnancies as antibody level rises, and anti-Rh D IgG must be given to a nonsensitized Rh-negative mother within 72 h of delivery or termination (abortion) of the first and of all subsequent pregnancies.

116. The answer is d. (_Cotran, 5/e, pp 172–173. Rubin, 2/e, p 101._) B cells possess surface membrane IgM and IgD, with monomeric IgM the antigen receptor of all B cells. B cells also express the pan-B-cell antigens CD19 and CD20, which is obviously of practical value in differentiating a chronic leukemia such as chronic lymphocytic leukemia (CLL) in which transformed B cells possess surface IgM and IgD and express CD19 and CD20 antigens, but not the early B cell antigen CD10. In contrast, CD8 and CD4 are on 30 percent and 60 percent of peripheral T cells, respectively. CD4 is a marker for T helper cells, and CD8 a marker for cytotoxic/suppressor T cells. B lymphocytes have receptors for fixed complement components C3b and C3d and for the Fc portion of IgG. Immunologic diagnosis of B-cell lymphoid tumors by immunofluorescence or flow cytometry shows the cell surface immunoglobulins and cluster differentiation antigens through detection by monoclonal antibodies; molecular biology techniques reveal Ig gene rearrangements on the altered B cells.

117. The answer is d. (_Henry, 19/e, pp 76–77. Cotran, 5/e, pp 200–201._) Diagnostic specificity is defined as the probability of a negative diagnostic test result in the absence of the disease the test is designed to detect, or, simply, the ability of a screening test to correctly identify a person who is free of the specific disease. Two clinically useful tests specific for systemic lupus erythematosus (SLE) are the detection of antibodies to double-stranded DNA (anti-ds DNA) and to the nonhistone Smith (Sm) antigen, since these antibodies are rare in other autoimmune diseases. Positive testing for antinuclear antibody (ANA) occurs in virtually all patients with SLE (marked diagnostic sensitivity), but the test is not specific since positive results are frequent in other autoimmune diseases. In diffuse systemic sclerosis, positive antibodies to nucleolar RNA and Scl-70 antibody to nonhistone nuclear protein are specific. In the CREST syndrome of systemic sclerosis, an anticentromere antibody is specific. The best information from laboratory tests comes from their positive and negative predictive values (PVs) relating the results (+ or −) to prevalence of the disease in the population being studied.

118. The answer is b. (*Cotran, 5/e, pp 199–208.*) Renal failure, not heart disease, is the most common cause of death in SLE. Most cases show some renal abnormality (mild or marked) by immunofluorescence and by light and electron microscopy. Diffuse proliferative glomerulonephritis (GN) occurs in about 50 percent of cases and is the most common and most serious renal lesion. Subendothelial location of immune complex deposits is particularly characteristic of SLE. Membranous GN occurs in only 10 percent of cases and has a better prognosis, but may progress. Polyclonal B-cell activation occurs with increased production of autoantibodies and hypergammaglobulinemia. This B-cell activation may follow genetic B-cell abnormalities or loss of T-suppressor cell influence. Most of the tissue lesions are mediated by the immune complex (type III hypersensitivity). Nonerosive arthritis occurs in about 90 percent of cases and often involves small peripheral joints. Lack of deformity and of synovial proliferation distinguish arthritis of SLE from rheumatoid arthritis.

119. The answer is c. (*Cotran, 5/e, pp 208–210.*) Sjögren's syndrome is characterized by dryness of the mouth (xerostomia) and eyes (keratoconjunctivitis sicca). Secondary Sjögren's syndrome is associated with rheumatoid arthritis (RA), or SLE, or systemic sclerosis. The primary form shows increased frequency of HLA-DR3, while association with RA shows a positive correlation with HLA-DR4. Anti-SSB antibodies are fairly specific, anti-SSA less so, and both may occur in SLE; rheumatoid factor is often present.

Glomerular lesions are very rare but a mild tubulointerstitial nephritis is quite common and may result in renal tubular acidosis. In addition to the usual dense, lymphoplasmacytic infiltrate of salivary glands, the lymph nodes may show a "pseudolymphomatous" appearance. True B-cell lymphomas have developed with increased frequency in Sjögren's syndrome (relative risk of 44).

120. The answer is d. (*Cotran, 5/e, pp 219–231.*) AIDS is caused by infection with the retrovirus human immunodeficiency virus (HIV) (formerly called HTLV III/LAV). The virus infects T helper cells, preventing function, destroying cells, and increasing susceptibility to and incidence of infection. Cytotoxic/suppressor T cells may be normal, slightly increased, or decreased in number, although they show a proportional increase in comparison to helper T cells, which are markedly decreased. In AIDS, the ratio of helper to suppressor cells is inverted, being approximately 1:2, instead of the normal 2:1. Wide defects of immune function in AIDS include defects in natural killer cells, in monocytes, and in virus-specific cytotoxic T cells and B cells. B cells are polyclonally activated, resulting in hypergammaglobulinemia. Patients with AIDS have an increased incidence of certain malignancies, including Kaposi's sarcoma and B-cell non-Hodgkin's lymphoma.

121. The answer is b. (*Henry, 19/e, pp 1140–1143, 1173–1174. Cotran, 5/e, pp 337–338.*) The pneumococcus (*Streptococcus pneumoniae*) is a Gram-positive, encapsulated coccus, differentiated from other alpha-hemolytic streptococci by bile solubility or serologic typing. But inhibition of pneumococci by Optochin is easier and has about 90 percent specificity. Capsular polysaccharides form the basis for division into serotypes; when exposed to type-specific antisera they show a positive precipitin reaction or capsular swelling, the quellung reaction. Detection of pneumococcal capsular polysaccharides in sputum or body fluids by immunologic methods (CIE or latex agglutination) are other methods for presumptive diagnosis of infection, but cross reactions between pneumococci and other bacteria occur. So, immunologic diagnosis is less specific than bacteriologic diagnosis by capsular typing by the quellung reaction. Capsular polysaccharides protect pneumococci from phagocytosis and are virulence factors. M protein occurs in the cell walls of pathogenic group A beta-hemolytic streptococci (*S. pyogenes*) and functions as the principal virulence factor by inhibiting phagocytosis.

122. The answer is c. *(Henry, 19/e, pp 1148–1149. Cotran, 5/e, p 309. Rubin, 2/e, p 283.)* Listeriosis is a food-borne illness (e.g., via milk products, coleslaw) usually occurring in the immunocompromised, in pregnant women and their fetuses, and in the debilitated elderly. *Listeria monocytogenes* is a gram-positive, motile bacillus, often found within circulating lymphocytes (similar to Legionella). Maternal infection is mild; fetal infection is severe. Meningitis is predominant in neonatal infections and in opportunistic adult disease, and *Listeria monocytogenes* is responsible for about 2 percent of bacterial meningitis cases in this country. True epithelioid granulomas are rare, although macrophages may appear late, following neutrophil infiltration or abscesses in organs or lymph nodes.

123. The answer is e. *(Rubin, 2/e, pp 386–387, 390–396.)* Lymphogranuloma venereum, usually transmitted by sexual contact, is caused by obligate intracellular parasites that contain both RNA and DNA and belong to the genus Chlamydia (*C. trachomatis*). Chlamydial agents, originally thought to be viruses because they form inclusion bodies in infected cells, also cause trachoma, inclusion conjunctivitis, and psittacosis-ornithosis. The other infections listed are caused by spirochetes and are nonvenereal.

124. The answer is e. *(Cotran, 5/e, pp 307, 698–699.)* Mycoplasma pneumoniae, the causative agent of primary atypical interstitial pneumonia, belongs to the mycoplasma group of tiny pleuropneumonia-like organisms (PPLOs, or Eaton agents), which lack cell walls and are beyond the resolution of light microscopy. *M. pneumoniae* can cause up to 50 percent of pneumonias in college students and mainly affects adolescents and young adults. The interstitial pneumonia with mononuclear response is similar to viral pneumonia; pharyngitis and tracheobronchitis with persistent cough are common. Serum immunoglobulins that agglutinate human type O red cells at 4°C (cold agglutinins) are often present; this test is nonspecific but suggestive of *M. pneumoniae*.

125. The answer is e. *(Cotran, 5/e, pp 365–367.)* Lepromatous and tuberculoid leprosy, the major forms, are caused by *Mycobacterium leprae* and nerve involvement is most typical of the lepromatous form. Numerous bacilli in packets occupy histiocytes or lepra cells in the lesions of lepromatous leprosy. Polyclonal hypergammaglobulinemia often occurs in lepromatous leprosy, in which patients do not have the adequate cellular immune response of the tuberculoid form. Large amounts of anti-lepra antibody occur in the lepromatous form with frequent formation of antigen-antibody complexes and resultant disorders such as erythema nodosum. A "clear" zone between infiltrate and overlying epidermis is characteristic of lepromatous leprosy, unlike the encroachment on basal epidermis of the tuberculoid infiltrate.

126. The answer is d. (*Damjanov, 10/e, pp 1013–1021.*) Eggs of the roundworm Ascaris are found in contaminated soil in the southeastern United States. When swallowed, these eggs hatch, reach the small intestinal vessels, and travel to the lungs, where they may produce clinical bronchial asthma and pneumonitis. The New World hookworm, *Necator americanus*, penetrates exposed skin through exposure to larvae-containing soil; these infective filariform larvae reach the pulmonary circulation via the lymphatic and vascular systems and cause alveolar hemorrhages and temporary bronchopneumonia. Rhabditiform Strongyloides soil larvae also gain access to the vascular system and pulmonary circuit through penetration of exposed skin and also cause intra-alveolar pneumonitis and hemorrhages. *Wuchereria bancrofti* filariae gain access to the human lymphatics (endolymphangitis, elephantiasis) via bites of the *Culex* mosquito; this organism is not noted for producing a pulmonary phase, but it does produce characteristic spermatic cord granulomas.

127. The answer is c. (*Henry, 19/e, pp 179–181. Cotran, 5/e, p 1143.*) Parathyroid hormone (PTH), by affecting the kidneys, bones, and intestinal mucosa, is the principal regulator of plasma levels of phosphate and calcium. PTH, by its action on renal tubular cells, not only causes decreased phosphate reabsorption, it causes increased calcium reabsorption; these reciprocal processes result in a decrease in serum phosphate and a corresponding increase in extracellular calcium levels. Extracellular levels of calcium are also maintained by the release of calcium during PTH-induced osteocytic and osteoclastic osteolysis, a process that is regarded as the mobilization of calcium from bone. PTH also may induce the intestinal mucosa to absorb calcium derived from dietary sources.

128. The answer is e. (*Henry, 19/e, pp 287–288.*) An elevated serum amylase level is usually associated with acute pancreatitis; it is practically diagnostic if it is more than three times normal, and if salivary gland disease and intestinal perforation or infarction are excluded. There may be increased amylase with parotitis alone, but increased lipase (more sensitive and much more specific) only with pancreatitis. Elevated amylase may be associated with biliary tract disease, and also with renal disease because of decreased clearance. Low serum amylase has been noted with serum protein loss in congestive heart failure. Amylase can be produced by certain tumors (lung, breast, ovarian cancer). In these and in acidotic states, the amylase must be distinguished from that of pancreatitis by isoenzyme analysis. P isoamylases arise from the pancreas; S isoamylases arise from nonpancreatic sources, as in diabetic ketoacidosis.

129. The answer is d. (*Henry, 19/e, pp 277–278, 287–289.*) In polycythemia vera the serum alkaline phosphatase level is not increased. However, the neutrophil alkaline phosphatase is markedly elevated in 80 percent of patients with polycythemia vera, while this leukocyte alkaline phosphatase level is depressed in chronic myelogenous leukemia. Serum alkaline phosphatase is usually quite markedly elevated in such hepatobiliary diseases as obstructive jaundice, intrahepatic cholestasis, biliary cirrhosis, and infectious mononucleosis. Milder elevations occur in alcoholic cirrhosis and viral hepatitis. The placental alkaline phosphatase isoenzyme peaks during the third trimester and returns to normal post partum.

130. The answer is c. (*Cotran, 5/e, pp 1255–1259. Rubin, 2/e, pp 1335–1339.*) Hyperuricemia, prominent in gout, occurs most often secondary to disorders that increase production or reduce excretion of uric acid. These include myeloproliferative disorders and some cancers, such as leukemias and lymphomas, in which there is increased turnover of nucleic acid with resultant hyperuricemia. Reduced excretion of uric acid may arise from renal causes, or from competition by certain organic acids, as in starvation ketosis. Lesch-Nyhan syndrome, a rare X-linked disease caused by an absence of hypoxanthine-guanine phosphoribosyltransferase (HGPRT), is characterized by mental retardation, self-mutilation, hyperuricemia, and gouty arthritis. Chondrocalcinosis, or calcium pyrophosphate dihydrate (CPPD) deposition disease, is not associated with hyperuricemia.

131. The answer is c. (*Henry, 19/e, pp 284–285. Rubin, 2/e, p 528.*) Creatine kinase (CK) is an enzyme found mainly in skeletal muscle, the myocardium, and the brain. Diseases that produce skeletal muscle destruction, such as all types of muscular dystrophy, polymyositis, viral myositis, and rhabdomyolysis, produce elevated levels of CK in the blood. Neurogenic muscle diseases, such as myasthenia gravis, multiple sclerosis, poliomyelitis, and parkinsonism, have normal levels of CK because there is no destruction of the muscle. Total CK activity is increased following a myocardial infarction and also following cerebrovascular diseases with cerebral ischemia. Serum CK levels have an inverse relationship with thyroid activity; that is, levels are increased in hypothyroid patients, but are low-normal to decreased in amount in patients with hyperthyroidism.

132–133. The answers are: 132-a, 133-c. (*Cotran, 5/e, pp 60–64, 218–219. Rubin, 2/e, pp 1031–1032.*) The Chédiak-Higashi syndrome is an autosomal recessive disorder characterized by the abnormal fusion of phagosomes with lysosomes, which results in ineffective bactericidal capabilities of neutrophils and monocytes. These abnormal leukocytes develop giant intracytoplasmic lysosomes. Abnormal formation of melanosomes in these individuals results in oculocutaneous albinism. Most of these patients eventually develop an "accelerated phase" in which an aggressive lymphoproliferative disease, possibly the result of an Ebstein-Barr viral infection, results in pancytopenia and death.

In contrast, patients with chronic granulomatous disease have defective functioning of phagocytic neutrophils and monocytes due to an inability to produce hydrogen peroxide. That is, their phagocytic cells have a decreased oxidative or respiratory burst. This results in recurrent infections with catalase-positive organisms, such as *staphylococcus aureus*. The classic form of chronic granulomatous disease usually affects boys and causes death before the age of 10. Key findings in chronic granulomatous disease include lymphadenitis, hepatosplenomegaly, eczematoid dermatitis, pulmonary infiltrates that are associated with hypergammaglobulinemia, and defective ability of neutrophils to kill bacteria.

Both leukemoid reactions and chronic granulocytic leukemia are characterized by increased numbers of neutrophils in the peripheral blood. Letterer-Siwe disease, a malignant form of Langerhans's cell histiocytosis, is characterized by widespread infiltration of organs, particularly the skin, by malignant Langerhans' cells. Thrombocytopenia is a feature of Wiskott-Aldrich syndrome.

134–135. The answers are: 134-g, 135-c. (*Cotran, 5/e, pp 420–423. Chandrasoma, 3/e, pp 160–162. Rubin, 2/e, pp 330–332.*) Deficiencies of the water-soluble B vitamins may result from dietary deficiencies or other abnormalities. Vitamin B1 (thiamine) has three important functions. Thiamine participates in oxidative decarboxylation of alpha ketoacids; thiamine participates as a cofactor for transketolase in the pentose phosphate path; and thiamine participates in maintaining neural membranes. The causes of thiamine deficiency include poor diet, deficient absorption and storage, and accelerated destruction of thiamine diphosphate. This deficiency may be seen in alcoholics and prisoners of war because of poor nutrition, or it may be seen in individuals who eat large amounts of polished rice. Polishing rice removes the outer, thiamin-containing portion of the grain. Thiamin deficiency (called "beriberi") mainly affects two organ systems, the heart and the nervous system. If the heart is affected in a patient with beriberi, it may become dilated and flabby. Patients may also develop peripheral vasodilatation that leads to a high-output cardiac failure and marked peripheral edema. This combination of vascular abnormalities is called "wet beriberi." The peripheral nerves in beriberi may be damaged by focal areas of myelin degeneration, which leads to foot drop, wrist drop, and sensory changes (numbness and tingling) in the feet and lower legs. These symptoms are referred to as "dry beriberi." Thiamin deficiency may produce the central nervous system (CNS) symptoms of Wernicke-Korsakoff syndrome. Wernicke encephalopathy consists mainly of foci of hemorrhages and necrosis in the mammillary bodies and about the ventricular regions of the thalamus and hypothalamus, about the aqueduct in the midbrain, and in the floor of the fourth ventricle. Symptoms of Wernicke syndrome include progressive dementia (confusion), ataxia, and paralysis of the extraocular muscles—often with bilateral lateral rectus, or sixth nerve, palsies (ophthalmoplegia). Korsakoff psychosis is a thought disorder that produces retrograde memory failure and confabulation.

Niacin (vitamin B3) is required for the synthesis of both NAD and NADP, two enzymes that participate in many dehydrogenase enzymes. In general NAD-linked dehydrogenases catalyze reactions in oxidative pathways like the TCA cycle, while NADP-linked enzymes are found in reductive syntheses pathways, such as the pentose phosphate pathway. Deficiencies of niacin will produce pellagra, a disease that is characterized by the triad of dementia, dermatitis ("glove" or "necklace" distribution), and diarrhea. Decreased levels of niacin may result from diets that are deficient in niacin, such as diets that depend upon maize (corn) as the main staple, because niacin in maize is bound in a form that is not available. Part of the body need for niacin is supplied by the conversion of the essential amino acid tryptophan to NAD, and therefore a deficiency of tryptophan can also produce symptoms of pellagra. Deficiencies of tryptophan can be seen in individuals with Hartnup's disease, which is caused by the abnormal membrane transport of neutral amino acids and tryptophan in the small intestines and kidneys. Deficiencies of tryptophan can also be found in individuals whose diets are high in leucine (an amino acid that inhibits one of the enzymes necessary to convert tryptophan to NAD), in patients with carcinoid tumors (tumors that can convert tryptophan into serotonin), or patients with tuberculosis who receive isoniazid therapy (because isoniazid is a pyridoxine antagonist and pyridoxine is also necessary for the conversion of tryptophan to NAD).

In contrast to niacin, a deficiency of riboflavin (vitamin B2) is characterized by changes that occur around the mouth, namely cheilosis (inflammation and fissuring of the lips), angular stomatitis (cheilosis occurring at the corners of the mouth), and glossitis (atrophy of the mucosa of the tongue). Additionally, patients may develop seborrheic dermatitis of the face or genitalia, or blindness, which is the result of vascularization of the cornea (interstitial keratitis). Biotin (vitamin H) is an important cofactor for multisubunit enzymes that catalyze carboxylation reactions, an example of which is the synthesis and oxidation of fatty acids. A deficiency of biotin can lead to multiple symptoms, including depression, hallucinations, muscle pain, and dermatitis. Biotin is present in dietary food and is also produced by intestinal bacteria. Deficiencies of biotin are quite rare, but can occur in people who consume raw eggs. This is because egg white contains a heat-labile protein, avidin, which combines very tightly to biotin and prevents the absorption of biotin. Pyridoxine is a cofactor that participates in transamination reactions, decarboxylation reactions, and transsulfuration reactions. It is important in the synthesis of GABA and δ-ALA. Deficiencies of pyridoxine can lead to decreased synthesis of GABA, which can cause convulsions in infants or a polyneuropathy in adults, or decreased ALA, which produces a hypochromic, sideroblastic anemia. Patients also develop cheilosis, angular stomatitis, glossitis, and seborrheic dermatitis. Pyridoxine deficiency may result from pregnancy or certain drug therapy, such as isoniazid, methyldopa, or levodopa. A common cause of B6 deficiency is chronic alcoholism. Finally, selenium is an antioxidant that is part of glutathione peroxidase, an enzyme that is found in red cells and white cells. As such it prevents oxidative damage to both red blood cells and white cells. A deficiency of selenium leads to a form of dilated cardiomyopathy in children. This deficiency has been described in China and is called Keshan disease.

136–137. The answers are: 136-h, 137-g. (*Cotran, 5/e, pp 216–219.*) Some genetic diseases are associated with abnormalities of specific leukocytes causing susceptibility to recurrent infections. In patients with chronic granulomatous disease (CGD), the neutrophils and macrophages have deficient H_2O_2 production due to abnormalities involving the enzyme NADPH oxidase. These individuals have frequent infections that are caused by catalase-positive organisms, such as *Staphylococcus aureus*, because the catalase produced by these organisms destroys the little hydrogen peroxide that is produced.

In X-linked agammaglobulinemia of Bruton, B cells are absent but T-cell numbers and function are normal. This abnormality results from defective maturation of B lymphocytes beyond the pre-B stage. This maturation defect leads to decreased or absent numbers of plasma cells, and therefore immunoglobulin levels will be markedly decreased. Male infants with Bruton's disease will begin having trouble with recurrent bacterial infections at about the age of nine months, which is when maternal antibodies are no longer present in the affected infant. Therapy for Bruton's disease consists primarily of IV γ-globulin. The Wiskott-Aldrich syndrome is also an X-linked recessive disorder, but it is characterized by thrombocytopenia, eczema and immune deficiency The immune abnormalities are characterized by progressive loss of T cell function and decreased IgM. The other immunoglobulin levels are normal or increased in amount. There are decreased numbers of lymphocytes in the peripheral blood and paracortical (T-cell) areas of lymph nodes. Both cellular and humoral immunity are affected, and because patients fail to produce antibodies to polysaccharides, they are vulnerable to infections with encapsulated organisms.

Common variable immunodeficiency (CVI) represents a heterogeneous group of disorders that are characterized by hypogammaglobulinemia. In contrast to X-linked agammaglobulinemia of Bruton, patients with CVI may be of either sex. They also have normal numbers of B cells in the blood and lymphoid tissue, and their symptoms develop later in life. The B cells cannot differentiate into plasma cells, and this leads to hyperplasia of the lymphoid follicles and hypogammaglobulinemia. Patients are prone to recurrent bacterial and viral infections and have an increased incidence of lymphoma and autoimmune diseases. DiGeorge's syndrome is a T-cell deficiency disorder that results from hypoplasia of the thymus due to abnormal development of the third and fourth pharyngeal pouches. The parathyroid glands are also abnormal, and these individuals develop hypocalcemia and tetany. Congenital heart defects are also present. Isolated deficiency of IgA is probably the most common form of immunodeficiency. It is due to a block in the terminal differentiation of B lymphocytes. Most patients are asymptomatic, but some patients will develop chronic sinopulmonary infections. Patients are prone to developing diarrhea (Giardia infection) and also have an increased incidence of autoimmune disease, such as Hashimoto's thyroiditis.

HEMATOLOGY

Questions

DIRECTIONS: Each question below contains five suggested responses. Select the **one best** response to each question.

138. Which of the following red cell abnormalities is most indicative of hemolysis?

a. Target cells
b. Acanthocytes
c. Schistocytes
d. Basophilic stippling
e. Heinz bodies

139. The graph below depicts the results of a red cell osmotic fragility test. The broken-line curve represents which of the following?

a. Glucose-6-phosphate dehydrogenase deficiency
b. Thalassemia
c. Hereditary spherocytosis
d. Drug-induced hemolytic anemia
e. Normal response

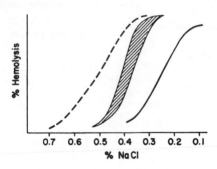

140. Two days after receiving the antimalarial drug primaquine, a 27-year-old black man developed sudden intravascular hemolysis resulting in a decreased hematocrit, hemoglobinemia, and hemoglobinuria. Examination of the peripheral blood revealed erythrocytes with a membrane defect forming "bite" cells; when crystal violet stain was applied, many Heinz bodies were seen. The most likely diagnosis is

a. Hereditary spherocytosis
b. Glucose-6-phosphate dehydrogenase deficiency
c. Paroxysmal nocturnal hemoglobinuria
d. Autoimmune hemolytic anemia
e. Microangiopathic hemolytic anemia

141. Which of the following laboratory findings is LEAST likely to be present in a patient with sickle cell anemia?

a. Normochromic anemia
b. Increased number of target cells
c. Elevated reticulocyte count
d. Elevated erythrocyte sedimentation rate
e. Increased hemoglobin F

142. Which one of the following gene abnormalities is associated with a relative excess production of β-globin chains?

a. Promoter region mutation of β-globin chain gene
b. Chain terminator mutation of β-globin chain gene
c. Splicing mutation of α-globin chain gene
d. Deletion of one β-globin chain gene
e. Deletion of three α-globin chain genes

143. A 49-year-old female presents with signs of anemia, and states that every morning her urine is dark. Work-up reveals that her red blood cells lyse in vitro with acid (positive Ham's test). What is the best diagnosis for this patient?

a. Warm autoimmune hemolytic anemia
b. Paroxysmal nocturnal hemoglobinuria
c. Paroxysmal cold hemoglobinuria
d. Isoimmune hemolytic anemia
e. Cold agglutinin autoimmune hemolytic anemia

144. A 25-year-old woman with known systemic lupus erythematosus presents with jaundice, splenomegaly, peripheral blood schistocytes, and a reticulocyte count of 24 percent. The antibody most likely to be responsible for this complex reacts in vitro at

a. 5°C
b. 20°C
c. 25°C
d. 37°C
e. 56°C

145. The neutrophil in the photomicrograph shown below was obtained from peripheral blood and is most likely to be found in association with

a. Folic acid deficiency
b. Infection
c. Iron deficiency
d. Malignancy
e. Ingestion of a marrow-toxic agent

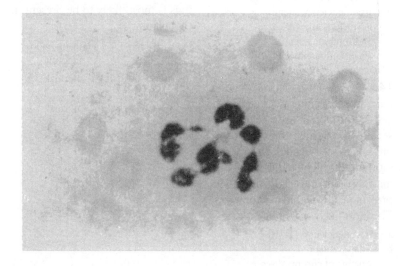

146. Megaloblasts are the result of impaired synthesis of

a. DNA
b. RNA
c. Glutathione
d. β-globin chains
e. Decay accelerating factor

147. An anemic patient has the following red cell indexes: mean corpuscular volume, 70 μm^3; mean corpuscular hemoglobin, 22 pg; and mean corpuscular hemoglobin concentration, 34 percent. These values are most consistent with a diagnosis of

a. Folic acid deficiency anemia
b. Iron deficiency anemia
c. Pernicious anemia
d. Sideroblastic anemia
e. Thalassemia minor

148. An anemic patient is found to have hypochromic, microcytic red cells. Additional tests reveal the serum iron levels, the total iron-binding capacity, and the transferrin saturation to all be reduced. A bone marrow biopsy reveals the iron to be present mainly within macrophages. The most likely diagnosis is

a. Iron deficiency
b. Thalassemia trait
c. Anemia of chronic disease
d. Sideroblastic anemia
e. Pernicious anemia

149. The most common type of disordered porphyrin metabolism (porphyria) is

a. Intermittent acute porphyria
b. Variegate porphyria
c. Protoporphyria
d. Congenital erythropoietic porphyria
e. Porphyria cutanea tarda

150. A 62-year-old man with a plethoric face and pruritus is being evaluated for recurrent thrombosis. This patient is not dehydrated, but laboratory examination reveals a peripheral neutrophilic leukocytosis and thrombocytosis. Which set of additional laboratory findings is most likely to be present in this patient?

	RBC mass	erythropoietin amount
a.	normal	normal
b.	normal	↑
c.	↓	normal
d.	↓	↑
e.	↑	↓

151. An 11-year-old Jamaican boy develops a massive benign enlargement of the cervical lymph nodes associated with fever and leukocytosis. Which of the following lymph node disorders could account for these findings?

a. Toxoplasmosis
b. Histiocytic medullary reticulosis
c. Burkitt's disease
d. Sinus histiocytosis with massive lymphadenopathy (SHML)
e. Angioimmunoblastic lymphadenopathy with dysproteinemia

152. A person taking an oral sulfonamide is found to have a markedly decreased peripheral blood neutrophil count, but the number of platelets and erythrocytes are normal. If the peripheral neutropenia is the result of antineutrophile antibodies being produced in response to taking the sulfonamide, then this patient would be expected to have

a. An atrophic spleen
b. Decreased vitamin B12 levels
c. Hypoplasia of the bone marrow myeloid series
d. Hyperplasia of the bone marrow myeloid series
e. A monoclonal large granular lymphocyte proliferation in the peripheral blood

153. During a viral infection, a 23-year-old female develops enlarged lymph nodes at multiple sites (lymphadenopathy). A biopsy from one of these enlarged lymph nodes reveals a proliferative of reactive T immunoblasts, cells that have prominent nucleoli. These reactive T cells are most likely to be found in which one of the following regions of the lymph node?

a. Hilum
b. Medullary sinuses
c. Paracortex
d. Primary follicles
e. Secondary follicles

154. The photomicrograph below was taken from a soft tissue swelling in the cheek and mandible of a 17-year-old girl. The cytoplasmic vacuoles would react with which one of the following?

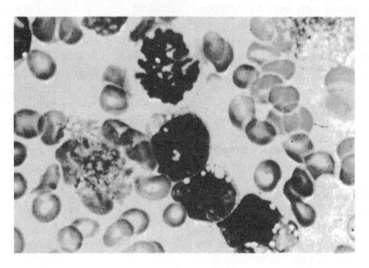

a. Myeloperoxidase
b. Oil red O
c. Nonspecific esterase
d. Chloracetate esterase
e. Periodic acid-Schiff (PAS)

155. A 20-year-old man presents in the emergency room with a lymphoma involving the mediastinum that is producing respiratory distress. The lymphocytes are most likely to have cell surface markers characteristic of which of the following?

a. B cells
b. T cells
c. Macrophages
d. Dendritic reticulum cells
e. Langerhans cells

156. The non-Hodgkin's lymphoma pictured in the photomicrograph below may be characterized by which of the following?

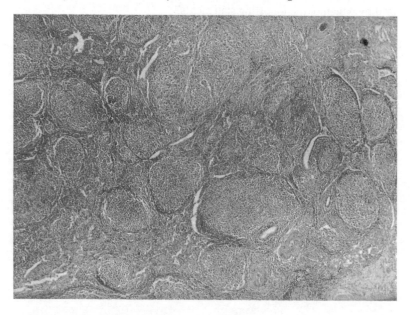

a.   Increased frequency in adolescents
b.   Lymphoblastic lymphoma
c.   B lymphocytes
d.   Tingible-body macrophages within nodules
e.   Well-differentiated lymphocytic lymphoma

157. True statements regarding nodular sclerosing Hodgkin's disease include that it

a.   Is more common in males
b.   Usually affects elderly people
c.   Is characterized by the presence of lacunar cells
d.   Is characterized by the presence of "popcorn" cells
e.   Usually involves infradiaphragmatic lymph nodes

158. The binucleate or bilobed giant cell with prominent acidophilic "owl-eye" nucleoli shown in the photomicrograph below is correctly characterized by which of the following statements?

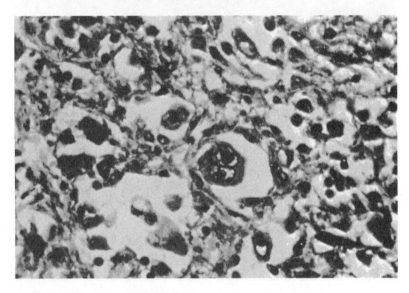

a. It is a rapidly proliferating tumor cell seen in middivision
b. It is sometimes referred to as the lacunar cell
c. It is necessary but not sufficient for the diagnosis of Hodgkin's disease
d. It is diagnostic of cytomegalic inclusion disease
e. It is diagnostic of giardiasis

159. A 28-year-old male presents with widespread ecchymoses and bleeding gums. Physical examination reveals enlargement of his spleen and liver. Laboratory examination of his peripheral blood reveals a normochromic, normocytic anemia, along with a decreased number of platelets, and increased number of white blood cells. Coagulation studies reveal prolonged prothrombin and partial thromboplastin times, and increased fibrinogen degradation products. Examination of his bone marrow reveals the presence of numerous granular-appearing blast cells with numerous Auer rods. These immature cells comprise about 38 percent of the nucleated cells in the marrow. The diagnosis for this patient is

a. Acute erythroid leukemia
b. Acute lymphoblastic leukemia
c. Acute monocytic leukemia
d. Acute myelomonocytic leukemia
e. Acute progranulocytic leukemia

160. A 4-year-old female is being evaluated for the sudden onset of multiple petechiae and bruises. She is found to have a peripheral leukocyte count of 55,000, 86 percent of which are small, homogeneous cells that have nuclei with immature chromatin. Indistinct nucleoli are also present. Initial tests on these immature cells are as follows: TdT positive, PAS positive, acid phosphatase positive, and myeloperoxidase negative. Based on these findings, the immature cells most likely originated from

a. Myeloblasts
b. Monoblasts
c. Megakaryoblasts
d. Lymphoblasts
e. Erythroblasts

161. Chronic myeloid leukemia is LEAST likely to be associated with

a. Splenomegaly
b. Basophilia
c. Translocation t (8;14)
d. Thrombocytosis
e. Low leukocyte alkaline phosphatase (LAP)

162. The photomicrograph below is of peripheral blood from a patient with splenomegaly, anemia, and pancytopenia. If hairy cell leukemia is suspected, which of the following would be useful in establishing the diagnosis?

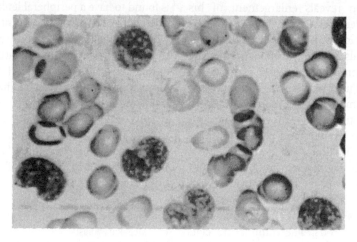

a. Myeloperoxidase stain
b. Sudan black B
c. Acid phosphatase stain
d. Leukocyte alkaline phosphatase
e. Nonspecific esterase

163. A 72-year-old male presents with increasing fatigue. Physical examination reveals an elderly male in no apparent distress (NAD). He is found to have multiple enlarged, non-tender lymph nodes along with an enlarged liver and spleen. Laboratory examination of his peripheral blood reveals a normocytic normochromic anemia, a slightly decreased platelet count, and a leukocyte count of 72,000 cells/microliter. An example of his peripheral blood is seen in the associated picture. What is your diagnosis?

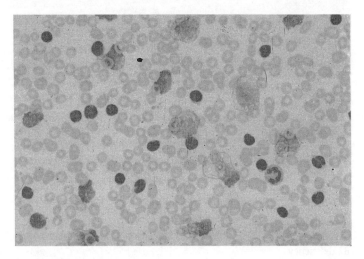

   a.   Acute lymphoblastic leukemia
   b.   Atypical lymphocytosis
   c.   Chronic lymphocytic leukemia
   d.   Immunoblastic lymphoma
   e.   Prolymphocytic leukemia

164. The cells seen in the photomicrograph below were removed from an anemic patient and stained with an iron stain. This patient is most likely to have

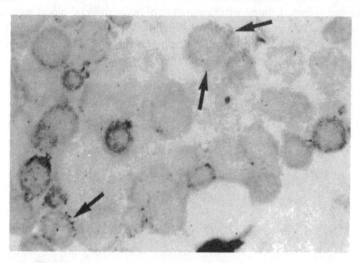

a. Iron deficiency anemia
b. Acute blood loss
c. B12 deficiency
d. B2 deficiency
e. Pyridoxine deficiency

165. In polycythemia rubra vera (PRV),

a. The bone marrow shows selective erythroid hyperplasia
b. Hemorrhagic phenomena are uncommon
c. Pruritus is common
d. The platelet count is typically <150,000/mm3
e. Leukocyte alkaline phosphate levels are decreased

166. The bone marrow biopsy shown below was performed because of splenomegaly and anemia in an adult. On the basis of the appearance of the bone marrow core, choose the most likely diagnosis.

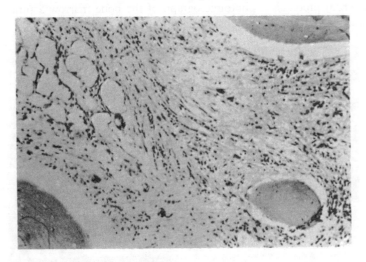

a. Chronic myeloid leukemia (CML)
b. Aplastic anemia
c. Acute leukemia
d. Myeloid metaplasia with myelofibrosis
e. Microangiopathic hemolytic anemia

167. A bone marrow aspirate was obtained from a 70-year-old man whose symptoms included weakness, weight loss, and recurrent infections. Laboratory findings included proteinuria, anemia, and an abnormal component in serum proteins. A photomicrograph of the bone marrow aspirate is shown below. The most probable diagnosis is

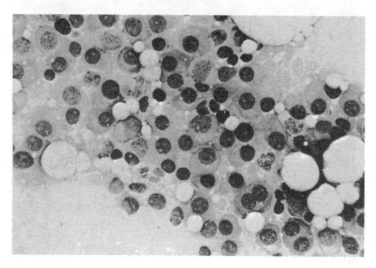

a. Monomyelocytic leukemia
b. Histiocytic leukemia
c. Multiple myeloma
d. Gaucher's disease
e. Leukemic reticuloendotheliosis

168. The presence in serum of a mu heavy-chain protein is associated with which of the following diseases?

a. Chronic lymphocytic leukemia
b. Lymphoblastic lymphoma
c. Poorly-differentiated lymphocytic lymphoma
d. Plasma cell myeloma
e. Multiple myeloma

169. A 5-year-old girl is brought to your office by her mother, who states that the girl has been drinking a lot of water lately. Your physical examination reveals a young girl whose eyes protrude slightly. Further work-up reveals the presence of multiple lytic bone lesions involving her calvarium and the base of her skull. What is the most likely diagnosis for this young girl?

a. Letterer-Siwe disease
b. Hand-Schuller-Christian disease
c. Dermatopathic lymphadenopathy
d. Unifocal Langerhans cell histiocytosis
e. Sarcoidosis

170. A 7-year-old girl presents with fever, abdominal pain, and painful joints (arthralgia). After taking a careful history you discover that she had a sore throat about two weeks prior to the onset of these signs and symptoms. If this young patient had developed a hypersensitivity vasculitis, then which one of the following skin lesions would be most indicative of cutaneous hemorrhage secondary to vasculitis?

a. Petechiae
b. Palpable purpura
c. Nonpalpable purpura
d. Ecchymoses
e. Telangiectasis

171. Acute idiopathic thrombocytopenic purpura (ITP) is characterized by

a. An insidious onset
b. Being more common in females of childbearing age
c. A history of recent viral infection
d. megakaryocytic hypoplasia in the bone marrow
e. A high mortality

172. A 37-year-old woman who has a clinical picture of fever, splenomegaly, varying neurologic manifestations, and purplish ecchymoses of the skin is found to have a hemoglobin level of 10.0 g/dL, a mean corpuscular hemoglobin concentration (MCHC) of 48, peripheral blood polychromasia with stippled macrocytes, and spherocytes, with a blood urea nitrogen level of 68 mg/dL. The findings of coagulation studies and the patient's fibrindegraded products are not overtly abnormal. Which of the following is most closely identified with these findings?

a. Idiopathic thrombocytopenic purpura
b. Thrombotic thrombocytopenic purpura
c. Disseminated intravascular coagulopathy
d. Submassive hepatic necrosis
e. Waterhouse-Friderichsen syndrome

173. A woman who is 5 weeks post partum (normal delivery, healthy child) develops bleeding episodes with oliguria and hematuria. No fever or neurologic manifestations are present. The blood urea nitrogen level is 65 mg/dL; a peripheral blood smear is presented in the photomicrograph below. This patient most likely has

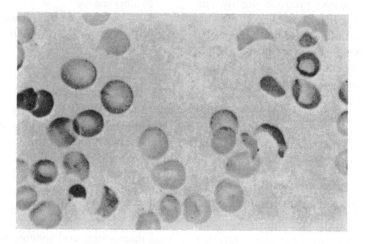

a. Thrombotic thrombocytopenic purpura
b. Autoimmune thrombocytopenic purpura
c. Hemolytic uremic syndrome
d. Disseminated intravascular coagulopathy
e. Sickle cell crisis

174. A 27-year-old female in the last trimester of her first pregnancy presents with the sudden onset of multiple skin hemorrhages. She states that for the past several days she has not felt the baby move. Work-up reveals an increase in the PT and PTT, while fibrin degradation products (FDP) are increased in her blood. Her platelet count is found to be 43,000/μL. What is the most likely diagnosis for this patient?

a. Autoimmune thrombocytopenia purpura (autoimmune ITP)
b. Isoimmune thrombocytopenia purpura (isoimmune ITP)
c. Thrombotic thrombocytopenia purpura (TTP)
d. Hemolytic uremic syndrome (HUS)
e. Disseminated intravascular coagulation (DIC)

175. A 45-year-old male with an artificial heart valve is given oral Coumadin (Warfarin) to prevent the formation of thrombi on his artificial valve. Which combination of laboratory tests is most likely to be found in this individual?

	tourniquet test	bleeding time	platelet count	PTT	PT
a.	positive	prolonged	normal	normal	normal
b.	normal	normal	normal	prolonged	normal
c.	positive	prolonged	decreased	normal	normal
d.	normal	normal	normal	normal	prolonged
e.	normal	prolonged	normal	prolonged	normal

176. Intravascular hemolysis results in all the following EXCEPT

a. Elevated plasma hemoglobin (hemoglobinemia)
b. Hemoglobinuria
c. Hemosiderinuria
d. Jaundice
e. Splenomegaly

177. The causes of secondary aplastic anemia include all the following EXCEPT

a. Whole body irradiation
b. Alkylating agents
c. Chloramphenicol
d. Myelophthisic anemia
e. Viral hepatitis

178. The photomicrograph below is from the bone marrow of a patient with weakness. All the following may be associated with this abnormality EXCEPT

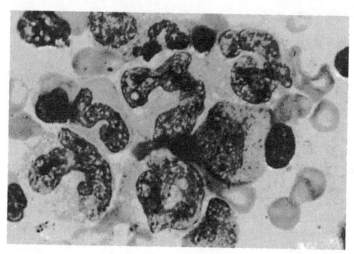

a. Pernicious anemia
b. Hyperthyroidism
c. Celiac disease
d. HTLV
e. Alcoholism

179. Transferrin shows all the following characteristics EXCEPT

a. Normally about 33 percent saturation with iron
b. Increased saturation in hemochromatosis
c. Increased saturation in severe liver disease
d. Decreased saturation in marrow hypoplasia
e. Decreased saturation in iron deficiency anemia

180. True statements regarding hemochromatosis include all the following EXCEPT

a.   It characteristically causes a micronodular pigment cirrhosis

b.   It is complicated by carcinoma of the liver in 15 to 30 percent of cases with cirrhosis

c.   It causes diabetes with severity unrelated to the degree of pancreatic iron deposition

d.   it can be diagnosed by liver biopsy showing raised amounts of hemosiderin

e.   It is associated with skin pigmentation due entirely to deposition of hemosiderin

181. An elderly woman enters the hospital with an abdominal mass, anemia, and weakness. At surgery, an infiltrating retroperitoneal mass is found involving the mesenteric lymph nodes and right kidney. A biopsy specimen from one of the lymph nodes is shown and is compatible with large-cell immunoblastic lymphoma. This neoplasm is associated with all the following EXCEPT

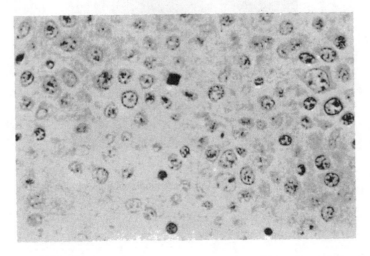

a.   Predominant B-cell origin

b.   Prior immunologic disorder

c.   Typical "starry sky" pattern

d.   Rapid death if untreated

e.   Plasmacytoid or polymorphous features

182. In the disorder depicted below in which multiple, focal osteolytic skull lesions occur, all the following are common EXCEPT

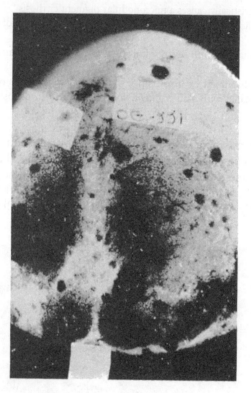

a. A normal serum alkaline phosphatase level
b. Increased production of monoclonal immunoglobulin
c. Lymphadenopathy
d. Bone pain
e. Hypercalcemia

183. All the following are known to cause splenomegaly EXCEPT

a. Sickle cell disease
b. Hodgkin's disease
c. Chronic lymphocytic leukemia (CLL)
d. Hairy cell leukemia
e. Polycythemia vera

184. True statements concerning the hemolytic-uremic syndrome (HUS) in young children include all the following EXCEPT

a. Endothelial injury is an initiating pathologic event
b. Prior infection with *E. coli* is common
c. Hypertension exists in about half the patients
d. Involvement of the CNS is a dominant feature
e. Acute, anuric renal failure occurs in over 50 percent of cases

185. Typical findings in a patient with von Willebrand's disease include all the following EXCEPT

a. Decreased levels of factor VIII
b. Normal platelet count
c. Prolonged bleeding time
d. Frequent hemarthrosis and spontaneous joint hemorrhage
e. Menorrhagia

DIRECTIONS: Each group of questions below consists of lettered headings followed by a set of numbered items. For each numbered item select the one lettered heading with which it is most closely associated. Each lettered heading may be used once, more than once, or not at all.

Questions 186–187

Match each of the following descriptions of cells or clinical scenarios with the type of cell with which it is associated.

a.   Basophil
b.   Eosinophil
c.   Macrophage
d.   Monocyte
e.   Neutrophil
f.   B lymphocyte
g.   T lymphocyte

186. This cell processes antigen during the initiation of the immune response. Upon further activation it may become an epithelioid cell.

187. A patient presents with fever, weakness, and pain and tenderness over the left deltoid muscle. A biopsy of this area reveals *Trichinella spiralis*. Examination of his peripheral blood reveals elevated levels of a particular type of leukocyte.

Questions 188–189

For each of the following questions select the appropriate test or clinical procedure.

a.   Blood cultures
b.   Bone marrow biopsy
c.   Coombs test
d.   Lymph node biopsy
e.   Metabisulfite test
f.   Monospot test
g.   Osmotic fragility test
h.   Schilling test
i.   Sucrose hemolysis test
j.   Treatment with ampicillin

188. A 19-year-old man presents with a sore throat, malaise, and cervical lymphadenopathy. The peripheral lymphocyte count is 6,100/μL. Examination of the peripheral smear reveals that many lymphocytes have atypical nuclei and abundant basophilic cytoplasm. These cytoplasm of these lymphocytes is indented by the red blood cells in the smear. What is the most appropriate course of action?

189. A 22-year-old African-American male wants to know if he has sickle cell trait. He has no previous history of the signs or symptoms of sickle cell anemia. What method or test can be used to detect the presence of hemoglobin S?

Questions 190–191

Match each of the following clinical scenarios with the coagulation factor that is deficient or abnormal.

a. Factor I
b. Factor V
c. Factor VIII
d. Factor IX
e. Factor XI
f. Factor XII
g. Factor XIII
h. Plasma fibrinogen
i. Prothrombin time
j. Ristocetin cofactor

190. A 20-year-old female presents with metromenorrhagia and recurrent bleeding from the gums. She relates a history of excessive bleeding from minor trauma to the skin. A prolonged bleeding time is discovered, and her peripheral platelet count is 220,000/μL.

191. An 11-month-old boy who has just begun walking is being evaluated because of a history of easy bruising. Physical examination reveals a swollen left knee and several intramuscular hematomas. A family history reveals that his mother's brother also suffered from severe bleeding problems. Laboratory tests reveal a normal PT, but an abnormal (prolonged) PTT.

HEMATOLOGY

Answers

138. The answer is c. (*Henry, 19/e, pp 576–582. Rubin, 2/e, pp 1012–1013.*)
Abnormalities of red cells can help to identify a disease process. Schistocytes, which are red cell fragments, indicate the presence of hemolysis, and
they can occur in hemolytic anemia, megaloblastic anemia, or severe burns.
Red cell shapes characteristic of hemolysis include triangular cells and helmet cells. Target cells—red cells with a central dark area—are the result of
excess cytoplasmic membrane material and are found in patients with liver
disease, such as obstructive jaundice, or in any of the hypochromic anemias. Acanthocytes are irregularly spiculated red cells found in patients
with abetalipoproteinemia or liver disease. Echinocytes, in contrast, have
regular spicules (undulations) and may either be artifacts (crenated cells) or
found in hyperosmolar diseases such as uremia. Basophilic stippling of red
cells—irregular basophilic granules within erythrocytes—vary from fine
granules, seen in young reticulocytes (polychromatophilic cells), to coarse
granules, seen in diseases with impaired hemoglobin synthesis, such as lead
poisoning and megaloblastic anemia. Heinz bodies are formed by denatured
hemoglobin and are not seen with routine stains. They are found in patients
with glucose-6-phosphatase dehydrogenase deficiency and the unstable he-
moglobinopathies.

139. The answer is c. (*Henry, 19/e, pp 633–634. Cotran, 5/e, pp 589–591.*)
Spherocytes in a peripheral blood smear show a smaller diameter than normal and an apparent increase in hemoglobin concentration because of a decrease in cell surface, with consequent deeper staining for hemoglobin.
Spectrin lacks the ability to bind protein 4.1 in this autosomal dominant
disorder, yielding a skeleton defect of the red cell membrane. Other proteins
that help maintain the shape of the red cell include protein 3 and ankyrin,
which bridges the spectrin and the cell membrane protein 3. The disorder
can be diagnosed in the laboratory by the osmotic fragility test (the shaded
area in the graph reflects a normal response to a hypotonic solution). Sphe-

rocytes will lyse at a higher concentration of sodium chloride than will normal red cells. Flat hypochromic cells, as those in thalassemia, have a greater capacity to expand in dilute salt solution and thus lyse at a lower concentration (which is seen in the unbroken curve to the far right). The longer the incubation of the red cells in these salt concentrations, the greater the response to osmotic change.

140. The answer is b. (*Cotran, 5/e, pp 589–592, 601–603.*) Glucose-6-phosphate dehydrogenase (G6PD) is an enzyme of the hexose monophosphate shunt pathway that maintains glutathione in a reduced (active) form. Glutathione normally protects hemoglobin from oxidative injury. If the erythrocytes are deficient in G6PD, as occurs in G6PD deficiency, exposure to oxidant drugs, such as the antimalarial drug primaquine, denatures hemoglobin, which then precipitates with erythrocytes as Heinz bodies. Macrophages within the spleen remove these bodies, producing characteristic "bite" cells. These red cells then become less deformable and are trapped and destroyed within the spleen (extravascular hemolysis). The gene for G6PD is located on the X chromosome and has considerable pleomorphism at this site. Two variants are the A type, which is found in 10 percent of African-Americans and is characterized by milder hemolysis of younger red cells, and the Mediterranean type, which is characterized by a more severe hemolysis of red cells of all ages. Hereditary spherocytosis (HS), an autosomal dominant disorder, is characterized by an abnormality of the skeleton of the red cell membrane that makes the erythrocyte spherical, less deformable, and vulnerable to splenic sequestration and destruction (extravascular hemolysis). In HS, there is a defect in the spectrin molecule, which then has less binding to protein 4.1. This disorder can be diagnosed in the laboratory by the osmotic fragility test. Paroxysmal nocturnal hemoglobinuria (PNH), an acquired clonal stem cell disorder, is characterized by abnormal red cells, granulocytes, and platelets. The red cells are abnormally sensitive to the lytic activity of complement due to a deficiency of GPI (glycosyl phosphatidyl inositol) linked proteins, namely decay-accelerating factor (DAF, or CD55), membrane inhibitor of reactive lysis (CD59), or CD59 (a C8 binding protein). Complement is activated by acidosis, such as with exercise or sleep, which can produce a red morning urine. Complications of PNH include the development of frequent thromboses and possibly acute leukemia. Autoimmune hemolytic anemia is caused by anti-red cell antibodies and is diagnosed using the Coombs antiglobulin test. Microangiopathic hemolytic anemia refers to hemolysis of red cells caused by narrowing within the microvasculature and is seen in patients with prosthetic heart valves or those with disseminated intravascular coagulation, thrombotic thrombocytopenic purpura, or hemolytic-uremic syndrome.

141. The answer is d. (*Lee, 9/e, pp 30–31, 1077–1078.*) Blood from patients who have sickle cell anemia exhibits a low erythrocyte sedimentation rate (ESR). The irregular shape of sickle cells prevents the rouleaux formation that is prerequisite for a normal ESR. Sickle cell anemia is classified as a normocytic, normochromic, and hemolytic anemia in which target cells, found in increased numbers, can compose up to 30 percent of peripheral blood cells, and in which reticulocytosis—as a reflection of an increased rate of erythropoiesis in the hyperplastic bone marrow—is persistently 10 percent above normal. In addition, electrophoretic findings reveal an elevation of hemoglobin F up to 40 percent, the presence of hemoglobin S in a range of 60 to 99 percent, and the absence of hemoglobin A.

142. The answer is e. (*Cotran, 5/e, pp 596–601. Rubin, 2/e, pp 1020–1022.*) The thalassemia syndromes are characterized by a decreased or absent synthesis of either the α- or the β-globin chain of hemoglobin A (α2β2). β-Thalassemias result from reduced production of β-globin chains, while α-thalassemias result from reduced synthesis of α-globin chains. β-Thalassemias are associated with a relative excess production of α-globin chains, while a-thalassemias are associated with a relative excess production of non-α-globin chains. In the fetus these are γ-globin chains, but in the adult they are β-globin chains. Most of the β thalassemias result from point mutations involving the β-globin gene, while α thalassemias result from deletions of one or more of the four α-globin genes. The amount of β-globin produced depends upon the location of the point mutation. Promoter region mutations result in decreased production of β-globin. This is called β+ thalassemia. Chain terminator mutations generally produce no functional β-globin. This is called β0 thalassemia. Splicing mutations may result in either β0 or β+ thalassemia. The severity of α thalassemia depends on the number of a genes deleted. Deletion of three α-globin genes results in excess production of β-globin chains, which then form β tetramers (HbH); this disease is called hemoglobin H disease.

143. The answer is b. (*Cotran, 5/e, pp 601–603.*) Paroxysmal nocturnal hemoglobinuria (PNH) is an acquired clonal stem cell disorder that is characterized by abnormal red cells, granulocytes, and platelets. The red blood cells (RBC's) are abnormally sensitive to the lytic activity of complement due to a deficiency of GPI (glycosyl phosphatidyl inositol) linked proteins, namely decay-accelerating factor (DAF, or CD 55), membrane inhibitor of reactive lysis (CD55), or CD59 (a C8 binding protein). Complement is normally activated by acidotic states, such as occurs with exercise or sleep. In patients with PNH, the acidotic condition that develops during sleep (which is usually at night) causes hemolysis of red blood cells and results in a red urine in the morning. The erythrocytes of these patients lyse in vitro with acid (Ham's test) or sucrose (sucrose lysis test). Complications of PNH include the development of frequent thromboses, particularly of the hepatic, portal, or cerebral veins. Since PNH is a clonal stem cell disorder, patients are at an increased risk of developing aplastic anemia or acute leukemia.

Antibody-mediated destruction of red cells may be due to autoimmune reactions or isoimmune reactions. The latter is due to antibodies from one person which react with RBC's from another person. This isoimmune destruction is seen with blood transfusions and hemolytic disease of the newborn. The autoimmune hemolytic anemias (AIHA) are hemolytic anemias that are due to the presence of antibodies that destroy red cells. The AIHA's are divided into two main types: those secondary to "warm" antibodies and those reactive at cold temperatures. Warm-antibody autoimmune hemolytic anemias react at 37 degrees C in vitro, are composed of IgG, and do not fix complement. Instead, immunoglobulin-coated RBC's are removed by splenic macrophages that recognize the Fc portion of the immunoglobulin. These warm IgG antibodies are found in patients with malignant tumors, especially leukemia-lymphoma; they are associated with the use of such drugs as a methyldopa; and are also found in the autoimmune diseases, especially lupus erythematosus. Cold-antibody autoimmune hemolytic anemia (cold AIHA) is subdivided into two clinical categories based on the type of antibody that is involved. These two types of cold antibodies are cold agglutinins and cold hemolysins. Cold agglutinins are monoclonal IgM antibodies that react at 4 to 6 degrees C. They are called agglutinins because the IgM can agglutinate red cells due to its large size (pentamer). Additionally, IgM can activate complement, which may result in IV hemolysis. Two diseases are classically associated with cold agglutinin formation. They are mycoplasma pneumonitis and infectious mononucleosis. In contrast, cold hemolysins are seen in patients with PCH (paroxysmal cold hemoglobinuria). These cold hemolysins are unique because they are biphasic anti-erythrocyte autoantibodies. These antibodies are IgG that is directed against the "P" blood group antigen. They are called biphasic because they attach to red cells and bind complement at low temperatures, but the activation of complement does not occur until the temperature is increased. This antibody, called the Donath-Landsteiner antibody, was previously associated with syphilis, but may follow various infections, such as mycoplasmal pneumonia.

144. The answer is d. (*Cotran, 5/e, pp 601–603.*) The autoimmune hemolytic anemias are important causes of acute anemia in a wide variety of clinical states and can be separated into two main types: those secondary to "warm" antibodies and those reactive at cold temperatures. Warm-antibody autoimmune hemolytic anemias react at 37°C in vitro, are composed of IgG, and do not fix complement. They are found in patients with malignant tumors, especially leukemia-lymphoma; with use of such drugs as alpha methyldopa; and in the autoimmune diseases, especially lupus erythematosus. Cold-antibody autoimmune hemolytic anemia reacts at 4 to 6°C, fixes complement, is of the IgM type, and is classically associated with mycoplasma pneumonitis (pleuropneumonia-like organisms). These antibodies are termed cold agglutinins and may reach extremely high titers and cause intravascular red cell agglutination.

145. The answer is a. (*Cotran, 5/e, pp 603–605.*) In contrast to a normal, mature neutrophil, which has from two to five nuclear lobes, the neutrophil shown has at least six lobes and is an illustration of neutrophilic hypersegmentation. Granulocytic hypersegmentation is significant and among the first hematologic findings in the peripheral blood of patients who have megaloblastic anemia in its developmental stages. Neutrophilic hypersegmentation is generally considered a sensitive indicator of megaloblastic anemia, which can be caused by a deficiency either in vitamin B12, in folate, or in both.

146. The answer is a. (*Cotran, 5/e, pp 591, 596, 601, 603–605.*) Deficiency of either vitamin B12 or folate will result in megaloblastic anemia. Their deficiency impairs DNA synthesis and delays mitotic division. This in turn causes the nuclei to be enlarged. The synthesis of RNA and cytoplasmic elements is not affected, however, so there is nuclear-cytoplasmic asynchrony. These cellular changes affect all rapidly proliferating cells in the body, but in the bone marrow, they result in enlarged erythroid precursors, which are referred to as megaloblasts. These abnormal cells produce abnormally enlarged red cells, which are called macroovalocytes. These megaloblasts also undergo autohemolysis within the bone marrow, resulting in ineffective erythropoiesis. Granulocyte precursors are also enlarged and are called giant metamyelocytes. These abnormal cells produce enlarged hypersegmented neutrophils. The megakaryocytes are large and have nuclear abnormalities, but although the platelet count is decreased, the platelets are not enlarged. Abnormalities of glutathione production are seen in patients with glucose-6-phosphate dehydrogenase deficiency, while decreased synthesis of β-globin chains is seen in patients with β thalassemia. Abnormalities of decay accelerating factor are seen in patients with paroxysmal nocturnal hemoglobinuria.

147. The answer is e. (*Henry, 19/e, pp 78–79, 657–659.*) Both thalassemia minor and iron deficiency anemia are microcytic disorders in which the mean corpuscular hemoglobin is usually found to be reduced. Red blood cell indexes may be useful in differentiating the two disorders, for while the mean corpuscular hemoglobin concentration (MCHC) is often normal or only slightly reduced in association with thalassemia minor, the MCHC is often definitely reduced in association with iron deficiency anemia. Both pernicious and folate deficiency anemias lead to megaloblastic changes in erythrocytes.

148. The answer is c. (*Henry, 19/e, pp 618–620, 626–627, 630–631, 657–659.*) The four main causes of microcytic/hypochromic anemias are iron deficiency, anemia of chronic disease (AOCD), thalassemia, and sideroblastic anemia. Additional laboratory tests can differentiate between these four diseases. The serum iron and percentage of saturation are decreased in both iron deficiency anemia and AOCD, increased in sideroblastic anemia, and may be normal or increased in thalassemia. The total iron-binding capacity (TIBC) is increased only in iron deficiency. It is normal or decreased in the other diseases. An additional differentiating test for these four diagnoses is evaluation of the bone marrow iron stores. In iron deficiency, iron stores are decreased or absent. In AOCD, iron is present, but is restricted to and increased within macrophages. It is decreased in amount within marrow erythroid precursors. Marrow iron is increased in patients with sideroblastic anemia. The iron levels in patients with thalassemia trait are generally within normal limits. Approximately one-third of the normoblasts in the normal bone marrow contain ferritin granules and are called sideroblasts. In sideroblastic anemia, because of the deficiency of pyridoxine and ferritin, the production of globin or heme is markedly reduced, and ferritin granules accumulate within the mitochondria that rim the nucleus. This produces the characteristic ring sideroblast.

149. The answer is e. *(Lee, 9/e, pp 1272–1290.)* The porphyrias are inherited or acquired disorders of heme biosynthesis with varied patterns of overproduction, accumulation, and excretion of heme synthesis intermediates. Major characteristics include intermittent neurologic dysfunction and skin sensitivity to sunlight, but intermittent acute porphyria shows no skin photosensitivity, unlike the other types. Porphyria cutanea tarda is the most common type and has chronic skin lesions (face, forehead, forearms) and frequent hepatic disease. Excess urinary porphobilinogen excretion occurs in variegate porphyria and intermittent acute porphyria. Detection of porphobilinogen in the urine forms the basis for a positive Watson-Schwartz reaction in the diagnosis of variegate and intermittent acute porphyria.

150. The answer is e. *(Cotran, 5/e, pp 616, 658–660.)* Polycythemia refers to an increased concentration of red blood cells (RBC) in the peripheral blood. This is manifested by an increase in the red blood cell count, the hemoglobin concentration, or the hematocrit. An increase in the red blood cell count, reported clinically as number of cells/microliters, is not the same thing as the RBC mass, which is a radioactive test that is reported in ml/kg. The RBC count and the RBC mass do not always parallel each other. For example, a decreased plasma volume increases the RBC count, but it does not affect the RBC mass. An increased red blood cell concentration may be relative polycythemia or an absolute polycythemia. A relative polycythemia is due to a decrease in the plasma volume (hemoconcentration), causes of which include prolonged vomiting, diarrhea, or the excessive use of diuretics. An absolute polycythemia is due to an increase in the total red cell mass and may be primary, due to a defect in myeloid stem cells (polycythemia rubra vera), or secondary, due to an increase in the production of erythropoietin (EPO). In patients with primary polycythemia, a myeloproliferative disorder, the red cell mass is increased but the levels of erythropoietin are normal or decreased. The EPO level is low because the total oxygen content of the blood is increased, and there is no stimulus for increasing the secretion of EPO. The marked increased red cell mass in patients with P. vera predisposes them to thrombotic complications and hemorrhages. The high cell turnover from the increase in the red cell mass predisposes these patients to develop hyperuricemia and symptoms of gout. Patients also develop increased numbers of basophils and eosinophils in the peripheral blood. The increased histamine release from these basophils may result in intense pruritus and peptic ulceration. Bleeding from the latter may lead to an iron-deficiency anemia. In patients with secondary polycythemia, the increased erythropoietin may be appropriate or inappropriate. Appropriate causes of increased erythropoietin include lung disease, cyanotic heart disease, living at high altitudes, or abnormal hemoglobins with increased oxygen affinity. Inappropriate causes of increased erythropoietin include erythropoietin-secreting tumors, such as renal cell carcinomas, hepatomas, or cerebellar hemangioblastomas.

151. The answer is d. (*Damjanov, 10/e, pp 1125–1144. Rubin, 2/e, p 1033.*) Clinicians and pathologists alike should be familiar with the benign syndrome of lymph node enlargement called sinus histiocytosis with massive lymphadenopathy. This is a self-limiting, invariably benign disorder found classically in young, black, African and Caribbean patients, but it has been found in others as well. It is characterized clinically by profound enlargement of regional cervical lymph nodes, fever, and leukocytosis. Histologically, the lymph nodes show marked histiocytic proliferation within the sinuses, with engulfment of lymphocytes within the histiocytes. There may be skin involvement, and histiocytes containing phagocytosed lymphocytes may be present in the skin biopsy specimen. The patients predictably revert to normal within a period of months. Histiocytic medullary reticulosis is a disease in which a form of malignant histiocytes is found in lymph node sinuses, with engulfed red cells found within the neoplastic histiocytes (erythrophagocytosis). Primitive, round lymphoblastic tumor cells are found in tissue taken from patients with Burkitt's lymphoma.

152. The answer is d. (*Cotran, 5/e, pp 630–631.*) Decreased numbers of neutrophils in the peripheral blood, neutropenia, may be due to decreased production of neutrophils in the bone marrow or increased peripheral destruction of neutrophils. Decreased production may be caused by megaloblastic anemia, certain drugs, or stem cell defects, such as aplastic anemia, leukemias, or lymphomas. Drug-induced destruction of neutrophil precursors is the most common cause of peripheral neutropenia. With all of these different causes of decreased neutrophil production, the bone marrow will be hypoplastic and there will be a decrease in the number of granulocytic precursors. Some causes of neutropenia will also cause a decrease in the numbers of platelets and erythrocytes (pancytopenia).

In contrast to decreased production, cases of neutropenia secondary to peripheral destruction causes a hyperplasia of the bone marrow, with an increase in the number of granulocytic precursors. Causes of increased destruction of neutrophils include sequestration in the spleen due to hypersplenism (not splenic atrophy), increased utilization, such as with overwhelming infections, and immunologically mediated destruction (immune destruction). Causes of the immune destruction include Felty's syndrome and certain drug reactions, such as aminopyrine and some sulfonamides. Drugs may cause decreased production or increased destruction of neutrophils. In the latter, antibodies are formed against neutrophils, and then these cells are destroyed peripherally. Felty's syndrome refers to the combination of rheumatoid arthritis, splenomegaly, and neutropenia. A significant number of patients with Felty's syndrome will have a monoclonal proliferation of CD8 large granular lymphocytes, unrelated to drug use.

153. The answer is c. (*Cotran, 5/e, pp 632–633. Chandrasoma, 3/e, pp 433–443.*) Lymph nodes may be enlarged (lymphadenopathy) secondary to reactive processes, which can be either acute or chronic reactions. Acute reaction (acute nonspecific lymphadenitis) can result in focal or generalized lymphadenopathy. Focal lymph node enlargement is usually the result of bacterial infection. Sections from involved lymph nodes will reveal infiltration by neutrophils. In contrast, generalized acute lymphadenopathy is usually the result of viral infections and will usually produce a proliferation of reactive T lymphocytes called T immunoblasts. These reactive T cells tend to have prominent nucleoli and can be easily mistaken for malignant lymphocytes or malignant Hodgkin cells.

Reactive processes involving lymph nodes typically involve different and specific portions of the lymph nodes depending upon the type of cell that is reacting. For example, reactive B lymphocytes typically result in hyperplasia of the lymphoid follicles and germinal centers (follicular hyperplasia). Examples of diseases that are associated with follicular hyperplasia include chronic inflammation caused by organisms, rheumatoid arthritis, and AIDS. Lymph nodes from patients with AIDS have characteristic changes that initially show follicular hyperplasia with loss of mantle zones, intrafollicular hemorrhage ("follicle lysis"), and monocytoid B cell proliferation. Subsequently there will be depletion of lymphocytes (CD4+ lymphocytes) in both the follicles and the interfollicular areas. In contrast to reactive B cell processes, reactive T lymphocytes typically result in hyperplasia involving the T cell areas of the lymph node, namely the interfollicular regions and the paracortex. Examples of clinical situations associated with a T lymphocyte response include patients with viral infections, vaccinations, some drugs (particularly Dilantin), and systemic lupus erythematosus. Finally, the sinusoidal pattern of reaction involves expansion of the sinuses by benign macrophages as seen in reactive proliferations of the mononuclear-phagocytic system. Stellate microabscesses, irregular areas composed of central necrotic cellular and neutrophil debris surrounded by palisading macrophages, are characteristic of cat-scratch disease, lymphogranuloma venereum, and tularemia.

154. The answer is b. (*Henry, 19/e, pp 695–699. Cotran, 5/e, p 641.*) Burkitt's lymphoma, or undifferentiated lymphoma, is characterized by a rapid proliferation of primitive lymphoid cells with thick nuclear membranes, multiple nucleoli, and intensely basophilic cytoplasm when stained with Wright's stain. The cells are often mixed with macrophages in biopsy, giving a starry-sky appearance. The vacuoles contain lipid and this would be reflected by a positive oil-red-O reaction. PAS stain is nonspecific but does mark neutrophils and acute lymphoblastic leukemia cells. Nonspecific esterase is found predominantly within monocytes but also in megakaryocytes. Chloracetate esterase and myeloperoxidase are primarily found within the lysosomes of granulocytes, including neutrophils, promyelocytes, and faintly in rare monocytes.

155. The answer is b. (*Cotran, 5/e, p 641.*) T-cell lymphomas occurring in the thoracic cavity in young patients usually arise in the mediastinum and have a particularly aggressive clinical course with rapid growth in the mediastinum impinging upon the trachea or mainstem bronchi and leading to marked respiratory deficiency, which can in turn lead to death in a relatively short period of time if not treated. These unique lymphomas are characterized by rapid cell growth and spread into the circulation, where they produce elevated total white counts reflected by circulating lymphoma cells. As T cells they have characteristics of rosette formation with sheep blood cells. T cells also have subtypes and subsets, which can be delineated by monoclonal antibodies as CD4 helper, CD8 suppressor (cellular differentiation) T-cell surface antigens. The tumor cells also express IL-2 receptor. FC receptors occur on B cells and macrophages. Class II HLA antigens can be found on macrophages, Langerhans cells, and dendritic reticulum cells.

156. The answer is c. (*Cotran, 5/e, pp 634–636. Rubin, 2/e, pp 1074–1076. Silverberg, 2/e, pp 383–384.*) The Rappaport classification has separated NHL into nodular and diffuse categories; this is of major importance since the nodular pattern, independent of the cytologic subtype, is associated with a much better prognosis than is the diffuse type. The nodular lymphomas are composed of neoplastic B cells. Unlike the diffuse lymphomas, which often occur in children and adolescents, nodular lymphomas are rare in those under 20. They affect males and females equally, while diffuse lymphomas are much more common in males. Well-differentiated lymphocytic lymphoma and lymphoblastic lymphoma occur only in the diffuse form. Tingible-body macrophages are present within germinal centers of reactive, nonneoplastic lymph nodes.

157. The answer is c. (*Cotran, 5/e, pp 643–648.*) Hodgkin's disease is broadly divided into four histologic subtypes, the most common of which is the nodular sclerosis variant. This is characterized morphologically by the presence of the lacunar variant of Reed-Sternberg (RS) cells and by bands of fibrous tissue that divide the lymph node into nodules. Unlike the other subtypes of Hodgkin's disease, it is more common in females. Young adults are classically affected and the disease typically involves the cervical, supraclavicular, or mediastinal lymph nodes. Involvement of extranodal lymphoid tissue is unusual. Variant RS cells with a multilobed, puffy nucleus ("popcorn" cell) are seen in the lymphocyte-predominant subtype.

158. The answer is c. (*Cotran, 5/e, pp 643–648.*) The diagnosis of Hodgkin's disease depends on the total histologic picture and the presence of binucleated or bilobed giant cells with prominent acidophilic "owl-eye" nucleoli known as Reed-Sternberg (RS) cells. However, cells similar in appearance to RS cells may also be seen in infectious mononucleosis, mycosis fungoides, and other conditions. Thus, while RS cells are necessary for histologic confirmation of the diagnosis of Hodgkin's disease, they must be present in the appropriate histologic setting of lymphocyte predominance, nodular sclerosis, mixed cellularity, or lymphocyte depletion.

159. The answer is e. (*Cotran, 5/e, pp 649–654.*) The leukemias are malignant neoplasms of the hematopoietic stem cells that are characterized by diffuse replacement of the bone marrow by neoplastic cells. These malignant cells frequently spill into the peripheral blood. The leukemias are divided into acute and chronic forms, and then further subdivided based on lymphocytic or myelocytic (myelogenous) forms. Thus, the four basic patterns of acute leukemia are: acute lymphocytic leukemia (ALL), chronic lymphocytic leukemia (CLL), acute myelocytic leukemia (AML), and chronic myelocytic leukemia (CML).

Acute leukemias are characterized by a decrease in the mature forms of cells and an increase in the immature forms (leukemic blasts). Acute leukemias, both ALL and AML, have an abrupt clinical onset and present with symptoms due to failure of normal marrow function. Symptoms include fever (secondary to an infection), easy fatigability (due to anemia), and bleeding (due to thrombocytopenia). The peripheral smear in patients with acute leukemia reveals the white cell count to usually be increased. The peripheral smear also reveals signs of anemia and thrombocytopenia. More importantly, however, there are blasts in the peripheral smear. The diagnosis of acute leukemia is made by finding more than 30 percent blasts in the bone marrow.

AML primarily affects adults between the ages of 15 and 39 and is characterized by the neoplastic proliferation of myeloblasts. Myeloblasts, characterized by their delicate nuclear chromatin, may contain 3 to 5 nucleoli. Myeloblasts in some cases of AML have distinct intracytoplasmic rod-like structures that stain red and are called Auer rods. These are abnormal lysosomal structures (primary granules) that are considered pathognomonic of myeloblasts. AML is divided into seven types by the French-American-British (FAB) classification:

M1 - myeloblastic leukemia without maturation (cells are mainly blasts)

M2 - myeloblastic leukemia with maturation (some promyelocytes are present)

M3 - hypergranular promyelocytic leukemia (numerous granules and many Auer rods)

M4 - myelomonocytic leukemia (both myeloblasts and monoblasts)

M5 - monocytic leukemia (infiltrates in the gingiva are characteristic)

M6 - erythroleukemia (Di Guglielmo's disease)

M7 - acute megakaryocytic leukemia (associated with myelofibrosis)

Acute promyelocytic leukemia (M3 AML) is characterized by several specific features that are found in no other types of acute leukemia. There are numerous abnormal promyelocytes present that have numerous cytoplasmic granules and numerous Auer rods. If these numerous granules are released from dying cells, which may occur with treatment, they may activate extensive, uncontrolled intravascular coagulation and cause the development of DIC (disseminated intravascular coagulation). This abnormality is characterized by increased fibrin degradation products in the blood. M3 AML is also characterized by the translocation t(15;17), which results in the fusion of the retinoic acid receptor-alpha gene on chromosome 17 to the PML unit on chromosome 15. This produces an abnormal retinoic acid receptor and provides the basis for treatment of these patients with all-trans-retinoic acid.

160. The answer is d. (*Cotran, 5/e, pp 649–651.*) Acute lymphoblastic leukemia (ALL) is primarily a disease of children and young adults that is characterized by the presence of numerous lymphoblasts within the bone marrow. These malignant cells may spill over into the blood and other organs. In contrast to myeloblasts, lymphoblasts do not contain myeloperoxidase, but they do stain positively with the PAS stain, acid phosphatase stain, and for the enzyme TdT. The French-American-British (FAB) classification of ALL divided ALL into three types based on the morphology of the proliferating lymphoblasts. L1 ALL, seen in about

85 percent of the cases of ALL, consists of small homogeneous blasts. L2 ALL, seen in only 15 percent of cases of ALL, but more common in adults, consists of lymphoblasts that are larger and more heterogeneous (pleomorphic) than L1 blasts. These cells also may contain nuclear clefts. The final type of FAB ALL is the L3 type, which is seen in less than 1 percent of the cases of ALL. This form is essentially the leukemic form of Burkitt's lymphoma. Like the malignant cells of Burkitt's lymphoma, these L3 ALL cells are large blasts with cytoplasmic vacuoles that stain positively with the oil-red-O lipid stain.

In contrast to the FAB classification of ALL, the immunologic classification of ALL is based on the developmental sequence of maturation of B lymphocytes and T lymphocytes. First it is necessary to determine whether the blasts have B cell or T cell markers. Most cases of ALL are of B cell origin; that is, the lymphoblasts express both CD19 and DR. A few cases of ALL are of T cell origin; the lymphoblasts lack CD19 and DR and instead express T cell antigens CD2, 5, and 7. Many patients with T-ALL have a mediastinal mass and are clinically similar to cases of lymphoblastic lymphoma. To subclassify B-ALL, first determine if surface immunoglobulin (sIg) is present. Mature B-ALL cells (L3 ALL or Burkitt's lymphoma) have surface immunoglobulin, which is not found in the other types of B-ALL. These mature cells typically lack TdT, which is a marker for more immature cells. Next determine if there is cytoplasmic μ present. Cytoplasmic μ chains are specific for pre-B ALL cells, which has a characteristic translocation t(1;19). Finally the B-cell ALL cells that lack both surface Ig and cytoplasmic μ are called early pre-B ALL and are separated into the CALLA (CD10) positive and CALLA negative types.

161. The answer is c. (*Cotran, 5/e, pp 264–265, 654–655.*) Chronic myeloid leukemia (CML) is one of the four chronic myeloproliferative disorders, but, unlike myeloid metaplasia or polycythemia vera, CML is associated with the Philadelphia chromosome translocation t (9;22) in over 90 percent of cases. Association with the translocation t (8;14) is characteristic of Burkitt's lymphoma. In differentiating CML from a leukemoid reaction, several other features are important: lack of alkaline phosphatase in granulocytes, increased basophils and eosinophils in the peripheral blood, and, often, increased platelets in early stages followed by thrombocytopenia in late or blast stages. Other well-known features of CML include marked splenomegaly, leukocyte counts greater than 50,000/mm^3, and mild anemia.

162. The answer is c. (*Cotran, 5/e, pp 656–658.*) Hairy cell leukemia, a type of chronic B-cell leukemia, should be suspected in patients with splenomegaly; pancytopenia, including thrombocytopenia; bleeding; fatigue; and leukemic lymphocyte-like cells in the peripheral blood demonstrating cytoplasmic projections at the cell periphery ("hairy" cells). These cells stain for acid phosphatase, and the reaction is refractory to treatment with tartaric acid (tartrate-resistant acid phosphatase, or TRAP).

163. The answer is c. (*Cotran, 5/e, pp 655–656.*) Chronic lymphocytic leukemia (CLL) is the most common leukemia and is similar in many aspects to small lymphocytic lymphoma. It is typically found in patients who are older than 60 years of age. Histological examination of the peripheral smear reveals a marked increase in the number of mature-appearing lymphocytes. These neoplastic lymphocytes are fragile and easily damaged. This fragility produces the characteristic finding of numerous smudge cells in the peripheral smear of patients with CLL. About 95 percent of the cases of CLL are of B cell origin (B-CLL) and are characterized by having pan B cell markers, such as CD19. These malignant cells characteristically also have the T cell marker CD5. The remaining 5 percent of cases of CLL are mainly of T cell origin. Patients with CLL tend to have an indolent course and are associated with long survival in many cases. The few symptoms that may develop are related to anemia and the absolute lymphocytosis of small, mature cells. Splenomegaly may be noted. In a minority of patients, however, the disease may transform into prolymphocytic leukemia or a large cell immunoblastic lymphoma (Richter's syndrome). Prolymphocytic leukemia is characterized by massive splenomegaly and a markedly increased leukocyte count consisting of enlarged lymphocytes having nuclei with mature chromatin and nucleoli.

164. The answer is e. (*Henry, 19/e, pp 630–631, 685.*) Seen in the photomicrograph are sideroblasts that are demonstrating distinctive rings of Prussian blue-positive granules that indicate iron. Approximately 35 percent of normoblasts in normal bone marrow contain ferritin granules under normal conditions of iron metabolism. Heme synthetase mediates the attachments of iron onto protoporphyrin for the synthesis of hemo-globin. In sideroblastic anemia the production of globin or of heme is markedly reduced because of the deficiency of pyridoxine and ferritin, which contains iron accumulations with sideroblasts without progression into hemoglobin. The accumulation of these ferritin granules takes place in the mitochondria, where heme synthetase is located, and then can be seen rimming the nucleus of the normoblast—hence the name ring sideroblasts. This is the opposite abnormality from iron deficiency anemia. This type of anemia may be seen in patients suffering from alcoholism, se-lective deficiencies of pyridoxine, and myelodysplastic syndromes (MDS).

165. The answer is c. (*Cotran, 5/e, pp 658–660.*) Polycythemia rubra vera (PRV) is one of the myeloproliferative diseases characterized by excessive proliferation of erythroid, granulocytic, and megakaryocytic precursors derived from a single stem cell. In PRV the erythroid series dominates, but there is hyperplasia of all elements. There is plethoric congestion of all organs. The liver and spleen are typically moderately enlarged and may show extramedullary hemopoiesis. Thrombotic complications are an important cause of morbidity and mortality, and major and minor hemor-rhagic complications are also frequent. The red cell count is elevated with hematocrit >60 percent. The white cell count and platelet count are also elevated. Leukocyte alkaline phosphatase (LAP) activity is elevated in contrast to chronic myeloid leukemia, where it is reduced. Pruritus and peptic ulceration are common, possibly in relation to increased histamine release from basophils.

166. The answer is d. (*Cotran, 5/e, pp 660–662.*) Myeloid metaplasia with myelofibrosis is a myeloproliferative disorder in which the bone marrow is hypocellular and fibrotic and extramedullary hematopoiesis occurs, mainly in the spleen (myeloid metaplasia). Marked splenomegaly with trilineage proliferation of normoblasts, immature myeloid cells, and large megakaryocytes occurs. Giant platelets and poikilocytic (teardrop) red cells are seen in the peripheral smear. Clinically, myeloid metaplasia may be preceded by polycythemia vera or chronic myeloid leukemia. Biopsy of the marrow is essential for diagnosis. In contradistinction to chronic myeloid leukemia, levels of leukocyte alkaline phosphatase are elevated or normal in myeloid metaplasia; in CML, levels are low or absent. In 5 to 10 percent of cases of myeloid metaplasia, acute leukemia occurs. In aplastic anemia the marrow is very hypocellular, but consists largely of fat cells, not fibrosis. There is no splenomegaly. Microangiopathic and other hemolytic anemias that result from trauma to red cells show many erythrocytic abnormalities (helmet and burr cells, triangle cells, and schistocytes) in the peripheral smear.

167. The answer is c. (*Cotran, 5/e, pp 663–665.*) The bone marrow aspirate exhibits a proliferation of plasma cells that are characterized by well-defined perinuclear clear zones and by dense cytoplasmic basophilia due to increased RNA accumulations. Weakness, weight loss, recurrent infections, proteinuria, anemia, and abnormal proliferation of plasma cells in the bone marrow are findings that highly suggest the presence of multiple myeloma, a plasma cell dyscrasia. The more definitive diagnostic criteria are findings of M-component in the results of serum electrophoresis and plasma cell levels above 20 percent in the bone marrow. Multiple myeloma, which occurs more commonly in males than in females, shows an increasing incidence with increasing age, and most patients are in their seventies.

168. The answer is a. (*Cotran, 5/e, p 666. Silverberg, 2/e, pp 452–453.*) The finding of mu heavy-chain proteins in the serum is diagnostic generally of macroglobulinemia and specifically of mu heavy-chain disease. This form of macroglobulinemia has been detected in patients with chronic lymphocytic leukemia without findings of lymphadenopathy or bone marrow infiltrates of lymphocytes and plasma cells, which are typical of Waldenström's macroglobulinemia. Hepatomegaly and splenomegaly are usually present.

169. The answer is b. (*Cotran, 5/e, pp 666–667. Rubin, 2/e, pp 1034–1036.*) Langerhans' cell histiocytosis, previously known as histiocytosis X, refers to a spectrum of clinical diseases that are associated with the proliferation of Langerhans' cells. These cells, not to be confused with the Langhans-type giant cells found in caseating granulomas of tuberculosis, have Fc receptors, HLA-D/DR antigens, and react with CD1 antibodies. These cells have distinctive granules seen by electron microscopy that are rod-shaped organelles resembling tennis rackets. They are called LC (Langerhans' cells) granules, pentilaminar bodies, or Birbeck granules. There are three general clinical forms of Langerhans' histiocytosis. Acute disseminated Langerhans cell histiocytosis (Letterer-Siwe disease) affects children before the age of three. These children have cutaneous lesions that resemble seborrhea, hepatosplenomegaly, and lymphadenopathy. The Langerhans' cells infiltrate the marrow, which leads to anemia, thrombocytopenia, and recurrent infections. The clinical course is usually rapidly fatal; however, with intensive chemotherapy 50 percent of patients may survive 5 years. Multifocal Langerhans cell histiocytosis (Hand-Schuller-Christian disease) usually begins between the second and sixth year of life. The characteristic triad consists of bone lesions, particularly in the calvarium and the base of the skull, diabetes insipidus, and exophthalmos. These lesions are the result of proliferations of Langerhans' cells. Lesions around the hypothalamus lead to decreased ADH production and signs of diabetes insipidus. Unifocal Langerhans cell histiocytosis (eosinophilic granuloma), seen in older patients, is usually a unifocal disease, most often affecting the skeletal system. The lesions are granulomas that contain a mixture of lipid-laden Langerhans cells, macrophages, lymphocytes, and eosinophils.

Sarcoidosis is characterized by a proliferation of activated macrophages that form granulomas. It is not a proliferation of Langerhans' cells. Dermatopathic lymphadenitis refers to a chronic lymphadenitis that affects the lymph nodes draining the sites of chronic dermatologic diseases. The lymph nodes have hyperplasia of the germinal follicles and accumulation of melanin and hemosiderin pigment by the phagocytic cells.

170. The answer is b. (*Cotran, 5/e, pp 98, 616–617. Isselbacher, 13/e, pp 305–306.*) Hemorrhages into the skin may produce lesions of varying sizes. Petechiae measure less than two mm in size, purpuric lesions measure two mm to one cm, and ecchymoses are larger than one cm. Both erythema and telangiectasis do not involve hemorrhage outside of blood vessels. They can be differentiated from true hemorrhages into the skin by the fact that they will blanch if direct pressure is applied to them. True purpura may be caused by hemostatic defects or non-hemostatic defects. Hemostatic defects are caused by platelet or coagulation abnormalities, while non-hemostatic defects generally involve the blood vessels. These vascular abnormalities can be separated into palpable and nonpalpable purpura. The latter may be caused by excess corticosteroids (Cushing's syndrome), vitamin C deficiency (scurvy), infectious agents, and abnormal connective tissue diseases (Ehlers-Danlos syndrome). Causes of palpable purpura include diseases that cause cutaneous vasculitis, such as collagen vascular diseases and Henoch-Schonlein purpura. The latter, also known as anaphylactoid purpura, is a type of hypersensitivity vasculitis found in children. It usually develops one to three weeks following a streptococcal infection, but it may also occur in relation to allergic food reactions. Cross-reacting IgA or immune complexes are deposited on the endothelium of blood vessels. Patients may develop fever, purpura, abdominal pain, arthralgia, arthritis, and glomerulonephritis.

171. The answer is c. *(Cotran, 5/e, pp 617–619.)* In acute idiopathic thrombocytopenic purpura (ITP), which occurs predominantly in children under 8 years of age, there is an acute onset about 2 weeks after a viral infection (rubella, viral hepatitis, infectious mononucleosis). There is no female predominance as seen in chronic ITP, which is most frequent in women 20 to 50 years old and is characterized by an insidious onset. Both acute and chronic forms are associated with increased platelet destruction and normal or increased megakaryocytes in bone marrow. Most patients with acute ITP make a spontaneous recovery in 4 to 6 weeks.

172. The answer is b. *(Cotran, 5/e, pp 117–121, 619–620, 981.)* A fulminating septic state should always be considered whenever the constellation of fever, deteriorating mental status, skin hemorrhages, and shock develops. Such conditions can be seen in gram-negative rod septicemia caused by any of the coliforms (gram-negative endotoxic shock) or fulminant meningococcemia (Waterhouse-Friderichsen syndrome). However, a form of nonbacterial vasculitis termed thrombotic thrombocytopenic purpura (TTP) is notorious for producing a clinical syndrome very similar to fulminating infective states. It is characterized by arteriole and capillary occlusions by fibrin and platelet microthrombi and is usually unassociated with any of the predisposing states seen in disseminated intravascular coagulopathy (DIC), such as malignancy, infection, retained fetus, and amniotic fluid embolism. Macrocytic hemolytic anemia, variable jaundice, renal failure, skin hemorrhages, and central nervous system dysfunction are all seen in TTP and are related to the fibrin thrombi, which can be demonstrated with skin, bone marrow, and lymph node biopsies. There is less coagulopathy in TTP than is found in DIC, and hemolytic anemia is generally not found in idiopathic or autoimmune thrombocytopenic purpura. The condition of patients with TTP may be improved by plasmapheresis, with 80 percent survival.

173. The answer is c. *(Damjanov, 10/e, pp 1089, 1716, 1751, 1823. Cotran, 5/e, pp 619–620, 980–981.)* A woman who manifests a hemorrhagic diathesis following childbirth should be considered to have intravascular coagulopathy until proof to the contrary is obtained—for instance, the condition may be due to retained products of conception. However, the peripheral blood smear depicted in the question shows, in addition to thrombocytopenia (three to four platelets are normally present in every high-power field), remarkably misshapen red blood cells (poikilocytosis) in the form of schistocytes (fragments of red cells), spherocytes, and, importantly, "helmet" red cells, so named because of their similarity in shape to military or football helmets. Helmet cells imply the presence of microangiopathic hemolytic anemia and are thought to form through hemolytic-mechanical red cell membrane disruption by passing through arteriole-capillary beds that have fibrin thrombin meshes. Disorders that cause microangiopathic hemolytic anemia are childhood and adult hemolytic uremic syndrome and thrombotic thrombocytopenic purpura (TTP). The lack of jaundice and neurologic symptoms in this case rules out TTP. The combination of microangiopathic hemolytic anemia and renal insufficiency strongly suggests hemolytic uremic syndrome.

174. The answer is e. *(Cotran, 5/e, pp 623–626.)* Disseminated intravascular coagulation (DIC) is a severe thrombohemorrhagic disorder that results from extensive activation of the coagulation sequence. With DIC there is widespread fibrin deposits in the microcirculation, which leads to hemolysis of the red cells (microangiopathic hemolytic anemia), ischemia, and infarcts in multiple organs. Continued thrombosis leads to consumption of platelets and the coagulation factors, which will subsequently lead to a bleeding disorder. The excessive clotting also activates plasminogen and increases plasmin levels, which will cleave fibrin and increase serum levels of fibrin split products. DIC is never a primary disorder, but instead is always secondary to other diseases that activate either the intrinsic or the extrinsic coagulation system. Activation of the intrinsic pathway results from the release of tissue factor into circulation. Examples include obstetric complications, from the release of placental tissue factor, and cancers, from the release of the cytoplasmic granules of the leukemic cells of acute promyelocytic leukemia or from release of mucin from adenocarcinomas. Coagulation may also result from the activation of the extrinsic pathway by widespread injury to endothelial cells, such as with the deposition of antigen-antibody complexes (vasculitis) or endotoxic damage by microorganisms.

175. The answer is d. (*Cotran, 5/e, pp 616–623. Henry, 19/e, pp 725–726, 729–736, 740–743.*) Abnormalities of blood vessels (capillary fragility) or platelets can be detected by either the tourniquet test or the bleeding time. These tests do not test the coagulation cascade. In contrast, the platelet count and platelet morphology are both useful in evaluating platelet abnormalities, while the prothrombin time (PT) and the partial thromboplastin time (PTT) measure the coagulation cascade. The PT measures the extrinsic pathway, while the PTT measures the intrinsic coagulation pathway.

An abnormal tourniquet test and bleeding time with a normal PTT and PT may be caused by either blood vessel abnormalities or platelet abnormalities. Blood vessel abnormalities and abnormal platelet function have normal platelet counts (choice "A" in table). Causes of blood vessel abnormalities include decreased vitamin C (scurvy) and vasculitis, while causes of platelet dysfunction include the Bernard-Soulier syndrome and Glanzmann's thrombasthenia. A decrease in the platelet count (choice "C" in the table) indicates thrombocytopenia and can be seen in patients with ITP. Normal platelet counts with normal bleeding times are suggestive of abnormalities of the coagulation cascade. A prolonged PTT only (choice "B" in the table) is seen with abnormalities of the intrinsic pathway, such as hemophilia A or B. A prolonged PT only (choice "D" in the table) is seen with abnormalities of the extrinsic pathway, such as a deficiency of factor VII. A prolongation of both PTT and PT is seen with liver disease, vitamin K deficiency, and DIC. Deficiencies of the vitamin K-dependent factors, such as induced with Coumadin therapy or broad-spectrum antibiotic therapy, are associated with a normal tourniquet test, bleeding time, and platelet count, but there will be a markedly increased PT, and the PTT may be increased or normal (also choice "D" in the table). Therefore, the PT is used as a screening test to monitor patients taking oral Coumadin. A prolonged bleeding time with a normal platelet count, but a prolonged PTT (choice "E" in table) is highly suggestive of von Willebrand disease.

176. The answer is e. (*Cotran, 5/e, pp 587–589.*) Destruction of red cells, hemolysis, may occur within the vascular compartment (intravascular hemolysis) or within the mononuclear-phagocyte system (extravascular hemolysis). In both cases, the hemolysis will lead to anemia, and the breakdown of hemoglobin will lead to jaundice, which is increased indirect bilirubin. Intravascular hemolysis releases hemoglobin into the blood (hemoglobinemia), which then binds to haptoglobin. When haptoglobin levels are depleted, free hemoglobin is oxidized to methemoglobin, and then both hemoglobin and methemoglobin are secreted into the urine (hemoglobinuria and methemoglobinuria). Within the renal tubular epithelial cells, hemoglobin is reabsorbed, hemosiderin is formed, and when these cells are shed into the urine, hemosiderinuria results. Since extravascular hemolysis does not occur within the vascular compartment, hemoglobinemia, hemoglobinuria, methemoglobinuria, and hemosiderinuria do not occur. The breakdown of the red cells within the phagocytic cells causes anemia and jaundice, just as with intravascular hemolysis, and since hemoglobin escapes into the blood from the phagocytic cells, plasma haptoglobin levels are also reduced. Unlike intravascular hemolysis, the erythrophagocytosis causes hypertrophy and hyperplasia of the mononuclear phagocytic system, which in turn may lead to splenomegaly.

177. The answer is d. (*Cotran, 5/e, pp 613–615.*) Hematopoietic stem cell failure occurs in aplastic anemia, probably because of defective stem cells or their immunologic suppression. Pancytopenia results, although selective suppression with pure red cell aplasia, agranulocytosis, or thrombocytopenia may occur. In 50 percent of cases, aplastic anemia is idiopathic or primary, but there are many physical and chemical causes of secondary aplastic anemia. Whole body irradiation is the major physical cause. Chemical causes include many drugs, such as alkylating agents, antimetabolites, and the antibiotic chloramphenicol. Severe aplastic anemia may occur following viral hepatitis C (non-A, non-B) or following infectious mononucleosis. An inherited form of aplastic anemia is seen in patients with Fanconi's anemia. In myelophthisic anemia, marrow failure is due to marrow replacement by metastatic tumor or other lesions, but no association with stem cell defects exists.

178. The answer is d. (*Cotran, 5/e, pp 603–610.*) The photomicrograph in the question shows the presence of megaloblasts accompanied by unusually large neutrophils and precursors. These abnormalities may be caused by either a deficiency or lack of absorption of vitamin B12 or of folic acid. In addition to diets deficient in these two substances, any condition leading to poor absorption of them will also lead to megaloblastic anemia. Thus malabsorption (as in celiac disease), gastrectomy, infiltrative disorders of the bowel (including lymphoma and collagen vascular disease such as scleroderma), infections by the fish tapeworm, and metabolic disorders (such as hyperthyroidism and increased demand for folic acid as in advanced stages of malignancy) all will lead to reduced levels of vitamin B12 and folic acid. A deficiency of either vitamin B12 or folic acid will lead to maturational arrest of the red cell precursors, which yields large and apparently immature red cell precursors—hence the name megaloblastic. The nuclei of red cell precursors are in an immature stage for the maturation of the cytoplasm, which results in an unusually large nucleus.

179. The answer is d. *(Henry, 19/e, pp 189–190, 243, 246. Cotran, 5/e, pp 610–613.)* Intravascular iron is bound to transferrin, which is usually about 33 percent saturated with iron. Increased saturation occurs in states of iron overload (hemochromatosis), in severe liver disease, hemolytic conditions, and marrow hypoplasia (reduced iron utilization). Iron deficiency is associated with low serum iron levels, increased iron-binding capacity, and decreased saturation.

180. The answer is e. *(Cotran, 5/e, pp 861–863.)* Hemochromatosis is a generic term for disorders of iron overload marked by increases in total body iron and deposition of ferritin and hemosiderin in various organs with morphologic and functional damage to those organs. The pathogenesis is not fully understood but involves altered intestinal handling of iron with decreased post-absorption excretion, and alterations in iron metabolism and storage in reticuloendothelial cells. It causes a micronodular pigment cirrhosis with hemosiderin deposition in parenchymal, Kupffer, and bile duct epithelial cells, which is highlighted on Prussian blue staining. Hepatocellular carcinoma is a frequent (15 to 30 percent) complication of pigment cirrhosis. The pancreas shows intense pigmentation with atrophy and loss of parenchymal cells and diffuse interstitial fibrosis. Diabetes is a major feature of the clinical syndrome but is poorly correlated to the degree of iron deposition in the islets. Other tissues and organs that suffer major deposition of iron include the myocardium, the endocrine glands, skin (melanin and hemosiderin), and testes. Various tests useful in diagnosis reveal increased serum ferritin and plasma iron and decreased iron-binding capacity, reflecting increased body iron load. Liver biopsy is definitive when it shows elevated hemosiderin content. Skin pigmentation is mainly due to increased amounts of melanin, seen with various types of cirrhosis.

181. The answer is c. (Cotran, 5/e, pp 640–642.) The large-cell immunoblastic lymphoma is one of the three high-grade lymphomas, which also include lymphoblastic lymphoma and small, noncleaved lymphomas, such as Burkitt's lymphoma. Lymphoblastic lymphoma occurs predominantly in adolescents, is closely related to T-cell acute lymphoblastic leukemia, and, in addition to a mediastinal mass, disseminates early to bone marrow and blood. In contrast, large-cell immunoblastic lymphoma is predominantly of B-cell origin (5 to 10 percent are T cell) and occurs in much older people, many of whom had a prior immune or lymphoproliferative disorder (Sjögren's syndrome, AIDS, or renal transplant immunosuppression). Bone marrow involvement is uncommon except in late stages; extranodal tumor (retroperitoneum) is common. The tumor is aggressive and rapidly fatal if untreated. The cells appear plasmacytoid (B immunoblasts) or show multilobed, polymorphous nuclei (T immunoblasts), but molecular studies are essential to differentiate T-cell receptor gene rearrangement from the immunoglobulin gene rearrangements of B immunoblasts. A "starry sky" pattern is produced by the digestion of cellular debris by benign macrophages and is typically seen in both lymphoblastic lymphoma and Burkitt's lymphoma.

182. The answer is c. (Cotran, 5/e, pp 662–666.) Multiple myeloma has a peak incidence at 50 to 60 years of age and presents a classic triad of marrow plasmacytosis; a serum or urine M (monoclonal) protein or both, which represent the immunoglobulin molecule (or heavy or light chain) produced by the tumor cells; and lytic bone lesions. Myeloma is a monoclonal malignancy of the B-lymphocyte system with bone pain the most common symptom; osteolytic, punched-out bone lesions are characteristic, especially in the skull. Since the process is lytic, alkaline phosphatase is usually not raised. Lymphadenopathy occurs in Waldenström's macroglobulinemia, another malignancy of lymphoplasmacytoid cells, but myeloma is not associated with lymphadenopathy. Hypercalcemia from bone resorption is frequent, as are recurrent infections

because of severe suppression of normal immunoglobulins. In about 55 percent of patients, the abnormal M component is IgG and in 25 percent it is IgA.

183. The answer is a. (*Cotran, 5/e, pp 592–596.*) Homozygous expression of hemoglobin S results in nearly all the hemoglobin in the red blood cell's being of the S type. Thus, most of the circulating red cells have the abnormal sickling forms that are sequestered by the spleen and produce sludging within the splenic capillaries and consequent multiple and continuing infarctions. Eventually the spleen becomes small as it is replaced by fibrous tissue. This is sometimes referred to as "autosplenectomy." Multiple crises contribute to this event. Massive enlargements of the spleen may be found in neoplastic blood disorders. Chronic lymphocytic leukemia (CLL) produces some very large spleens late in the disease, but massives plenomegaly has been seen in many examples of leukemias and lymphomas, including hairy cell leukemia. Even conversion from cutaneous T-cell lymphoma (mycosis fungoides) may result in a transformed immunoblastic-like sarcoma state.

184. The answer is d. (*Damjanov, 10/e, pp 1716, 1751. Cotran, 5/e, pp 979–981.*) Endothelial injury is considered to be an initiating pathologic event, especially in HUS associated with gram-negative infections, predominantly infection with verocytotoxin-producing *E. coli*. The verocytotoxins of *E. coli*, which infects up to 75 percent of the patients, are cytotoxic to endothelium and are similar to the shigatoxins produced by Shigella. Hypertension exists in about 50 percent of the patients, but the relative lack of CNS involvement helps to distinguish HUS from thrombotic thrombocytopenic purpura in which there is usually more general involvement with thrombi formed in several organs.

185. The answer is d. (*Lee, 9/e, pp 1432–1437. Cotran, 5/e, p. 622.*) In contrast to factor VIII deficiency, hemarthroses are uncommon in patients who have von Willebrand's disease. Von Willebrand's disease is characterized by quantitative or qualitative abnormalities of von Willebrand's factor. A prolonged bleeding time affects most of the patients, and there is a moderate deficiency in coagulation factor VIII. Decreased retention of platelets in glass bead filters, normal numbers of platelets, and menorrhagia are usual findings, but petechiae rarely occur. The most common symptoms include epistaxis, increased susceptibility to bruises, and excessive bleeding from wounds.

186–187. The answers are: 186-c, 187-b. *(Cotran, 5/e, pp 173, 631–632. Rubin, 2/e, pp 1030–1033. Anderson, 9/e, pp 494–495.)* While the exact interactions between different cells are not totally understood, there is current evidence that an initiating antigen is first processed by a macrophage. The macrophage interacts with helper T cells and B cells in a conceptual triangular fashion with helper T cells functioning in the recognition of the carrier component of the antigen on the macrophage as well as recognizing the major histocompatibility complex (MHC) marker (Ia) on the macrophage surface. The macrophage appears to concentrate the antigen, thereby orchestrating interactions between itself and the T and B lymphocytes. After stimulation, the B cell may differentiate into antibody-producing plasma cells. Eosinophils and basophils function in type I reactions (anaphylaxis) by degranulation and binding of IgE.

Leukocytosis, increased numbers of leukocytes in the peripheral blood, is a reaction seen in many different disease states. The type of leukocyte that is mainly increased may be an indicator of the type of disease process present. Eosinophilia is associated with cutaneous allergic reactions; allergic disorders, such as bronchial asthma or hay fever; Hodgkin's disease; some skin diseases, such as pemphigus, eczema, and dermatitis herpetiformis; and parasitic infections, such as trichinosis, schistosomiasis, and strongyloidiasis. The most common cause of eosinophilia is probably allergy to drugs such as iodides, aspirin, and sulfonamides, but eosinophilia is also seen in collagen vascular diseases. Marked eosinophilia occurs in hypereosinophilic syndromes (Loeffler's syndrome and idiopathic hypereosinophilic syndrome), which may be treated with corticosteroids. Neutrophilic leukocytosis (neutrophilia) may be the result of acute bacterial infections or tissue necrosis, such as is present with myocardial infarction, trauma, or burns. Basophilia is most commonly seen in immediate-type (type I) hypersensitivity reactions. Both eosinophils and basophils may be increased in patients with any of the chronic myeloproliferative syndromes. Monocytosis is seen in chronic infections, such as tuberculosis, some collagen vascular diseases, neutropenic states, and some types of lymphomas. Lymphocytosis may be seen along with monocytosis in chronic inflammatory states or in acute viral infections, such as viral hepatitis or infectious mononucleosis.

188–189. The answers are: 188-f, 189-e. (*Cotran, 5/e, pp 347–349.* *Henry, 19/e, pp 623–624, 635, 641–642, 771–772, 1096–1098.*) Infectious mononucleosis is a benign lymphoproliferative disorder caused by the Epstein-Barr virus (EBV). It typically occurs in young adults and presents with systemic symptoms, lymphadenopathy, and pharyngitis. Hepatosplenomegaly may be present. Peripheral blood shows an absolute lymphocytosis, and many lymphocytes are atypical with irregular nuclei and abundant basophilic vacuolated cytoplasm. These represent CD8+ T-killer cells induced by EBV-transformed B lymphocytes. These atypical lymphocytes are usually adequate for diagnosis, along with a positive heterophil or monospot test (increased sheep red cell agglutinin). Administration of ampicillin for a mistaken diagnosis of streptococcal pharyngitis results in a rash in many patients.

The metabisulfite test is used to detect the presence of hemoglobin S, but it does not differentiate the heterozygous sickle cell trait from the homozygous sickle cell disease. The test is based on the fact that erythrocytes with a large proportion of hemoglobin S sickle in solutions of low oxygen content. Metabisulfite is a reducing substance that enhances the process of deoxygenation. The osmotic fragility test is a diagnostic test for hereditary spherocytosis. Spherocytes will lyse at a higher concentration of salt than will normal cells, thus causing an increased osmotic fragility. The direct antiglobulin test (DAT), or Coombs test, is used to differentiate autoimmune hemolytic anemia (AIHA) due to the presence of anti-red cell antibodies from other forms of hemolytic anemia. In this test, antibodies to human immunoglobulin cause the agglutination (clotting) of red cells if these anti-red cell antibodies are present on the surface of the red cells. In patients with paroxysmal nocturnal hemoglobinuria, the erythrocytes are excessively sensitive to complement-mediated lysis in low ionic environments (the basis for the sucrose hemolysis test) or in acidotic conditions, such as sleep, exercise, or the Ham acid hemolysis test. The Schilling test, which measures intestinal absorption of vitamin B12 with and without intrinsic factor, is used to diagnose decreased vitamin B12 caused by pernicious anemia, which is characterized by a lack of intrinsic factor.

190–191. The answers are: 190-j, 191-c. (*Cotran, 5/e, pp 621–623.* *Henry, 19/e, pp 725–726, 729–731.*) Von Willebrand's disease is not as rare as once thought, and numerous subtypes, which are delineated by two-dimensional electrophoresis, have been described. The disease is characterized clinically by mucocutaneous bleeding, menorrhagia, and epistaxis. Milder forms of the disease may not be diagnosed until the patient is older. Factor VIII is a complex of several components that can be discerned electrophoretically. Of all the factor VIII components, factor VIII:R, or ristocetin cofactor, is most apt to be abnormal in von Willebrand's disease. The coagulant (C) and the related antigen (Ag) forms of factor VIII may sometimes be normal in various autosomal dominant types. Most patients even with the milder forms will have decreased factor VIII:R. Prothrombin time, fibrinogen levels, and factors IX and XIII are not affected in this disorder.

Hemophilia A is an X-linked disorder that results from a deficiency of coagulation factor VIII. Clinically patients with hemophilia exhibit a wide range of severity of symptoms that depends upon the degree that the factor VII activity is decreased. Petechiae and small ecchymoses are characteristically absent, but large ecchymoses and subcutaneous and intramuscular hematomas are common. Other types of bleeding that are characteristic include massive hemorrhage following trauma or surgery, and "spontaneous" hemorrhages in parts of the body that are normally subject to trauma, such as the joints (hemarthroses). Intra-abdominal hemorrhage and intracranial hemorrhage also occur. The latter is a major cause of death for these individuals. Because of the decreased factor VIII activity, patients with hemophilia A have a prolonged PTT, which measures the intrinsic coagulation cascade. Other clinical tests, including bleeding time, tourniquet test, platelet count, and PT, are normal. Treatment is with factor VIII concentrates, but this carries a risk for the transmission of viral hepatitis and AIDS.

CARDIOVASCULAR SYSTEM

Questions

DIRECTIONS: Each question below contains five suggested responses. Select the **one best** response to each question.

192. Type II hyperlipidemia (familial hypercholesterolemia) results from a defect in

a. Lipoprotein lipase
b. Low-density lipoprotein (LDL) receptor
c. Apolipoprotein E
d. Apolipoprotein CII
e. Lipoprotein(a)

193. A factor that stimulates the proliferation of smooth muscle cells and also relates to the pathogenesis of atherosclerosis is

a. Platelet-derived growth factor (PDGF)
b. Transforming growth factor β (TGF-β)
c. Interleukin 1 (IL-1)
d. Interferon α
e. Tumor necrosis factor (TNF)

194. The form of vascular disease responsible for malignant hypertension is

a. Medial calcific sclerosis
b. Arteriosclerosis obliterans
c. Hyperplastic arteriolosclerosis
d. Hyaline arteriolosclerosis
e. Thromboangiitis obliterans

195. An 82-year-old woman complaining of headaches, visual disturbances, and muscle pain has a biopsy of the temporal artery. The changes revealed by the biopsy specimen are shown in the photomicrograph below. The next course of action is to

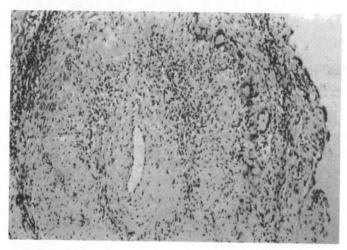

a.   Administer corticosteroids
b.   Verify with a repeat biopsy
c.   Administer anticoagulants
d.   Perform angiography
e.   Order a test of the erythrocyte sedimentation rate (ESR)

196. The necrotizing inflammation of the small gastrointestinal artery shown in the photomicrograph below is most likely due to

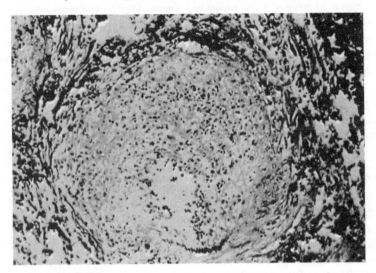

a. Myasthenia gravis
b. Polyarteritis nodosa
c. Atherosclerosis
d. Dissecting aneurysm
e. Syphilis

197. In a patient with vasculitis, the finding of serum antineutrophil cytoplasmic autoantibodies (ANCA's) that react by immunofluorescence staining in a perinuclear pattern is most suggestive of

a. Giant cell arteritis
b. Classic polyarteritis nodosa
c. Wegener's granulomatosis
d. Churg-Strauss syndrome
e. Microscopic polyangiitis

198. During a routine physical examination A 60-year-old white male is found to have a 5 cm pulsatile mass in his abdomen. Angiography reveals a marked dilatation of his aorta distal to his renal arteries. This aneurysm is most likely the result of

a. Atherosclerosis
b. A congenital defect
c. Hypertension
d. A previous syphilitic infection
e. Trauma

199. A 56-year-old male presents with the sudden onset of excruciating pain. He describes the pain as beginning in the anterior chest, radiating to the back, and then moving downward into the abdomen. His blood pressure is found to be 160/115. Your differential diagnosis includes myocardial infarction; however, no changes are seen on his EKG, and you consider this to be less of a possibility. You obtain an X-ray of this patient's abdomen and discover a "double barrel" aorta. This abnormality is most likely a result of

a. A microbial infection
b. Loss of elastic tissue in the media
c. A congenital defect in the wall of the aorta
d. atherosclerosis of abdominal aorta
e. Abnormal collagen synthesis

200. A 2-year-old girl is being evaluated from marked swelling of her neck. During the work-up of this patient, a karyotype reveals that she is monosomic for the X chromosome. Which one of the listed abnormalities is most likely responsible for the swelling of this young girl's neck?

a. Bacillary angiomatosis
b. Capillary hemangioma
c. Cystic hygroma
d. Glomus tumor
e. Spider angioma

201. A 56-year-old woman died in a hospital where she was being evaluated for shortness of breath, ankle edema, and mild hepatomegaly. Because of the gross appearance of the liver at necropsy in the photograph below, one would also expect to find

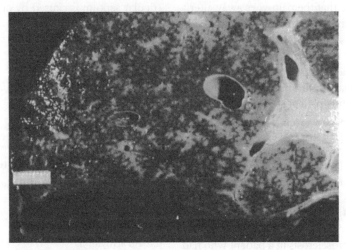

a. A pulmonary saddle embolus
b. Right heart dilatation
c. Portal vein thrombosis
d. Biliary cirrhosis
e. Splenic amyloidosis

202. An elderly man treated for congestive heart failure for years with digitalis and furosemide dies of pulmonary edema. A postmortem examination of the heart would most likely show

a. Severe left ventricular hypertrophy
b. Right and left ventricular hypertrophy
c. Right ventricular infarction
d. Aortic and mitral valve stenosis
e. A dilated, globular heart with thin walls

203. A 64-year-old male presents with recurrent chest pain that develops whenever he attempts to mow the grass in his yard. He relates that the pain goes away after a couple of minutes if he stops and rests. He also states that the pain has not increased in frequency or duration in the last several months. What is the most likely diagnosis for this patient?

a. Stable angina
b. Unstable angina
c. Atypical angina
d. Prinzmetal angina
e. Myocardial infarction

204. If the coronary arteries on dissection at autopsy show severe atherosclerosis in a patient who had clinically acute (60-h) myocardial infarction, you would expect to find

a. Gross evidence of myocardial scarring
b. Coronary thrombosis in 90 percent of cases
c. Coronary thrombosis in 65 percent of cases
d. A plaque with ulceration, fissure, or hemorrhage
e. Rupture of a papillary muscle

205. A posterior myocardial infarction that involves the posterior portion of the left ventricle and the posterior one-third of the interventricular septum is caused by occlusion of the

a. Left coronary artery
b. Right coronary artery
c. Circumflex artery
d. Left anterior descending (LAD) artery
e. Posterior descending artery

206. The mortality from myocardial infarction is most closely related to the occurrence of

a. A pericardial effusion
b. Pulmonary edema
c. Coronary artery thrombosis
d. An arrhythmia
e. Systemic hypotension

207. Unexpected sudden cardiac death is a very rare complication of

a. Severe coronary artery disease
b. Myocarditis
c. Cardiac tamponade
d. Mitral valve prolapse
e. Dilated or hypertrophic cardiomyopathy

208. The pathology evident in the photomicrograph below usually first appears after which of the following lengths of time following a myocardial infarction?

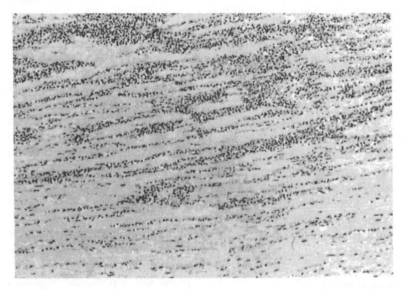

a. 12 h
b. 3 days
c. 7 days
d. 14 days
e. 28 days

209. Following development of an acute myocardial infarction (MI), the LEAST likely complication is

a. Cardiac arrhythmia
b. Cardiogenic shock
c. Sudden cardiac death
d. Cardiac rupture
e. Thromboembolism

210. A 39-year-old female presents with increasing shortness of breath. She states that for the past 6 months she has been taking an unauthorized appetite suppressant to try to lose weight. Physical examination reveals signs of right heart failure. She is admitted to the hospital to work-up her symptoms, but she dies suddenly. A section from her heart at the time of autopsy reveals marked thickening of the right ventricle, but the thickness of the left ventricle is within normal limits. The endocardium does not appear to be increased in thickness or fibrotic, and the cardiac valves do not appear abnormal. Neither ventricular cavity is dilated. Which one of the following best describes this cardiac pathology?

a. Carcinoid heart disease
b. Cor pulmonale
c. Eccentric hypertrophy
d. Systemic hypertensive heart disease
e. Volume overload to the heart

211. The most frequent cause of aortic valve incompetence and regurgitation is

a. Latent syphilis
b. Infective endocarditis
c. Rheumatic fever
d. Aortic dissection
e. Congenital

212. The most characteristic feature of chronic rheumatic heart disease is

a. Endocarditis
b. Myocarditis
c. Pericarditis
d. Mitral valvulitis
e. Pulmonic valvulitis

213. A 31-year-old female presents with fever, intermittent severe pain in her left upper quadrant of her abdomen, and painful lesions involving her fingers and nailbeds. History reveals that she had acute rheumatic fever as a child, and when she was around 20 years of age she developed a new cardiac murmur. At the present time one of three blood cultures submitted to the hospital lab grows out a particular organism. Which one of the following is most likely to be that organism?

a. *Staphylococcus aureus*
b. α-hemolytic viridans streptococci
c. *Candida* species
d. Group A streptococci
e. *Pseudomonas* species

214. A 23-year-old woman develops the sudden onset of congestive heart failure. Her condition rapidly deteriorates and she dies in heart failure. At autopsy, patchy interstitial infiltrates composed mainly of lymphocytes are found, some of which surround individual myocytes. The most likely cause of this patient's heart failure is

a. Viral myocarditis
b. Bacterial myocarditis
c. Giant cell myocarditis
d. Hypersensitivity myocarditis
e. Beriberi

215. A 37-year-old woman complained of prolonged cramps, nausea, vomiting, diarrhea, and episodic flushing of the skin. At autopsy, pearly-white, plaque-like deposits were found on the tricuspid valve leaflets. These cardiac lesions most likely were due to

a. Rheumatic heart disease
b. Amyloidosis
c. Iron overload
d. Hypothyroidism
e. Carcinoid heart disease

216. The heart in the gross photograph below came from a patient who

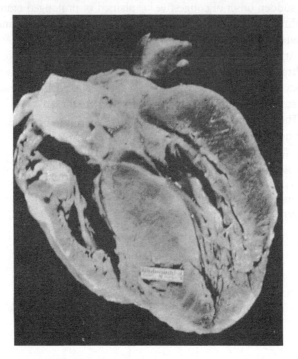

a.   Suffered from alcohol toxicity
b.   Had Libman-Sacks endocarditis
c.   May have had a family history of similar cardiac involvement
d.   Frequently had obstructive symptoms
e.   Had a hypocontractile heart

217. A 35-year-old European male, who is an avid beer drinker, presents with the sudden onset of signs of heart failure. If these symptoms are the result of cobalt put in his beer as a foam stabilizer, then gross examination of this patient's heart would most likely reveal

a.   No gross abnormalities
b.   Four chamber dilation with hypertrophy
c.   Asymmetric septal hypertrophy
d.   A stiff, hypocontracting heart
e.   Constrictive cardiomyopathy

218. A 17-year-old high school student died suddenly while playing basketball. At autopsy asymmetric hypertrophy of the interventricular septum was discovered. Histologic sections from this area revealed disorganization of the myofibers, which were thicker than normal and had hyperchromatic nuclei. What is the most likely diagnosis?

a. Hypertrophic cardiomyopathy
b. Dilated cardiomyopathy
c. Constrictive cardiomyopathy
d. Secondary cardiomyopathy
e. Endomyocardial fibrosis

219. A elderly patient who becomes acutely short of breath presents with the combination of hypotension, elevated jugular venous pressure, and muffled heart sounds. This triad of symptoms is most suggestive of

a. Chronic pericarditis
b. Chronic pericardial effusion
c. Cardiac tamponade
d. Dissecting aortic aneurysm
e. Right heart failure

220. Which one of the following is the most common congenital heart defect to cause an initial left-to-right shunt?

a. Tetralogy of Fallot
b. Coarctation of the aorta
c. Ventricular septal defect
d. Atrial septal defect
e. Patent ductus arteriosus

221. Complete obliteration of the aortic lumen by a coarctation proximal to the ductus arteriosus is fatal unless

a. The foramen ovale is closed
b. The ductus is ligated
c. Pulmonary stenosis coexists
d. The ductus remains patent
e. The tricuspid valve is incompetent

222. Atherosclerosis, the most prevalent form of arterial disease in humans, is first manifested by an innocuous fatty streaking of the intima and is characterized by all the following EXCEPT

a. Onset in mid-life
b. Formation of essential lesions in the intima
c. Disintegration of the internal elastic lamina in advanced lesions
d. Relatively numerous lesions in larger arteries and fewer in smaller arteries
e. Plaque formations that cause little reduction in the luminal size of large arteries

223. Major risk factors associated with development of coronary and generalized atherosclerosis (AS) include all the following EXCEPT

a. Cigarette smoking
b. Elevated high-density lipoprotein (HDL) levels
c. Diabetes mellitus
d. Hypertension
e. Hypercholesterolemia

224. The biopsy specimen shown below reveals a dermal vascular tumor with angular, slitlike spaces and spindle cells in the dermal stroma. This lesion is associated with all the following EXCEPT

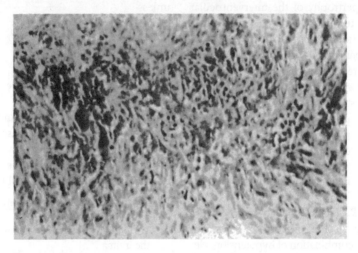

a. Several clinically distinct forms
b. Immunosuppression
c. Depletion of T-suppressor cells
d. Early histologic resemblance to granulation tissue
e. Tumor origin from vascular endothelium

225. Severe mitral stenosis, as shown in the photograph below, is frequently accompanied by all the following EXCEPT

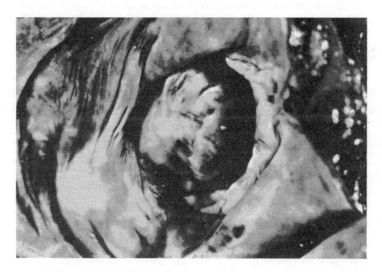

a.   aortic valve disease
b.   Antecedent rheumatic fever
c.   Left atrial enlargement with atrial fibrillation
d.   Pulmonary valvular stenosis
e.   Chronic passive pulmonary congestion

226. Manifestations of rheumatic fever that are of major diagnostic value include all the following EXCEPT

a.   Subcutaneous nodules
b.   Migratory arthritis of large joints
c.   Fever
d.   Erythema marginatum
e.   Chorea minor

227. Features of tetralogy of Fallot include all the following EXCEPT

a.   Obstruction to the pulmonary outflow
b.   Hypertrophy of the right ventricle
c.   Aortic dextroposition in 50 percent of cases
d.   Development of cyanosis before 1 year of age
e.   Ventricular septal defect

DIRECTIONS: Each group of questions below consists of lettered headings followed by a set of numbered items. For each numbered item select the *one* lettered heading with which it is *most* closely associated. Each lettered heading may be used *once, more than once, or not at all.*

Questions 228–229

Match each of the following clinical scenarios with the correct diagnosis from the following list.

a. Buerger's disease
b. Cystic medial necrosis
c. Giant cell arteritis
d. Goodpasture's disease
e. Hyaline arteriolosclerosis
f. Hyperplastic arteriolosclerosis
g. Kawasaki's syndrome
h. Microscopic polyarteritis nodosa
i. Mönckeberg's arteriosclerosis
j. Takayasu's disease

228. A 3-year-old Japanese boy presents with a high fever, conjunctival and oral erythema, a diffuse skin rash, and enlarged, painful lymph nodes. Work-up reveals focal dilations of the coronary arteries (aneurysms).

229. A 57-year-old female presents with signs of hyperthyroidism, and physical examination reveals her thyroid gland to be enlarged (goiter). Tissue taken from her thyroid reveals hyperplastic thyroid follicles. In addition, several of the larger blood vessels have large areas of calcification within the media of their wall. What is the proper diagnosis for her blood vessel pathology?

Questions 230–231

Match each of the following clinical scenarios with the correct diagnosis from the following list.

a. Angiosarcoma
b. Capillary hemangioma
c. Cystic hygroma
d. Glomus tumor
e. Kaposi's sarcoma
f. Lipoma
g. Myxoma
h. Papillary fibroelastoma
i. Rhabdomyoma
j. Rhabdomyosarcoma

230. A 25-year-old female presents with a painful lesion located under the nail of her second finger of her left hand. A section from this lesion reveals vascular spaces lined by nests of uniform cells. What is the most accurate diagnosis for this lesion?

231. A 45-year-old male presents with trouble breathing and is found to have signs and symptoms of mitral valve disease. Prior to complete work-up, he dies suddenly. Gross examination of his heart at the time of autopsy reveals a 5 cm mass attached to the wall of the left atrium. The mass appears to be freely movable, enough to obstruct the mitral valve. Histologic sections from this mass reveal stellate cells in a loose myxoid background. "Spider cells" are not found. What is the most accurate diagnosis for this lesion?

CARDIOVASCULAR SYSTEM

Answers

192. The answer is b. *(Cotran, 5/e, pp 135–137, 481–483.)* Lipids are transported in the blood complexed to proteins called apolipoproteins. Abnormalities of this lipid transport or metabolism result in hyperlipoproteinemias, which are responsible for most syndromes of premature atherosclerosis. The hyperlipidemias are divided into five distinct electrophoretic patterns. Type I hyperlipoproteinemia, caused by a mutation in the lipoprotein lipase gene, results in increased chylomicrons and triglycerides. Type II hyperlipoproteinemia, perhaps the most frequent mendelian disorder, is caused by a mutation in the low-density lipoprotein (LDL) receptor gene. This results in increased LDL and cholesterol. Homozygotes for this gene defect have markedly increased plasma cholesterol levels and develop severe atherosclerosis at an early age. Mutations in the apolipoprotein E gene result in type III hyperlipoproteinemia, which is characterized by increased intermediate-density lipoproteins (IDL), triglycerides, and cholesterol. Type IV hyperlipoproteinemia causes increased very low-density lipoproteins (VLDL) and triglycerides. The genetic defect causing this is presently unknown. Type V hyperlipoproteinemia, caused by a mutation in apolipoprotein CII, results in increased VLDL, chylomicrons, triglycerides, and cholesterol. Lipoprotein(a) is an altered form of LDL that contains the apolipoprotein B100 linked to apolipoprotein(a). Increased levels of lipoprotein(a) are associated with an increased incidence of coronary and cerebral vascular disease, independent of the total LDL level.

193. The answer is a. *(Cotran, 5/e, pp 479–481. Rubin, 2/e, pp 466–470.)* The pathogenesis of atherosclerosis depends in part on the inflammatory function of macrophages, which involves the release of numerous cytokines. Platelet-derived growth factor (PDGF) is mitogenic and chemotactic for smooth muscle cells. This may explain the recruitment and proliferation of smooth muscle cells in atherosclerosis. Other macrophage products participate in the pathophysiology of atherosclerosis by other means. Interleukin 1

(IL-1) and tumor necrosis factor (TNF) transform the normally anticoagulant endothelial surface into a procoagulant surface by stimulating endothelial cells to produce platelet activating factor (PAF), tissue factor (TF), and plasminogen activator inhibitor (PAI). Interferon α and transforming growth factor β inhibit cell proliferation. This could explain the failure of endothelial cells to repair endothelial defects. These defects could then either provide entry areas for lipoproteins and plasma-derived factors or serve as an area where thrombi are formed.

194. The answer is c. (*Cotran, 5/e, pp 484, 488–489, 498, 976–978.*) Malignant hypertension refers to dramatic elevations in systolic and diastolic blood pressure often resulting in early death from cerebral and brainstem hemorrhages. Pathologically the renal vessels demonstrate a concentric obliteration of arterioles by an increase in smooth muscle cells, and protein deposition in a laminar configuration that includes fibrin material, which leads to total and subtotal occlusion of the vessels. Hyaline arteriolosclerosis as seen in diabetes is presumably caused by leakage of plasma components across the endothelium with or without hypertension. Medial calcific sclerosis (Mönckeberg's arteriosclerosis) is characterized by dystrophic calcification in the tunica media of muscular arteries. There is no narrowing of the lumen of the affected vessels. Thromboangiitis obliterans (Buerger's disease) is occlusion by a proliferative inflammatory process in arteries of heavy cigarette smokers and is often associated with HLA-A9, B5 genotypes.

195. The answer is a. (*Cotran, 5/e, pp 492–493. Rubin, 2/e, pp 488–489.*) Giant cell arteritis (temporal arteritis), although not a major public-health problem, is an important disease to consider in the differential diagnosis of patients of middle to advanced age who present with a constellation of symptoms that may include migratory muscular and back pains (polymyalgia rheumatica), dizziness, visual disturbances, headaches, weight loss, anorexia, and tenderness over one or both of the temporal arteries. The cause of the arteritis (which may include giant cells, neutrophils, and chronic inflammatory cells) is unknown, but the dramatic response to corticosteroids suggests an immunogenic origin. The disease may involve any artery within the body, but involvement of the ophthalmic artery or arteries may lead to blindness unless steroid therapy is begun. Therefore, if temporal arteritis is suspected, the workup to document it should be expedited and should include a biopsy of the temporal artery. Frequently, the erythrocyte sedimentation rate (ESR) is markedly elevated to values of 90 or greater. Whereas tenderness, nodularity, or skin reddening over the course of one of the scalp arteries, particularly the temporal, may show the ideal portion for a biopsy, it is important to recognize that the temporal artery may be segmentally involved or not involved at all even when the disease is present.

196. The answer is b. (*Cotran, 5/e, p 494.*) Classic polyarteritis nodosa—a necrotizing inflammation that occurs in episodes at random locations within or on the walls of medium-sized and small arteries—has been reported in about 0.1 percent of autopsies and affects, in order of increasing frequency, the arteries associated with peripheral and central nerves, skeletal muscles, pancreas, gastrointestinal tract, liver, heart, and kidneys. Proceeding in stages, the inflammatory reaction features acute necrosis, with fibrinoid deposition and neutrophilic infiltration, and leads to thrombosis of the lumen and destruction of the internal elastic membrane. Polyarteritis nodosa probably could be more accurately called "panarteritis nodosa," because all vascular coats are subject to inflammation. A remnant of the internal elastic membrane is visible in the photomicrograph.

197. The answer is e. (*Cotran, 5/e, pp 490–491. Rubin, 2/e, pp 489, 853–854.*) Antineutrophil cytoplasmic antibodies (ANCA) may be found in patients with certain inflammatory vascular diseases or glomerular diseases, and their presence is of clinical importance for diagnosing these diseases. Immunofluorescence reveals ANCA to have two different patterns. One is directed toward myeloperoxidase of neutrophils and is found in a perinuclear location (P-ANCA). This pattern is seen in patients with microscopic polyarteritis nodosa (PAN) or idiopathic crescentic glomerulonephritis without systemic disease. The other pattern reveals the antibodies to be directed against neutral leukocyte protease (proteinase 3) and results in a cytoplasmic staining pattern (C-ANCA). This pattern is seen in patients with Wegener's granulomatosis, and Churg-Strauss syndrome.

198. The answer is a. (*Cotran, 5/e, pp 499–504.*) An aneurysm is an abnormal dilatation of any vessel. The causes of aneurysms are many, but the two most important are atherosclerosis and cystic medial necrosis. Atherosclerotic aneurysms, the most common type of aortic aneurysm, usually occur distal to the renal arteries and proximal to the bifurcation of the aorta. Many atherosclerotic aneurysms are asymptomatic, but if they rupture they will produce sudden, severe abdominal pain, shock, and a risk of death. Prior to rupture, physical examination reveals a pulsatile mass in the abdomen. Cystic medial necrosis refers to the focal loss of elastic and muscle fibers in the media of vessels and is seen in patients with hypertension, dissecting aneurysms, and Marfan's syndrome. Trauma may also lead to the formation of dissecting aneurysms.

Berry aneurysms, found at the bifurcation of arteries in the circle of Willis, are due to congenital defects in the vascular wall. Syphilitic (luetic) aneurysms are caused by obliterative endarteritis of the vasa vasorum of the aorta. These luetic aneurysms are part of the tertiary manifestation of syphilis and become evident 15 to 20 years after persons have contracted the initial infection with *Treponema pallidum*. Elastic tissue and smooth muscle cells of the media undergo ischemic destruction as a result of the treponemal infection (obliterative endarteritis). As a consequence of ischemia in the media, musculoelastic support is lost and fibrosis occurs. Grossly the aorta has a "tree-bark" appearance. Luetic aneurysm almost always occurs in the thoracic aorta and may lead to luetic heart disease by producing insufficiency of the aortic valve (aortic regurgitation).

199. The answer is b. (*Cotran, 5/e, pp 133–135, 499–504, 936, 1312–1313.*) Dissecting aneurysms are usually the result of cystic medial necrosis of the aorta. This abnormality results from loss of elastic tissue in the media and is associated with hypertension and Marfan's syndrome. Most cases of dissecting aneurysms have a transverse tear in the intima and are located in the ascending aorta, just above the aortic ring. The pain caused by a dissecting aneurysm is similar to the pain caused by a myocardial infarction, but it extends into the abdomen as the dissection progresses. Additionally, the blood pressure is not decreased with a dissecting aneurysm unless the aorta itself has ruptured.

Berry aneurysms, found at the bifurcation of arteries in the circle of Willis, are due to congenital defects in the vascular wall. Rupture of these aneurysms may produce a fatal subarachnoid hemorrhage. Berry aneurysms have been noted in about one-sixth of patients with adult polycystic renal disease and account for death in about 10 percent of patients with this type of polycystic renal disease. Syphilitic (luetic) aneurysms occur in the thoracic aorta and may lead to luetic heart disease by producing insufficiency of the aortic valve. Mycotic (infectious) aneurysms result from microbial infection during septicemia, usually secondary to bacterial endocarditis. They are prone to rupture and hemorrhage. Ehlers-Danlos syndromes (EDS's) are a group of eight syndromes characterized by defects in collagen synthesis. In EDS IV there is deficient synthesis of type III collagen and a tendency to rupture of muscular arteries, including dissecting aneurysms of the aorta.

200. The answer is c. (*Cotran, 5/e, pp 160–161, 506–509, 512.*) Benign tumors of vessels may originate from either blood vessels or lymphatics. Hemangiomas are benign tumors of blood vessels that histologically reveal the presence of red blood cells (erythrocytes) within the lumens of the proliferating vessels. Hemangiomas may be subclassified into capillary hemangiomas or cavernous hemangiomas. The juvenile (strawberry) hemangioma is a fast-growing lesion that appears in the first few months of life, but completely regresses by the age of five. In contrast to hemangiomas, lymphangiomas are tumors that are derived from lymphatic vessels. Histologically they reveal dilated vessels lined by endothelial cells, but they lack red blood cells in their lumen. The absence of red blood cells helps to distinguish these lesions from hemangiomas. Cystic hygromas are cystic lymphangiomas that typically occur in the neck or axilla. They may grow to such a large size that the neck is deformed. These lesions may be found in patients with Turner's syndrome, an abnormality that results from complete or partial monosomy for the X chromosome. Swelling of the neck of these individuals occurs because of dilated lymphatic vessels (cystic hygroma). With time the swelling decreases, but the patients may develop bilateral neck webbing and loose skin on the back of the neck.

Glomangiomas, glomus tumors, are very painful tumors that are derived from the glomus body. These tumors are typically found in the distal regions of the fingers and toes, sometimes in a subungual location. Histologically they reveal vascular spaces that are lined by nests of uniform cells. Dilated blood vessels (vascular ectasia) may be congenital or acquired. "Birthmarks" may be caused by congenital vascular ectasia or capillary hemangiomas. "Port wine stains" are similar lesions that may be caused by vascular ectasia or cavernous hemangiomas of the skin. Spider angiomas are acquired vascular ectasias that are the result of increased estrogen levels. They are associated with pregnancy and liver disease. Bacillary angiomatosis is a non-neoplastic proliferation of blood vessels that is found in immunocompromised patients, particularly patients with AIDS. Histologically there are proliferating capillaries that are lined by protuberant endothelial cells. Additionally numerous neutrophils are present along with nuclear dust and purple granules. These latter granules are rickettsia-like bacteria that are the cause of this lesion, which responds to erythromycin.

201. The answer is b. (*Cotran, 5/e, pp 97–98, 520–523.*) The photograph shows the classic pattern of hepatic congestion around central veins, which leads to necrosis and degeneration of the hepatocytes surrounded by pale peripheral residual parenchyma. This is the pattern arising in the liver from chronic passive congestion as a result of right heart failure ("nutmeg liver"). Mitral stenosis with consequent pulmonary hypertension leads to right heart failure, as does any cause of pulmonary hypertension, such as emphysema (cor pulmonale). Right heart failure also leads to congestion of the spleen and transudation of fluid into the abdomen (ascites) and lower extremity soft tissues (pitting ankle edema) as a result of venous congestion. Portal vein thrombosis is most often seen in association with hepatic cirrhosis.

202. The answer is e. (*Cotran, 5/e, pp 520–523.*) The morphological changes of clinical congestive heart failure cannot always be correlated with necropsy findings of the heart because there may be hypertrophy, dilatation, a combination of both, or even an absence of both. Many patients with long-standing congestive heart failure after decompensation will have hearts that are maximally dilated, with thinned and unusually soft myocardium rather than hypertrophic ventricular myocardium. This thinning of the myocardium occurs after a long period of compensatory hypertrophy and reflects a state in which the capacity of the myocardium to compensate has been exceeded. The first response of the myocardium to a demand for increased work (load) is to undergo hypertrophy according to Starling's law, leading to an increase in stroke volume. Eventually, this mechanism is exceeded under states of increased oxygen demand or demand for more cardiac output, and cardiac decompensation results, with the worst complication being acute pulmonary edema as a consequence of left ventricular failure.

203. The answer is a. (*Cotran, 5/e, pp 527–528.*) One of the consequences of myocardial ischemia is chest pain, which is called angina. Angina is caused by a mismatch between the myocardial oxygen demand and the myocardial blood flow. There are three main types of angina. Typical angina (stable angina) is the most common type and is characterized by pain that results from exercise, stress, or excitement. The pain is promptly relieved by rest, which decreases oxygen demand, or nitroglycerin. This chemical is converted to nitric oxide, which is a vasodilator that increases perfusion to the heart. EKG changes in patients with stable angina are nonspecific and include T wave inversion and ST segment depression, which occurs secondary to ischemia of the subendocardium of the left ventricle. Prinzmetal angina (atypical angina) is caused by coronary artery vasospasm and is characterized by pain occurring at rest. This pain may be relieved by calcium channel blockers or nitroglycerin. The EKG in these patients reveals ST segment elevation, which is the result of transmural ischemia. The third type of angina is unstable angina, which is characterized by increasing frequency of pain, increased duration of the pain, or pain that is produced by less physical exertion. This final type of angina indicates that a myocardial infarction (MI) may be near, most likely due to the formation of a thrombus over an area of coronary artery atherosclerosis. In contrast to an MI, with angina there is no actual necrosis (infarction) of myocardial tissue, and therefore there are no increased cardiac enzymes, such as LDH and CPK, in the serum. Also, the pain of angina is not made worse with deep inspiration, a sign that is suggestive of pleural disease.

204. The answer is d. (*Cotran, 5/e, pp 529–530, 533, 536.*) At autopsy, coronary artery thrombosis has been found in less than 50 percent of cases of myocardial infarction (MI). However, when coronary angiography is done within 4 h of MI onset, a thrombosed artery is found in almost 90 percent of cases; occlusion is found in only about 60 percent when angiography is delayed for 12 to 24 h. Therefore, lysis occurs or there is relaxation of spasm, or both. Also, intravenous or intracoronary fibrinolysis restore flow to thrombosed arteries in more than 75 percent of recent MIs. These findings are proof of coronary thrombosis, whether it is found at autopsy or not. Ulcerated, fissured, or hemorrhagic atheromas are usually found beneath the thrombus, whether still attached or lysed. Following an infarction, granulation tissue forms at 10 days to 2 weeks, and this is followed by fibrous scarring.

205. The answer is b. (*Cotran, 5/e, pp 518–519. Rubin, 2/e, p 506.*) The right and left main coronary arteries originate around the sinuses of Valsalva of the aortic valve. The left coronary artery divides into the left anterior descending artery (LAD) and the left circumflex artery. The LAD supplies the anterior left ventricle, the anterior right ventricle, and the anterior two-thirds of the interventricular septum. The left circumflex artery supplies the lateral wall of the left ventricle. The right coronary artery supplies the remainder of the right ventricle, the posteroseptal portion of the left ventricle, and the posterior one-third of the interventricular septum. The posterior descending artery is usually a branch of the right coronary artery. This anatomic relationship is called a right coronary dominant distribution. Posterior (inferior or diaphragmatic) infarcts result from occlusion of the right coronary artery; anterior infarcts from occlusion of the LAD; and posterolateral infarcts from occlusion of the left circumflex artery.

206. The answer is d. (*Cotran, 5/e, pp 537–540.*) In myocardial infarction, life-threatening arrhythmias occur in approximately 45 percent of patients without shock and in more than 90 percent of patients with shock. The most common arrhythmias are expressed as ventricular extrasystoles, but atrial extrasystoles, sinus tachycardia, and sinus bradycardia also occur. Even without arrhythmias, nearly two-thirds of patients with acute myocardial infarcts develop heart failure and pulmonary edema. Sudden death (death within 24 h of onset of symptoms and signs) occurs in about 20 to 25 percent of acute attacks.

207. The answer is d. (*Cotran, 5/e, pp 541, 545–547. Rubin, 2/e, p 542.*) The most common cause of sudden death in the adult is cardiac arrhythmia (usually ventricular fibrillation) due to severe coronary artery disease, with or without acute myocardial infarction. Ventricular fibrillation is also often due to primary cardiomyopathy, myocarditis, or congestive heart failure. However, sudden death is a rare complication of mitral valve prolapse (MVP), floppy valve syndrome, or the systolic click-murmur syndrome. In MVP the major complication is mitral insufficiency with left ventricular failure; however, MVP is asymptomatic in the majority of patients. Echocardiography has shown MVP to be common (5 to 10 percent of the general population). It is usually of unknown cause, but 10 to 15 percent of cases are familial with autosomal dominant inheritance. It is fairly frequent in Marfan's syndrome or cystic medial necrosis. There is excess mitral valve tissue and elongated chordae and the echocardiogram shows posterior displacement of the posterior (rarely anterior) mitral leaflet late in systole.

Another interesting, but rare, noncardiac cause of sudden unexpected death is unrecognized anaphylaxis from insect stings. Postmortem sera should be examined for elevated venom-specific IgE antibodies, and laryngeal and pulmonary edema noted at autopsy.

208. The answer is b. *(Cotran, 5/e, pp 533–537.)* Usually by 3 days after a myocardial infarction, the predominant microscopic features that develop and that can be seen in a stained section of the affected myocardium include coagulation necrosis of fibers and evidence of extensive neutrophilic exudation. Interstitial edema may also be observed in microscopy, and the cross-striations of fibers may appear less recognizable. In gross examination 3 days after the infarction, the infarct has a hyperemic border surrounding a central portion that is yellow-brown and soft as the result of fatty change.

209. The answer is d. *(Cotran, 5/e, pp 537–538.)* Cardiac rupture, whether of free wall, septum, or papillary muscle, occurs in only 1 to 5 percent of cases following acute myocardial infarction. It occurs usually within the first week of infarction when there is maximal necrosis and softening (4 to 5 days) and is very rare after the second week. Rupture of the free wall results in pericardial hemorrhage and cardiac tamponade. Rupture of the interventricular septum causes a left-to-right shunt. Serious mitral valve incompetence results from rupture of anterior or posterior papillary muscles. Other common complications include arrhythmias such as heart block, sinus arrhythmias, or ventricular tachycardia or fibrillation. These occur in 90 percent of complicated cases. Next in importance, but not in frequency (only 10 percent), is cardiogenic shock from severe left ventricular contractile incompetence. Milder left ventricular failure with lung edema occurs in 60 percent, while mural thrombosis with peripheral emboli may occur in up to 40 percent. Ventricular aneurysm forms a "bulge" of the left ventricular chamber; it consists of scar tissue, does not rupture, but may contain thrombus. Sudden cardiac death occurs within 2 h in 20 percent of patients with acute myocardial infarction.

210. The answer is b. *(Cotran, 5/e, pp 541–543. Abenhaim L, N Engl J Med 335(9), 609–616. Connolly HM, N Engl J Med 337(9), 581–588.)* Hypertensive heart disease (HHD) can be divided into systemic HHD and pulmonary HHD. Systemic HHD is the result of systemic hypertension, which causes left ventricular (LV) hypertrophy. There is by definition no other cardiac disease present that could cause LV hypertrophy, such as aortic stenosis. Hypertension is a pressure overload on the heart, and as such it causes concentric LV hypertrophy without dilation. In contrast, eccentric hypertrophy is the result of volume overload on the heart. In systemic HHD the LV is stiff as there is decreased LV compliance. In a patient with uncontrolled hypertension, LV dilation would indicate LV failure. Pulmonary HHD indicates right ventricular hypertrophy that is the result of pulmonary disease. By definition this type of heart disease is called cor pulmonale. Pulmonary diseases that can cause cor pulmonale include diseases of the lung parenchyma, such as chronic obstructive pulmonary disease and interstitial fibrosis, and diseases of the pulmonary vessels, such as multiple pulmonary emboli and pulmonary vascular sclerosis. The latter has been associated with the use of the combination of diet drugs fenfluramine and phentermine. This combination has been referred to as "Fen-Phen."

211. The answer is c. *(Damjanov, 10/e, pp 1257–1272.)* Aortic regurgitation (AR) is rheumatic in origin in approximately 70 percent of cases. Much less frequently it is due to syphilis, ankylosing spondylitis (rarely), infective endocarditis, aortic dissection, or aortic dilatation from cystic medial necrosis. Congenital forms of aortic stenosis occur fairly frequently but AR is rarely congenital in origin. In chronic AR, patients remain asymptomatic for many years, but clinical manifestations will include exertional dyspnea, angina, and left ventricular failure. Owing to the rapidly falling arterial pressure during late systole and diastole, there is often wide pulse pressure, Corrigan's "water-hammer" pulse, capillary pulsations at the nail beds, and a pistol-shot sound over the femoral arteries. A blowing diastolic murmur is heard along the left sternal border. Volume overload of the heart is the basic defect and results in left ventricular dilatation and hypertrophy.

212. The answer is d. *(Cotran, 5/e, pp 547–550.)* Rheumatic fever (RF) produces both acute and chronic manifestations. Acute RF produces a pancarditis of all three layers of the heart. It is manifested by myocarditis, which is characterized by the Aschoff body; pericarditis, which is referred to as "bread and butter" pericarditis; and verrucous endocarditis. In contrast, chronic RF produces damage to cardiac valves. The mitral valve is most commonly involved, followed by the aortic valve. The stenotic valve has the appearance of a "fish mouth" or "buttonhole." An additional finding in chronic RF is a rough portion of the endocardium of the left atrium, called a MacCallum's patch.

213. The answer is b. (*Cotran, 5/e, pp 550–554. Chandrasoma, 3/e, pp 349–353.*) Infective endocarditis is the result of micro-organisms growing on any of the heart valves. These organisms may have either high virulence or low virulence. Highly virulent organisms, such as *Staphylococcus aureus* and group A streptococci, infect previously normal valves and produce severe symptoms within six weeks. This abnormality is referred to as acute bacterial endocarditis. In contrast, organisms of low virulence, such as α-hemolytic viridans streptococci and *Staphylococcus epidermis*, infect previously damaged valves, such as valves damaged by rheumatic fever. These organisms produce symptoms that last longer than six weeks. This abnormality is referred to as subacute bacterial endocarditis. Infective endocarditis in IV drug abusers, which normally occurs on the tricuspid valve, is caused by *Staphylococcus aureus*, group A streptococci, *Candida* species, and gram-negative bacilli like *Pseudomonas* species. Symptoms in patients with infective endocarditis are the result of bacteremia, emboli from the vegetations, immune complexes, and valvular disease. Bacteremia produces fever, positive blood cultures (several of which may be needed for confirmation), abscesses, and osteomyelitis. Embolization of parts of the large, friable vegetations can produce Roth spots in the retina, splinter hemorrhages in nail beds, and infarcts of the brain, heart, and spleen. Splenic infarcts will produce left upper quadrant (LUQ) abdominal pain. Immune complexes can deposit in multiple areas of the body and cause glomerulonephritis, vasculitis, tender nodules in the fingers and toes (Osler's nodes), and red papules in the palms and soles (Janeway lesions). Valvular disease can also result in perforation and valvular regurgitation.

214. The answer is a. (*Cotran, 5/e, pp 562–566. Rubin, 2/e, pp 543–545.*) Inflammation of the myocardium, myocarditis, has numerous causes, but most of the well-documented cases of myocarditis are of viral origin. The most common viral causes are coxsackieviruses A and B, ECHO virus, and influenza virus. Patients usually develop symptoms a few weeks after a viral infection. Most patients recover from the acute myocarditis, but a few may die from congestive heart failure or arrhythmias. Sections of the heart will show patchy or diffuse interstitial infiltrates composed of T lymphocytes and macrophages. There may be focal or patchy acute myocardial necrosis. Bacterial infections of the myocardium produce multiple foci of inflammation composed mainly of neutrophils. Giant cell myocarditis, which was previously called Fiedler's myocarditis, is characterized by granulomatous inflammation with giant cells and is usually rapidly fatal. In hypersensitivity myocarditis, which is caused by hypersensitivity reactions to several drugs, the inflammatory infiltrate includes many eosinophils, and the infiltrate is both interstitial and perivascular. Beriberi, one of the metabolic diseases of the heart, is a cause of high-output failure and is characterized by decreased peripheral vascular resistance and increased cardiac output. Patients have dilated hearts, but the microscopic changes are nonspecific. Hyperthyroid disease and Paget's disease are other causes of high-output failure.

215. The answer is e. (*Cotran, 5/e, pp 549, 555–556, 565–566.*) Plaques or vegetations are found in characteristic locations within the heart in several diseases. The carcinoid syndrome is characterized by episodic flushing, diarrhea, bronchospasm, and cyanosis. These symptoms are caused by the release of vasoactive amines, such as serotonin, from carcinoid tumors. These substances are inactivated by enzymes such as monoamine oxidase, which are found in the liver, lung, and brain. Therefore cardiac symptoms are found only in patients with liver metastases, which bypass the inactivation of the liver itself. The cardiac lesions are found on the right side of the heart since the active metabolites secreted by the tumor are inactivated in the lung and do not reach the left side of the heart. The cardiac lesions consist of fibrous plaques found on the tricuspid and pulmonic valves. In contrast, plaques in the left atrium are seen in chronic rheumatic heart disease and are called MacCallum's patches. Vegetations also occur in rheumatic heart disease; these are small and are found in a row along the lines of closure of the valve. Amyloid deposits may be found in the heart secondary to multiple myeloma, or as an isolated event, such as in senile cardiac amyloidosis. Grossly the walls of the heart may be thickened, and there may be multiple, small nodules on the left atrial endocardial surface. Iron overload can affect the heart as a result of hereditary hemochromatosis or hemosiderosis. Grossly the heart is a rust-brown color and resembles the heart in idiopathic dilated cardiomyopathy. In hypothyroidism the heart is characteristically flabby, enlarged, and dilated, which results in decreased cardiac output. This reduced circulation results in a characteristic symptom of hypothyroidism, cold sensitivity. Histologically there is an interstitial mucopolysaccharide edema fluid within the heart.

216. The answer is c. (*Cotran, 5/e, pp 560–561.*) The cardiomyopathy shown in the photograph is designated hypertrophic cardiomyopathy with the synonyms of idiopathic hypertrophic subaortic stenosis (IHSS), hypertrophic obstructive cardiomyopathy, and asymmetric septal hypertrophy (ASH). It is characterized by a prominent and hypertrophic interventricular septum that is out of proportion to the thickness of the left ventricle. Histologically the myocardial fibers have disarray, caused by wide fibers with unusual orientation, and prominent hyperchromatic nuclei. There is increased incidence within families and there is evidence that it may be an autosomal dominant disorder. Patients may have dyspnea, lightheadedness, and chest pain, especially upon physical exertion; however, many patients appear to be asymptomatic although a sudden, unexpected death occurs not infrequently, especially following or during physical exertion. There may be abnormalities of the coronary arteries. The mitral valve may be thickened and patients may experience endocarditis on it. Cardiac output can be markedly reduced in some patients because of reduced volume of the left ventricle. As the patient ages, however, cardiac dilatation often improves the reduced left ventricular volume. Chronic alcoholism and a flabby, hypocontractile heart occur with dilated (congestive) cardiomyopathy.

217. The answer is b. (*Cotran, 5/e, pp 557–562.*) The cardiomyopathies (CMP) may be classified into primary and secondary forms. The primary forms are mainly idiopathic (unknown cause). Most of these secondary cardiomyopathies result in a dilated cardiomyopathy that is characterized by congestion and four chamber dilation with hypertrophy. The walls are either of normal thickness or they may be thinner than normal. This results in a flabby, globular, banana-shaped heart that is hypocontracting. The microscopic appearance is not distinctive. The ventricles may have mural thrombi. The causes of secondary dilated CMP are many and include alcoholism (the most common cause in the United States), metabolic disorders, and toxins. Examples of the latter include cobalt, which has been used in beer as a foam stabilizer, anthracyclines, cocaine, and iron, the deposition of which is seen in patients with hemochromatosis. The anthracycline Adriamycin, which is used in chemotherapy, causes lipid peroxidation of myofiber membranes. One final form of DCM develops in the last trimester of pregnancy or the first six months after delivery. About 1/2 of these patients recover full cardiac function.

Other forms of cardiomyopathies include a hypertrophic form, a restrictive form, and an obliterative form. In hypertrophic CMP the major gross abnormality is within the interventricular septum, which is usually thicker than the left ventricle. Constrictive (restrictive) CMP is associated with amyloidosis, sarcoidosis, endomyocardial disease, or storage diseases. These abnormalities produce a stiff, hypocontracting heart.

218. The answer is a. (*Cotran, 5/e, pp 557–562.*) Cardiomyopathies can be separated into a dilated form, a hypertrophic form, a restrictive form, and an obliterative form. In hypertrophic cardiomyopathy, also called idiopathic hypertrophic subaortic stenosis (IHSS), and asymmetric septal hypertrophy (ASH), the major gross abnormality is within the interventricular septum. There is asymmetric hypertrophy of the septum, which is thicker than the left ventricle. Histologically, the myofibers in the septum are disorganized, hypertrophied, and have hyperchromatic nuclei. There is an increased incidence of hypertrophic cardiomyopathy within families, and there is evidence that it may be an autosomal dominant disorder. The disease is thought to result from a mutation in the cardiac β-myosin heavy chain gene. Patients may have dyspnea, light-headedness, and chest pain, especially upon physical exertion; however, many patients appear to be asymptomatic. Up to one-third of these patients die from sudden cardiac death, usually related to physical exertion. Cardiac output can be markedly reduced in some patients because of reduced volume of the left ventricle.

Patients with dilated (congestive) cardiomyopathy have a flabby, hypocontractile heart. Constrictive (restrictive) cardiomyopathy is associated in the United States with amyloidosis and endocardial fibroelastosis. It is so named because of the infiltration and deposition of material in the endomyocardium and the layering of collagen and elastin over the endocardium. This deposition affects the ability of the ventricles to accommodate blood volume during diastole. Endocardial fibroelastosis occurs mainly in infants during the first two years of life. It is associated with a prominent fibroelastic covering over the endocardium of the left ventricle. There may be associated aortic coarctation, ventricular septal defects, mitral valve defects, and other abnormalities. In contrast, endomyocardial fibrosis is a form of restrictive cardiomyopathy that is found mainly in young adults and children in Southeast Asia and Africa. It differs from endocardial fibroelastosis in the United States in that elastic fibers are not present.

219. The answer is c. (*Cotran, 5/e, pp 566–569.*) Accumulations of excess fluid within the pericardial cavity are called pericardial effusions. The sudden filling of the pericardial space with fluid is called pericardial tamponade. The three classic signs of pericardial tamponade, called Beck's triad, include hypotension, elevated jugular pressure, and muffled heart sounds. The latter is due to the dampening effect of the pericardial fluid on the heart sounds. Some patients may also demonstrate a decrease in systemic pressure with inspiration, which is called "paradoxic pulse." The decrease in cardiac output will produce dyspnea, shortness of breath, and hypotension. Decreased atrial filling results in elevated jugular venous pressure. There are several types of pericardial effusions. Serous pericardial effusion are caused most often by congestive heart failure, but they can also be caused by renal disease that produces uremia. Serosanguinous effusion are caused by trauma and cardiopulmonary resuscitation (CPR). Chylous effusion are caused by lymphatic obstruction, while cholesterol effusion are seen in patients with myxedema, which is caused by hypothyroidism. Finally hemopericardium, blood in the pericardial cavity, is most commonly caused by the rupture of a myocardial infarction.

220. The answer is c. (*Cotran, 5/e, pp 571–575. Rubin, 2/e, pp 511–515, 520.*) Congenital heart defects may or may not have shunting of blood between systemic and pulmonary circulations. Examples of defects with no shunts include coarctation of the aorta, Ebstein malformation (a downward displacement of an abnormal tricuspid valve into an underdeveloped right ventricle), and transposition of the great vessels. Examples of defects that initially involve a left-to-right shunt, from the higher pressure left side to the lower pressure right side, include ventricular septal defects (the most common of all heart defects), atrial septal defects, patent ductus arteriosus, and persistent truncus arteriosus. These defects initially are not cyanotic, but cyanosis may develop later (tardive cyanosis) if the shunt shifts to right to left because of increased pulmonary vascular resistance (Eisenmenger complex). A defect that initially involves a right-to-left shunt is the tetralogy of Fallot. This is the most common cyanotic congenital heart disease of older children and adults.

221. The answer is d. (*Cotran, 5/e, pp 577–578.*) Coarctation of the aorta occurs in 6 to 14 percent of cases of congenital heart disease. In its infantile form, coarctation takes place in the root of the aorta proximal to the ductus arteriosus, which, if patent, serves as a bypass to allow blood flow to the arterial system. Usually, surgical intervention is necessary for infants who have this anomaly, which may cause death soon after birth or within the first year of life.

222. The answer is a. (*Damjanov, 10/e, pp 1400–1410. Cotran, 5/e, pp 476–479.*) In atherosclerosis, primarily a disease of the arterial intima, disintegration of the internal elastic lamina is typical in advanced lesions, and necrosis commonly occurs at the base of the thickened intima. Essential lesions, occurring in the intima, are more numerous in larger than in smaller arteries. Although plaque formations cause little reduction in the size of the lumen of large arteries, atherosclerosis can lead to arterial dilatation and aneurysms. It is a progressive disease that begins early in life. Fatty streaks can be found in some children younger than 1 year of age and all children older than 10 years.

223. The answer is b. (*Damjanov, 10/e, pp 1405–1406. Cotran, 5/e, pp 474–476.*) Hypercholesterolemia (serum cholesterol greater than 200 to 230 mg/dL) is one of the major risk factors for development of atherosclerosis. Hypercholesterolemia is associated with elevated low-density lipoprotein (LDL), which contains a high proportion of cholesterol. Men with cholesterol levels above 240 mg/dL have a threefold risk of death from myocardial infarct compared with men with cholesterol below 200. However, in contrast to the LDL fraction, the HDL fraction is inversely related to the incidence of coronary heart disease (CHD). The Framingham heart study found that low plasma levels of HDL are a potent risk factor for coronary artery disease. HDL levels are increased by exercise, small amounts of alcohol, and administration of estrogens, but cigarette smoking depresses plasma HDL levels. Other major risk factors for atherosclerosis include hypertension, cigarette smoking, and diabetes.

224. The answer is c. (*Cotran, 5/e, pp 511–512.*) Kaposi's sarcoma (KS) comprises four distinct forms. The classic, or European, form has been known since 1862. It occurs in older men of Eastern European or Mediterranean origin (predominantly Italian or Jewish) and is characterized by purple maculopapular skin lesions of the lower extremities and visceral involvement in only 10 percent of cases. The African form occurs in younger people and is more aggressive; it often involves lymph nodes in children. The rare form in immunosuppressed recipients of renal transplants often regresses when immunosuppression stops. In the epidemic form associated with AIDS, skin lesions may occur anywhere and include dissemination to mucous membranes, GI tract, lymph nodes, and viscera. Histologic determination is difficult, but all four clinical types appear similar. Early, irregular, dilated epidermal vascular spaces, extravasated red cells, and hemosiderin (like granulation tissue or stasis dermatitis) are characteristic. Later, more characteristic lesions show spindle cells around slit-spaces that are angular and contain red cells—a picture like that of angiosarcoma. The tumor cells are almost certainly of vascular endothelial origin (blood vessel or lymphatic or both). This often multifocal disease is rarely fatal, but death may be caused by frequent opportunistic infections or, less often, lymphoma, leukemia, or myeloma. There is depletion of T-helper cells, but T-suppressor cells are normal or increased.

225. The answer is d. (*Damjanov, 10/e, pp 1263–1267.*) Mitral stenosis is most often associated with aortic valve disease and occasionally with tricuspid valve disease, especially in people with antecedent rheumatic fever. Occasionally, both aortic and mitral disease result from atherosclerosis. Pulmonary valvular stenosis is rarely caused by either aortic or mitral disease. Since severe mitral stenosis prevents significant regurgitation, left ventricular enlargement would not be expected. Left atrial enlargement and chronic pulmonary congestion are common in mitral disease.

226. The answer is c. (*Cotran, 5/e, pp 547–550.*) Rheumatic fever (RF) is a systemic disease with the major findings of migratory polyarthritis of large joints, carditis, erythema marginatum of skin (although skin involvement is not very common), subcutaneous nodules, and Sydenham's chorea, a neurologic disorder with involuntary, purposeless, rapid movements, most likely to occur in adolescent females and during pregnancy. There is no relation to Huntington's chorea. Fever is a minor characterization, although quite frequent. Rheumatic nodules may develop over pressure points during the later stages and seldom occur in cases without cardiac involvement. RF usually follows a pharyngeal infection with group A β-hemolytic streptococci because of an autoimmune mechanism based on cross-reactions between cardiac antigens and antibodies evoked by one of the many streptococcal antigens, e.g., streptococcal M protein. Immunofluorescence shows immunoglobulins and complement along sarcolemmal sheaths of cardiac myofibers, but Aschoff bodies seldom contain immunoglobulins or complement.

227. The answer is c. *(Cotran, 5/e, pp 575–576. Rubin, 2/e, p 517.)* Tetralogy of Fallot consists of subaortic ventricular septal defect, obstruction to right ventricular outflow, aortic override of the ventricular septal defect (aortic dextroposition), and moderate right ventricular hypertrophy. The obstruction to right ventricular outflow may be caused by infundibular stenosis of the right ventricle or stenosis of the pulmonic valve. A right-sided aorta occurs in about 25 percent of cases with tetralogy. Most patients are cyanotic from birth or develop cyanosis by the end of the first year of life, since even mild obstruction to right ventricular outflow is progressive. Tetralogy of Fallot is the most common cause of cyanosis after 1 year of age and causes 10 percent of all forms of congenital heart disease. Hypoxic attacks and syncope are serious complications, forming the commonest mode of death from this disease during infancy and childhood. Other complications include infectious endocarditis, paradoxical embolism, polycythemia, and cerebral infarction or abscess.

228–229. The answers are: 228-g, 229-i. *(Cotran, 5/e, pp 488–489, 498, 502–503. Rubin, 2/e, pp 483–486.)* Many of the symptoms produced by the inflammatory disorders of blood vessels are characteristic and depend upon the type of vessel that is affected. Takayasu's arteritis, or "pulseless disease," is seen in young women, affects large and medium arteries, especially the aortic arch and its larger branches, and results in decreased pulse and blood pressure in the upper extremities. Aneurysms are common in the abdominal and distal thoracic aorta, especially in older patients. There may be thrombosis of vessels that arise from the aortic arch, and many cases demonstrate the aortic arch syndrome. Marked weakening of the pulses in the upper extremities is noted. This arteritis has been known as aortic arch syndrome, primary aortitis, and giant cell arteritis of the aorta, in addition to other synonyms. The decreased blood flow may produce ocular problems, which can also be seen in patients with a different disorder called giant cell arteritis. This type of vasculitis most commonly affects the temporal artery (temporal arteritis). Visual symptoms may produce permanent blindness unless the patient is treated with corticosteroids. Patients also develop painful, tender nodules in the temporal area. Kawasaki's disease (mucocutaneous lymph node syndrome) predominately affects children, usually boys under the age of four. The disease was first recognized in Japan, but there have been several outbreaks in the continental US and in Hawaii. It is characterized by high fever, skin rash, conjunctival and oral erythema, and lymphadenitis. Coronary arteritis may result in aneurysms and is associated with myocarditis and sometimes infarction.

Microscopic polyarteritis commonly involves glomerular and pulmonary capillaries and may produce hematuria, hemoptysis, and renal failure. Patients are often positive for anti-neutrophil cytoplasmic antibodies (ANCA), mainly p-ANCA. Histologic sections reveal segmental fibrinoid necrosis. Patients with Wegener's granulomatosis may also develop similar symptoms; however, if the kidney is involved, the patients will be positive for c-ANCA. Medial calcific sclerosis (Mönckeberg's arteriosclerosis) is characterized by dystrophic calcification in the tunica media of muscular arteries. This calcification produces "pipestem" arteries and generally occurs in older persons. It does not lead to clinical symptoms, because the diameter of lumen of the effected vessel is not decreased in size. Thromboangiitis obliterans (Buerger's disease) is occlusion of arteries of the distal arms and legs by a proliferative inflammatory process. This abnormality occurs in young and middle-aged male cigarette smokers and is often associated with HLA-A9, B5 genotypes. Cystic medial necrosis is the focal loss of elastic and muscle fibers in the media of blood vessels. This degeneration produces spaces filled with myxoid material and is seen in patients with hypertension, dissecting aneurysms, and Marfan's syndrome. Malignant hypertension refers to dramatic elevations in systolic and diastolic blood pressure that produces symptomatic disease of the brain, heart, or kidney. At first the small muscular arteries display cell necrosis and deposition of plasma proteins in the vessel wall. This combination is called fibrinoid necrosis. It is followed by smooth muscle proliferation, which results in hyperplastic arteriolosclerosis. The effected blood vessels histologically have an "onion-skin" appearance. Hyaline arteriosclerosis is caused by the accumulation of plasma proteins in the vessel wall and is associated with benign hypertension, benign nephrosclerosis, diabetes, and the aging process.

230–231. The answers are: 230-d and 231-g. (*Cotran, 5/e, pp 506–512, 569–570. Rubin, 2/e, pp 551–552.*) Tumors of vessels may originate from either blood vessels or lymphatics and may be either benign or malignant.

Glomus tumors (glomangiomas) are exquisitely painful tumors derived from the glomus body and are found in the distal regions of the fingers and toes, possibly in a subungual location. Histologic section reveals vascular spaces that are lined by nests of uniform cells. Hemangiomas, benign tumors of blood vessels, may be subclassified into capillary hemangiomas and cavernous hemangiomas. "Birthmarks" are caused by capillary hemangiomas, while port wine stains are caused by cavernous hemangiomas of the skin. The juvenile (strawberry) hemangioma is a fast-growing lesion appearing in the first few months of life but it regresses completely by the age of 5. Cystic hygromas are cystic lymphangiomas, typically occurring in the neck or axilla. They may be found in patients with Turner's syndrome. Angiosarcomas are rare malignant tumors of blood vessels. In the liver they have been related to exposure to thorium dioxide (Thorotrast), arsenic, and vinyl chloride.

Most tumors involving the heart are secondary to metastases, most commonly from bronchogenic carcinoma or breast carcinoma, and usually involve the pericardium. Primary tumors of the heart are quite rare; the most common in the adult is the myxoma. These tumors occur most often in the left atrium, and if pedunculated they may interfere with the mitral valve by a "ball-valve" effect. Histologically, they are composed of stellate cells in a loose myxoid background. Rhabdomyomas are the most common primary cardiac tumor in infants and children and often occur in association with tuberous sclerosis. Histologically so-called spider cells may be seen. Papillary fibroelastomas usually are incidental lesions found at the time of autopsy and are probably hamartomas rather than true neoplasms.

RESPIRATORY SYSTEM

Questions

DIRECTIONS: Each question below contains five suggested responses. Select the **one best** response to each question.

232. Shown in the photomicrograph below is a section of alveolar tissue that was taken at autopsy of a 4-day-old premature infant. The pathologic process that is evident is consistent with

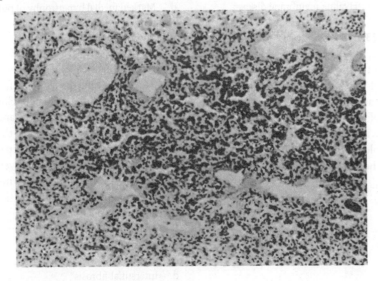

 a. Pneumococcal pneumonia
 b. Congenital pulmonary cystic malformation
 c. Extralobar pulmonary sequestration
 d. Primary fungal pneumonitis
 e. Respiratory distress syndrome (hyaline membrane disease)

233. A 7-year-old boy accidentally inhales a small peanut (he was trying to see if it would fit inside his nose), and the peanut lodges in one of his bronchi. A chest X-ray reveals the mediastinum to be shifted toward the side of the obstruction. The best description for the lung changes that result from this obstruction is

a. Absorptive atelectasis
b. Compression atelectasis
c. Contraction atelectasis
d. Patchy atelectasis
e. Hyaline membrane disease

234. A 47-year-old male dies suddenly five days following major surgery. At autopsy a large blood clot is found obstructing the bifurcation of the pulmonary arteries. No gross abnormalities are found within the heart. The pulmonary blood clot most likely originated in the

a. Femoral artery
b. Popliteal artery
c. Superficial leg veins
d. Deep leg veins
e. Tricuspid valve

235. A young woman succumbed after an 8-month course of severe dyspnea, fatigue, and cyanosis that followed an uneventful delivery of a healthy infant. At necropsy, small atheromas were present in the large and small branches of the pulmonary arteries. Which of the following findings can be predicted in the histologic slides of the lungs?

a. Diffuse hemorrhage and infarctions
b. Diffuse alveolar hyaline membranes
c. Severe atelectasis and edema
d. Marked medial hypertrophy of pulmonary arterioles
e. Multiple pulmonary emboli

236. A 19-year-old female presents with urticaria that developed after she took aspirin for a headache. She has a history of chronic rhinitis, and physical examination reveals the presence of nasal polyps. This patient is at an increased risk of developing which one of the following pulmonary diseases following the ingestion of aspirin?

a. Asthma
b. Chronic bronchitis
c. Emphysema
d. Interstitial fibrosis
e. Pulmonary hypertension

237. Alpha$_1$-antitrypsin deficiency is associated with

a. Thalassemia
b. Nephrotic syndrome
c. Panlobular emphysema
d. Centrilobular emphysema
e. Anthracosis

238. A 24-year-old man who is being evaluated for infertility complains of recurrent sinusitis and a productive cough. He is found to be sterile, and situs inversus of his organs is noted. The most likely diagnosis for his pulmonary disease is

a. Asthma
b. Bronchiolitis
c. Bronchiectasis
d. Chronic bronchitis
e. Emphysema

239. A 25-year-old female presents with fever, malaise, headaches, and muscle pain (myalgia). A chest X-ray reveals bilateral infiltrates. You draw a tube of blood in this patient (the tube contains anti-coagulant) and place the tube in a cup of ice. After the blood has cooled, you notice that the red cells have agglutinated (not clotted). This agglutination goes away after you warm up the tube of blood. This patient's illness is most likely due to infection with

a. Influenza A virus
b. *Mycoplasma pneumonia*
c. *Streptococcal pneumonia*
d. *Pneumocystis pneumonia*
e. *Mycobacteria tuberculosis*

240. Acute lymphoblastic leukemia was diagnosed in a 10-year-old child. When this child later developed a patchy pulmonary infiltrate and respiratory insufficiency, a lung biopsy was performed. The material obtained by biopsy was then stained with Gomori's methenamine-silver stain and is shown in the photomicrograph below. In consideration of the patient's signs and microscopic evaluations, the prognosis is now complicated by

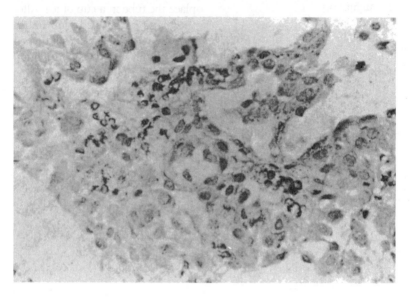

a. Pseudomonas pneumonia
b. Aspergillus pneumonia
c. *Pneumocystis carinii* pneumonia
d. Pneumococcal pneumonia
e. Influenza pneumonia

241. A routine chest X-ray performed on an asymptomatic adult male patient who works at sandblasting reveals a fine nodularity in the upper zones of the lungs and "eggshell" calcification of the hilar lymph nodes. His serum calcium level is 9.8 mg/dl, while his total protein is 7.2 g/dL. He denies any history of drug use or cigarette smoking. A biopsy from his lung reveals birefringent particles within macrophages. This material is most likely to be

a. Asbestos
b. Beryllium
c. Carbon
d. Silica
e. Talc

242. The photomicrograph of the bronchial washing specimen shown below depicts

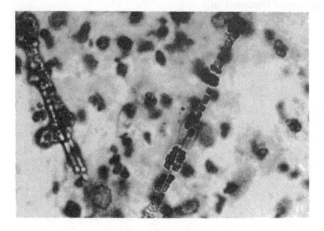

a. Schaumann bodies
b. Ferruginous bodies
c. Cholesterol crystals
d. *Candida* species
e. Silica particles

243. A 61-year-old male presents with increasing shortness of breath. A chest X-ray reveals a diffuse pulmonary infiltrate, while a transbronchial biopsy reveals fibrosis of the walls of the alveoli, many of which contain sheets of "desquamated" cells. Which of the following would be the best therapy for this patient?

a. Theophylline
b. Steroids
c. Antibiotics
d. Isoniazid
e. Symptomatic treatment only

244. Sections of the lung from a patient with Wegener's granulomatosis who presents clinically with hemoptysis are most likely to show

a. Atypical lymphocytes invading blood vessels
b. Granulomatous inflammation of blood vessels with numerous eosinophils
c. Granulomatous inflammation of bronchi with aspergillus
d. Large, serpiginous necrosis with peripheral, palisading macrophages
e. Necrotizing hemorrhagic interstitial pneumonitis

245. A 45-year-old man presents with shortness of breath, cough with mucoid sputum, and some weight loss and has diffuse, bilateral alveolar infiltrates on chest roentgenogram. Pulmonary function tests reveal decreased diffusing capacity and hypoxemia. The patient had worked for several years at grinding aluminum. The photomicrograph below is from a lung biopsy. Your diagnosis is

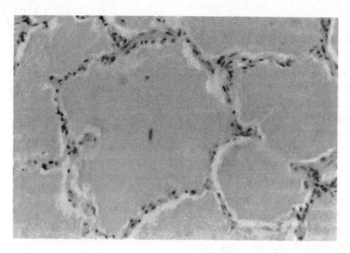

a. *Pneumocystis carinii* pneumonia
b. Diffuse alveolar damage (DAD)
c. Pulmonary edema
d. Pulmonary alveolar proteinosis (PAP)
e. Lipid pneumonia

246. A 34-year-old male presents with the sudden development of malaise along with dyspnea, fever, and a cough. You discover that approximately 5 hours prior to developing these symptoms he had been working with moldy hay, and this exposure led to the production of his symptoms. What is your diagnosis?

a. Farmer's lung
b. Bagassosis
c. Byssinosis
d. Progressive massive fibrosis
e. Pigeon breeder's disease

247. Horner's syndrome is associated with

a. Lymphangitis carcinomatosa
b. Bronchial carcinoid
c. Exophthalmos
d. Tumor of the superior sulcus
e. Thoracocervical venous dilatation

248. A 3 cm mass is found in the right upper lobe (RUL) of a 48-year-old male long-term smoker during a routine physical examination. Histologic examination of a transbronchial biopsy specimen reveals infiltrating groups of cells with scant cytoplasm. No glandular structures or keratin production are seen. The nuclei of these cells are small, round, and do not appear to have nucleoli. Electron microscopy reveals membrane-bound dense core neurosecretory granules. What is your diagnosis?

a. Adenocarcinoma
b. Hamartoma
c. Large cell undifferentiated carcinoma
d. Small cell carcinoma
e. Squamous cell carcinoma

249. A 49-year-old male presents with increasing shortness of breath, and a chest X-ray reveals bilateral pleural effusions. This fluid is tapped, and laboratory examination reveals a milky pleural fluid composed of finely emulsified fats. This fluid is most likely the result of

a. Congestive heart failure
b. A ruptured aortic aneurysm
c. Lymphatic obstruction by tumor
d. Suppurative infection of adjacent lung
e. Collagen-vascular disease

250. The condition seen below in the gross photograph of a sagittal section of the lung may occur in which of the following?

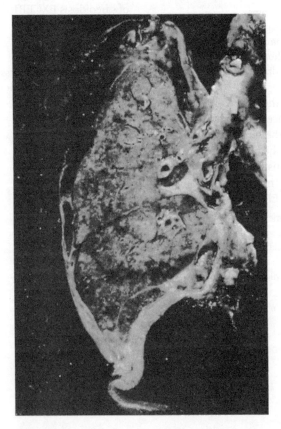

a. Squamous cell carcinoma
b. Oat cell carcinoma
c. Metastatic carcinoma
d. Benign spindle cell mesothelioma
e. Malignant mesothelioma

251. Common tumors or cysts in the superior mediastinum include

a. Schwannoma
b. Bronchogenic cyst
c. Thymoma
d. Neurofibroma
e. Pericardial cyst

252. All the following conditions can produce a histopathologic condition in the lungs of adults that is similar to the histopathology of respiratory distress syndrome of the newborn (hyaline membrane disease) EXCEPT

a. Viral pneumonia
b. Uremia
c. Pulmonary irradiation
d. Severe bacterial infection
e. Tuberculosis

253. All the following are presently used clinically for the diagnosis of sarcoidosis EXCEPT

a. Chest x-ray
b. Kveim skin test
c. Conjunctival biopsy
d. Cultures of affected tissue
e. Blood levels of angiotensin-converting enzyme

DIRECTIONS: Each group of questions below consists of lettered headings followed by a set of numbered items. For each numbered item select the **one** lettered heading with which it is **most** closely associated. Each lettered heading may be used **once, more than once, or not at all**.

Questions 254–255

Match each of the following clinical scenarios with the most likely organism that caused the abnormality.

a. *Actinomyces israelii*
b. *Corynebacterium diphtheriae*
c. *Gardnerella vaginalis*
d. *Klebsiella pneumoniae*
e. *Legionella pneumophila*
f. *Listeria monocytogenes*
g. *Nocardia asteroides*
h. *Pneumocystis carinii*
i. *Staphylococcus aureus*
j. *Streptococcus pneumoniae*

254. A 45-year-old male smoker presents with acute onset of fever, hemoptysis, and a nonproductive cough. A chest X-ray reveals a dense infiltrate in the right lower lobe that is consistent with a confluent bronchopneumonia. Sputum cultures were unremarkable, but direct immunofluorescence and silver staining of lung tissue reveal an aerobic bacillus. It was discovered that this individual's infection was acquired by the inhalation of infected aerosols from the air-conditioning system of the building where he worked.

255. A 33-year-old male in an underdeveloped country presents with a markedly edematous right foot that has multiple draining sinuses. A Gram stain from one of these draining sinuses reveal gram-positive filamentous bacteria that are partially acid fast.

Questions 256–257

Match each of the following clinical scenarios with the correct diagnosis from the following list.

a. Adenocarcinoma
b. Bronchioloalveolar carcinoma
c. Carcinoid
d. Fibroma
e. Hamartoma
f. Hemangioma
g. Large cell carcinoma
h. Leiomyoma
i. Lipoma
j. Small cell carcinoma
k. Squamous cell carcinoma

256. During a routine physical examination a 43-year-old male is found to have a 2.5 cm "coin" in the peripheral portion of his right upper lobe (RUL). Several sputum samples sent for cytology are unremarkable, and a bronchoscopic examination is also unremarkable. Surgery is performed and the mass is resected. Histologic examination reveals lobules of connective tissue that contain mature hyaline cartilage. These lobules are separated by clefts that are lined by respiratory epithelium.

257. A 39-year-old female presents with a cough and increasing shortness of breath. A chest X-ray is interpreted by the radiologist as showing a right lower lobe (RLL) pneumonia. No mass lesions are seen. She is treated with antibiotics, but her symptoms do not improve. On her return visit, the area of consolidation appears to be increased. Bronchoscopy is performed. No bronchial masses are seen, but a transbronchial biopsy is obtained in an area of mucosal erythema in the RLL. After the diagnosis is made, her RLL is removed and a section from this specimen reveals well-differentiated mucus-secreting columnar epithelial cells that infiltrate from alveolus to alveolus.

RESPIRATORY SYSTEM

Answers

232. The answer is e. *(Damjanov, 10/e, pp 1473–1483. Cotran, 5/e, pp 444–446.)* The photomicrograph shows classic hyaline membranes that are coating alveolar sacs and ducts and is diagnostic of the respiratory distress syndrome of the newborn. The eosinophilic, fibrin-like material is related to the alveolar surfactants. Atelectasis is usually also present, especially in premature infants. The deposited material appears not to form in utero, as it is found in infants who have breathed and is not found in stillborns. There is a direct correlation, however, between severity and the degree of prematurity.

233. The answer is a. *(Cotran, 5/e, pp 675–676.)* Atelectasis refers to lung collapse. It is divided into four types. Absorptive (obstructive) atelectasis results from airway obstruction, such as occurs with mucus, tumors, or foreign bodies. The air within the lungs distal to the obstruction is absorbed, the lung collapses, and the mediastinum then shifts toward the collapsed lung. With compression, atelectasis fluid within the pleural cavity, such as seen with congestive heart failure (CHF), causes increased pleural pressure, which collapses lung tissue. In this instance the mediastinum shifts away from the collapsed lung. In contraction atelectasis fibrosis causes collapse of lung tissue. Patchy atelectasis may result from loss of pulmonary surfactant, which is seen in hyaline membrane disease of the newborn.

234. The answer is d. *(Cotran, 5/e, pp 111–114, 679–680.)* An embolus is an intravascular solid, liquid, or gaseous mass that has been carried by the blood to a site away from where it was formed. Most emboli arise from thrombi and are called thromboemboli. These blood clots, most of which form in the deep veins of the lower extremities, may embolize to the lungs. The majority of small pulmonary emboli do no harm. If they are large enough, however, they may occlude the bifurcation of the pulmonary arteries and cause sudden death. This type of thromboembolus is called a saddle embolus. Arterial emboli most commonly originate within the heart from diseased valves (vegetations) or mural thrombi that are formed following myocardial infarctions. If there is a patent foramen ovale, a venous embolus may cross over through the heart to the arterial circulation producing an arterial (paradoxical) embolus.

There are several causes of non-thrombotic emboli. Fat emboli are associated with severe trauma and fractures of long bones. Fat emboli can be fatal because they can damage the endothelial cells and pneumocytes within the lungs, and produce adult respiratory distress syndrome (ARDS). Air emboli may be formed in decompression sickness, which is called Caisson's disease or the bends. Amniotic fluid emboli are associated with rupture of uterine venous sinuses and are a complication of childbirth. Amniotic fluid emboli may also lead to a fatal disease, disseminated intravascular coagulation (DIC), which is characterized by the combination of intravascular coagulation and hemorrhages. DIC results from the high thromboplastin activity of amniotic fluid.

235. The answer is d. (*Cotran, 5/e, pp 680–682.*) Many pathologic pulmonary changes can be found in the lungs of patients who expire under conditions of progressive, unexplained dyspnea, fatigue, and cyanosis. These changes range from pulmonary fibrosis to hypersensitivity pneumonitis and to recurrent, multiple pulmonary emboli. Furthermore, traditional hospital treatment modalities for progressive pulmonary deterioration (including high oxygen delivery, overhydration, lack of pulmonary ventilation, irregular ventilation by mechanical respiratory assistance [PEEP], and superimposed nosocomially acquired pneumonitis) can complicate pulmonary pathologic findings. However, unremitting, progressive dyspnea, cyanosis, and fatigue in a young woman should suggest the diagnosis of primary pulmonary hypertension. Pulmonary vascular sclerosis is always associated with pulmonary hypertension primary or secondary to other states, such as emphysema and mitral stenosis.

236. The answer is a. (*Cotran, 5/e, pp 683–692.*) Chronic obstructive pulmonary diseases (COPD) are characterized by obstruction to airflow somewhere along the airways. These diseases may affect the bronchus, the bronchiole, or the acinus. Asthma, bronchiectasis, and chronic bronchitis affect primarily the bronchus, while emphysema affects primarily the acinus. Asthma is a pulmonary disease that is caused by excessive bronchoconstriction secondary to airways that are hyper-reactive to numerous stimuli.

Asthma has been divided into extrinsic and intrinsic categories. The extrinsic category includes atopic (allergic) asthma, occupational asthma, and allergic bronchopulmonary aspergillosis. The intrinsic category includes non-reaginic asthma and pharmacologic asthma. The former is related to respiratory tract infections, while the latter is often related to aspirin sensitivity. These aspirin-sensitive patients often have recurrent rhinitis and nasal polyps. In these patients the aspirin initiates an asthmatic attack by inhibiting the cyclooxygenase pathway of arachidonic acid metabolism without affecting the lipoxygenase pathway. This causes the relative excess production of the leukotrienes, which are bronchoconstrictors.

237. The answer is c. (*Cotran, 5/e, pp 683–688.*) Patients who are homozygous for alpha$_1$-antitrypsin deficiency develop severe panlobular emphysema, often before the age of 40. This genetic disorder accounts for about 10 percent of cases of emphysema. Other factors in the pathogenesis of emphysema include air pollution and smoking. This disorder may result from variant alleles involving the Pi (proteinase inhibitor) locus on chromosome 14. Cigarette smoking greatly accelerates the emphysema in the homozygous (Pi ZZ) state.

238. The answer is c. (*Cotran, 5/e, pp 682–694.*) Chronic obstructive pulmonary disease (COPD) is a term that refers to a group of disorders characterized by dyspnea and airway obstruction. The spectrum of COPD includes all the diseases listed in the question. Patients with bronchiectasis have a persistent, productive cough due to abnormally dilated bronchi, which are the result of a chronic necrotizing infection. Patients with Kartagener's syndrome have the triad of bronchiectasis, recurrent sinusitis, and situs inversus. This syndrome is caused by abnormal motility of the cilia, which is due to abnormalities of the dynein arms. Males with this condition tend to be sterile because of the ineffective motility of the tail of the sperm. Patients with asthma suffer from episodic wheezing due to bronchial smooth muscle hyperplasia and excess production of mucus. Extrinsic (allergic) asthma may be related to IgE (type I) immune reactions; intrinsic (nonallergic) asthma may be triggered by infections or drugs. Clinically there is an elevated eosinophil count in the peripheral blood, and Curschmann's spirals and Charcot-Leyden crystals may be found in the sputum. Chronic bronchitis is characterized by a productive cough that is present for at least 3 months in at least 2 consecutive years. There is hyperplasia of mucous glands with hypersecretion due in large part to tobacco smoke. Emphysema is abnormal dilation of the alveoli due to destruction of the alveolar walls. Bronchiolitis is inflammation and scarring of bronchioles due mainly to tobacco smoke and air pollutants.

239. The answer is b. *(Cotran, 5/e, pp 694–699.)* Acute interstitial pneumonia refers to inflammation of the interstitium of the lung that is the result of infection, typically with either *Mycoplasma pneumoniae* or viruses, such as influenza A and B. This type of pneumonia is called primary atypical pneumonia because it is "atypical" when compared to the "typical" bacterial pneumonia, such as produced by *Streptococcal pneumonia.* These bacterial pneumonias are characterized by acute inflammation (neutrophils) within the alveoli. In contrast, acute interstitial pneumonia is characterized by lymphocytes and plasma cells within the interstitium, that is the alveolar septal walls. Viral cytopathic effects, such as inclusion bodies or multinucleated giant cells, may be seen histologically with certain viral infections. Certain viruses produce pneumonia in certain patient groups, that is, respiratory syncytial virus in infants, and adenovirus in military recruits. Infection with *Mycoplasma pneumonia* results in the production of a non-specific cold IgM antibody, which characteristically reacts with red cells having the I antigen. Since most adult red cells have I antigens, blood from a patient with mycoplasma pneumonia will hemagglutinate when cooled. This type of reaction is not seen with infection by either *Pneumocystis pneumonia* or *Mycobacteria tuberculosis.*

240. The answer is c. *(Damjanov, 10/e, pp 1006–1008. Cotran, 5/e, p 357, 694–698.)* Infection by the protozoan *Pneumocystis carinii* is characterized by the presence of oval and helmet-shaped organisms whose capsules are made more visible by use of Gomori's methenamine-silver staining technique. This organism, although it has low virulence, is opportunistic; it is often seen to attack severely ill, immunologically depressed patients. It is frequently the first opportunistic infection to be diagnosed in HIV-1 positive patients, and it is the leading cause of death in patients with AIDS.

241. The answer is d. *(Cotran, 5/e, pp 706–712.)* The pneumoconioses are pulmonary diseases that are caused by non-neoplastic lung reactions to several types of environmental dusts. Silicosis, seen in sandblasters and mine workers, is characterized by fibrosis. Early in the disease there are multiple, very small nodules in the upper zones of the lung, which produces a fine nodularity on X-ray. These areas histologically show fibrosis and birefringent particles. The fibrotic lesions may also be found in the hilar lymph nodes, which can become calcified and have an "eggshell" pattern on X-ray examination. Asbestos results in larger areas of fibrosis, and histologically asbestos (ferruginous) bodies are found. The reactions to coal (carbon) may result in anthracosis, simple coal workers pneumoconioses, which has multiple small nodules, or complicated coal workers pneumoconioses, which has fibrotic nodules that are larger than 2 cm (progressive massive fibrosis). In the chronic state, beryllium elicits a cell-mediated immunity response, seen histologically as noncaseating granulomas. Noncaseating granulomas are also seen in patients with sarcoidosis, a disease that may cause enlargement of the hilar lymph nodes ("potato nodes").

242. The answer is b. (*Damjanov, 10/e, pp 1536–1541. Cotran, 5/e, pp 709–714.*) The segmented or beaded, often dumbbell-shaped bodies are ferruginous bodies that are probably asbestos fibers coated with iron and protein. The term ferruginous body is applied to other inhaled fibers that become iron-coated; however, in a patient with interstitial lung fibrosis or pleural plaques, ferruginous bodies are probably asbestos bodies. The type of asbestos mainly used in America is chrysotile, mined in Canada, and it is much less likely to cause mesothelioma or lung cancer than is crocidolite (blue asbestos), which has limited use and is mined in South Africa. Cigarette smoking potentiates the relatively mild carcinogenic effect of asbestos. Laminated spherical (Schaumann) bodies are found in granulomas of sarcoid and chronic berylliosis.

243. The answer is b. (*Cotran, 5/e, pp 703–706, 714–715.*) Interstitial pulmonary fibrosis (IF) may be a slowly progressive disease with no recognizable etiology. This disease entity has many names, such as chronic interstitial pneumonitis and diffuse fibrosing alveolitis, but the common name is usual interstitial pneumonitis (UIP). The form of this disease that progresses very rapidly is called the Hamman-Rich syndrome. The pathogenesis of UIP involves damage to type I pneumocytes with the subsequent proliferation of type II pneumocytes and secretion of factors by macrophages that cause fibrosis. The end stage form of IF is characterized by large cysts with intervening fibrosis, which imparts the gross appearance of a "honeycomb lung." There are several subtypes of IF which are characterized by their histologic appearance. Lymphocytic interstitial pneumonitis (LIP) has numerous lymphocytes, Giant cell interstitial pneumonitis (GIP) has giant cells, and plasma cell interstitial pneumonitis (PIP) has numerous plasma cells. LIP is seen in patients with Sjögren's syndrome or AIDS and is associated with an increased risk of developing lymphoma. An important subtype is desquamative interstitial pneumonitis (DIP), which is characterized histologically by sheets of cells within the alveoli. This type of IF may respond to the use of steroids. UIP, in contrast, does not respond to therapy, and therefore treatment is symptomatic treatment only. Theophylline is used to treat asthma, antibiotics are used to treat bacterial infections, and INH is used in combination with other drugs to treat tuberculosis.

244. The answer is d. (*Cotran, 5/e, pp 496–497, 717–718.*) The pulmonary hemorrhagic syndromes are characterized by hemorrhage within the alveoli, which may be severe enough to produce hemoptysis. Several of these diseases are associated with blood vessel abnormalities, namely inflammation of the vessels (angiitis). Necrotizing granulomatous arteritis affecting the upper and lower respiratory tracts and the kidneys is seen in patients with Wegener's granulomatosis. These areas of necrosis are characteristically large, serpiginous, and have peripheral palisading of macrophages. In patients with Wegener's granulomatosis the nose, sinus, antrum, and trachea often exhibit ulcerations. Originally lethal, the prognosis is now much improved by immunosuppressive drugs. Eosinophilic granulomatous arteritis occurs is some patients with asthma who have eosinophilic pulmonary infiltrates. This abnormality is called Churg-Strauss syndrome. The areas of necrosis are not large and serpiginous like in Wegener's. Granulomatous inflammation centered around bronchi (bronchocentric granulomatosis) is often related to allergic pulmonary aspergillosis. Lymphomatoid granulomatosis is a disease of middle-aged people that is characterized by an angiocentric and angioinvasive infiltrate of atypical lymphoid cells. Goodpasture's syndrome is characterized by the development of a necrotizing hemorrhagic interstitial pneumonitis and rapidly progressing glomerulonephritis because of antibodies directed against the capillary basement membrane in alveolar septa and glomeruli. A linear IgG immunofluorescence pattern is present, which is characteristic of a type II hypersensitivity reaction. The prognosis for Goodpasture's syndrome has been markedly improved by intensive plasma exchange to remove circulating anti-basement membrane antibodies and by immunosuppressive therapy to inhibit further antibody production.

245. The answer is d. (*Cotran, 5/e, pp 718–719. Rubin, 2/e, pp 580–581.*) The alveolar spaces contain an intensely eosinophilic, proteinaceous, granular substance. Alveolar walls are relatively normal without inflammatory exudate or fibrosis, although type II pneumocytes may be hyperplastic. The process is often patchy, with groups of normal alveoli alternating with groups of affected alveoli. Acicular (cholesterol) clefts and densely eosinophilic bodies (necrotic cells) are found within the granular material. Distinction from edema fluid may be difficult, but PAP alveolar material stains with periodic acid-Schiff (PAS). At low power, alveolar material seen in *P. carinii* pneumonia may also mimic PAP, but with high power the foamy material seen with Pneumocystis is not present in PAP. In PAP the material is surfactant accumulation, either because of overproduction or failure of macrophage clearance. Causes of PAP include occupational exposure to silica or aluminum dusts. It also occurs in immunosuppressed patients and toxic drug reactions and is often associated with infections like nocardia, fungi, and TB (possible impaired macrophage killing). The treatment of choice is bronchoalveolar lavage to remove the proteinaceous debris.

246. The answer is a. (*Cotran, 5/e, pp 707–708, 715–716.*) Hypersensitivity pneumonitis refers to immunologically mediated interstitial lung diseases that are the result of exposure to specific antigens. Affected individuals have an abnormal sensitivity to the antigen. In contrast to asthma, hypersensitivity pneumonitis primarily involves the alveolus. A classic example of a hypersensitivity pneumonitis is Farmer's lung, which is caused by exposure to thermophilic actinomyces that grows on moldy hay. Byssinosis is a hypersensitivity that is caused by inhalation of cotton, flax, or hemp dust. Prolonged exposure causes chronic lung disease with chronic bronchitis, emphysema, and interstitial granulomas. Two other examples of hypersensitivity pneumonitis include byssinosis (caused by exposure to cotton), and Bird-breeder's lung (caused by exposure to bird droppings). Progressive massive fibrosis (PMF) is not a hypersensitivity reaction but is most commonly caused by exposure to coal (coal workers pneumoconioses) or silica.

247. The answer is d. (*Cotran, 5/e, pp 571, 725.*) Horner's syndrome occurs with apical (superior sulcus) tumors of any type (Pancoast tumor). The syndrome is characterized by enophthalmos, ptosis, miosis, and anhidrosis on the same side as the lesion due to invasion of the cervical sympathetic nerves. Involvement of the brachial plexus causes pain and paralysis in the ulnar nerve distribution. Venous dilatation of the upper thorax and neck is seen in the superior vena cava syndrome because of compression or invasion by lung cancer or lymphoma. Lymphangitic carcinomatosis usually results from spread of metastatic tumors within subpleural lymphatics.

248. The answer is d. *(Cotran, 5/e, pp 722–726.)* Lung cancers are classified according to their histologic appearance. First they are divided into two groups based on the size of the tumor cells, namely small-cell carcinomas and non-small cell carcinomas. Small cell carcinomas, also called "oat cell" carcinoma, have scant amounts of cytoplasm, and their nuclei are small, round, and rarely have nucleoli. These malignancies, which are of neuroendocrine origin and display neurosecretory granules on electron microscopy, may cause a variety of paraneoplastic syndromes, such as from the synthesis and secretion of hormones such as ACTH and serotonin. Other effects not well understood on the neuromuscular system include central encephalopathy and Eaton-Lambert syndrome, a myasthenic syndrome resulting from impaired release of acetylcholine and usually associated with pulmonary oat cell carcinoma. Oat cell carcinomas form 20 to 25 percent of primary lung tumors, occur most frequently in middle-aged or older men, have a strong association with cigarette smoking, and carry a poor prognosis. The non-small cell carcinomas are classified as to the differentiation of the tumor cells. Squamous cell carcinomas are characterized by keratin pearl formation, intracytoplasmic keratin, or the formation of intercellular bridges. Adenocarcinomas are characterized by the formation of glandular structures. They typically are found at the periphery of the lung (peripheral carcinomas) and sometimes may be found in an area of previous scar (scar carcinoma). Non-small cell carcinomas of the lung that do have form glands or squamous differentiation are called undifferentiated large cell carcinomas.

A hamartoma is the most common benign tumor of the lung. It is composed mainly of cartilage arranged in a haphazard fashion. Other benign neoplasms of the lung include fibromas (composed of fibroblasts), hemangiomas (composed of blood vessels), and leiomyomas (composed of smooth muscle).

249. The answer is c. *(Cotran, 5/e, pp 728–730.)* The causes of pleural effusions may be inflammatory or noninflammatory. The formation of noninflammatory edema is related to abnormalities involving the Starling forces and may result in the formation of noninflammatory pleural effusions. Increased hydrostatic pressure, such as seen with congestive heart failure, causes hydrothorax, which is a transudate. Decreased oncotic pressure, such as seen with renal disease associated with albuminuria, also causes hydrothorax. Increased intrapleural negative pressure produced by atelectasis causes hydrothorax, while decreased lymphatic drainage, which can be caused by a tumor obstructing lymphatics, produces chylothorax. Chylothorax is characterized by milky fluid that contains finely emulsified fats. An additional type of noninflammatory pleural effusion is hemothorax, which may be caused by trauma or ruptured aortic aneurysm. Inflammatory edema may be caused by increased vascular permeability. Inflammation in the adjacent lung, such as with collagen vascular diseases, produces a serofibrinous exudate. Suppurative inflammation in the adjacent lung may produce a suppurative pleuritis, which is called an empyema.

250. The answer is e. (*Cotran, 5/e, pp 730–732.*) Malignant mesothelioma and adenocarcinoma are two neoplasms that may involve the pleural surfaces as seen in the gross photograph. Malignant mesothelioma arises from the pleural surfaces and develops with significant and chronic exposure to asbestos, usually occupationally incurred. As the malignant mesothelioma spreads, it lines the pleural surfaces including the fissures through the lobes of the lungs and results in a tight and constricting encasement. This restricts the excursions of the lungs during ventilation. Adenocarcinoma of the lung also may invade the pleural surfaces and spread in an advancing manner throughout the pleural lining. The differential diagnosis histologically between an epithelial type of malignant mesothelioma and an adenocarcinoma may be difficult and sometimes impossible without special techniques. A characteristic feature seen by electron microscopy is numerous, long microvilli on the surface of cells from mesotheliomas. Oat cell carcinoma usually arises in the central portions of the lungs near the hilum and does not invade the pleura in a spreading fashion. Benign spindle (fibrous) mesothelioma of the lung arises as a discrete mass that is spherical to ovoid in shape in a subpleural configuration and expands as this localized mass without spread over the surfaces.

251. The answer is c. (*Cotran, 5/e, pp 727–728.*) The superior mediastinum consists of structures cephalad to the pericardial reflection of the heart. Metastatic carcinoma is fairly frequent in the superior mediastinum, arising often from lung or breast primaries, and less frequently from testis or kidney. Bronchogenic and pericardial cysts occur in the middle mediastinum, whereas neurogenic tumors such as neurofibroma and schwannoma are in the posterior mediastinum. Thymoma is found in the anterosuperior mediastinum. Lymphoma, especially Hodgkin's disease, is common in all mediastinal compartments and involves paratracheal lymph nodes in the superior mediastinum. Seminoma and metastatic choriocarcinoma from the testis are not uncommon. Parathyroid tumors and thyroid lesions occupy both the superior and anterior mediastinum. Retrosternal extension of a goiter, presenting as a superior mediastinal mass, is not unusual.

252. The answer is e. (*Damjanov, 10/e, pp 1503–1505. Cotran, 5/e, pp 676–679.*) The presence of hyaline membranes indicates a diagnosis of acute alveolar injury, which can occur in all the conditions mentioned except tuberculosis. Indeed, the alveoli-lining, fibrin-like material may be found in multiple conditions of circulatory compromise and in poor perfusion states, such as hypovolemia; it may also be seen where 100% oxygen has been used for longer than 32 h (e.g., "shock lung" of Vietnam casualties). At autopsy, the lungs are relatively airless and heavy, and this finding is frequently accompanied by pulmonary edema and hemorrhage.

253. The answer is b. (*Henry, 19/e, pp 271, 287, 360. Lever, 7/e, pp 252–256. Cotran, 5/e, pp 712–714.*) Sarcoidosis is a systemic disease characterized by noncaseating granulomas in multiple organs. The diagnosis of sarcoidosis depends upon finding these noncaseating granulomas in commonly affected sites. In 90 percent of cases, bilateral hilar lymphadenopathy or lung involvement is present and can be seen by chest x-ray or transbronchial biopsy. The eye and skin are next most commonly affected, so that both conjunctival and skin biopsies are clinical possibilities. Noncaseating granulomas may be found in multiple infectious diseases, such as fungal infections, but sarcoidosis is not caused by any known organism. Therefore, before the diagnosis of sarcoidosis can be made, cultures must be taken from affected tissues, and there must be no growth of any organism that may produce granulomas. Also in patients with sarcoid, blood levels of angiotensin-converting enzyme are increased, and this may be used as a clinical test. In the past, the Kveim skin test was used to assist in the diagnosis of sarcoid, but since it involves injecting into patients extracts of material from humans, it is no longer used.

254–255. The answers are: 254-e, 255-g. *(Cotran, 5/e, pp 309, 353–354, 694–698. Chandrasoma, 3/e, pp 488, 794, 882–883.)* Pulmonary infections may be caused by bacteria, fungi, viruses, or mycoplasma. Bacterial infections generally result in a polymorphonuclear (neutrophil) response. Bacterial infection of the lung (pneumonia) results in consolidation of the lung, which may be patchy or diffuse. Patchy consolidation of the lung is seen in bronchopneumonia (lobular pneumonia), while diffuse involvement of an entire lobe is seen in lobar pneumonia. Histologically, bronchopneumonia is characterized by multiple, suppurative, neutrophil-rich exudates that filled the bronchi and bronchioles, and spilled over into the adjacent alveolar spaces. In contrast, lobar pneumonia is characterized by four distinct stages: congestion, red hepatization, gray hepatization, and resolution. Legionnaire's disease is caused by the soil organism *Legionella pneumophila*, a weakly gram-negative aerobic bacillus. The disease results from inhalation of infectious aerosols from hot water or air-conditioning systems of buildings (including hospitals); these aerosols contain legionellae, which are deposited in the lung alveoli. Legionellosis ranges from the fulminant pneumonia of Legionnaire's disease (first recognized in Philadelphia, 1976) to the mild, flulike Pontiac fever. Diarrhea, nausea, and vomiting are early symptoms, as well as headache, fever, and often delirium. Chest X-ray shows dense infiltrates, with pulmonary gross findings of a confluent bronchopneumonia with alveoli containing neutrophils and mononuclear phagocytes with many intracytoplasmic bacilli that may be seen by silver staining. Organisms are also detected by immunofluorescent staining and culture of lung tissue, pleural fluid, or transtracheal aspirate, but not sputum culture since other organisms overgrow legionellae. Organisms cannot be visualized by routine stains, so instead a Dieterle silver stain is used. Erythromycin is the favored therapy.

Many other types of bacteria can infect the lungs. *Streptococcus pneumoniae* (pneumococcus) is the major cause of community-acquired pneumonia. It typically produces a lobar pneumonia and is the major cause of this type of pneumonia. Gram stain of the sputum of infected individuals reveals typical lancet-shaped gram-positive diplococci surrounded by an unstained capsule. *Staphylococcus aureus* is a gram-positive coccus that is associated with the formation of multiple abscesses within the lungs. *Klebsiella pneumoniae* has a prominent capsule and is characterized by its mucoid appearance. The most common infection in patients with AIDS is *Pneumocystis carinii*. Microscopically, in patients with *Pneumocystis carinii* pneumonia the alveoli are filled with a foamy protein rich fluid. The organisms are best seen with silver stains and appear as cup or boat-shaped cyst forms that have central dark dots.

Nocardia (*Nocardia asteroides*) and *Actinomyces* species are classified as filamentous soil bacteria, although they are often described among the fungi. *Actinomyces israelii* is a normal inhabitant of the mouth; it can be seen in the crypts of tonsillectomy specimens. Actinomyces is a branched, filamentous gram-positive bacteria. Two forms of disease produced by Actinomyces are cervicofacial actinomyces and pelvic actinomyces. The former consists of an indurated (lumpy) jaw with multiple draining fistulas or abscesses. Small yellow colonies may be seen in the draining material, these being called sulfur granules. Histologic section will reveal tangled masses of gram-positive filamentous bacteria. Cultures of actinomyces grow as white masses with a domed surface, which is called a "molar tooth" appearance. Another filamentous gram-positive bacteria is *Nocardia asteroides*. A characteristic that helps to differentiate these two is the fact that nocardia is partially acid fast. "Partial" means using weak mineral acids in the acid fast stain. Nocardiae are aerobic and acid-fast in contrast to Actinomyces, which are strict anaerobes and not acid-fast. Inhaled nocardial bacteria produce lung or skin infections. Progressive pneumonia with purulent sputum and abscesses is suggestive of nocardiosis, especially if dissemination to brain or subcutaneous tissue occurs. Nocardia is also one cause of mycetoma, a form of chronic inflammation of the skin that causes indurated abscesses with multiple draining sinuses. Patients developing nocardiosis are often immunosuppressed, and transplant rejection, steroid therapy, AIDS, and alveolar proteinosis are often antecedent. Organisms in sputum, pus, or bronchial lavage specimens are gram-positive. A modified acid-fast stain should be used for diagnosis.

Corynebacterium diphtheriae is a small, pleomorphic, gram-positive bacillus, which may have club-shaped swellings at either pole. These rods tend to arrange themselves at right angles producing characteristic V or Y configurations described as "Chinese characters." *C. diphtheriae* produces a toxin that blocks protein synthesis by causing irreversible inactivation of elongation factor 2 (EF-2). This toxin can produce a pseudomembrane covering the larynx, which is difficult to peel away without causing bleeding, and heart damage with fatty change. *Gardnerella vaginalis* is a gram-positive bacillus that is part of the normal vaginal flora. It is, however, a cause of nonspecific vaginitis and can produce a characteristic appearance in PAP smears in which vaginal epithelial cells are covered with bacteria. These cells are called "clue cells." Finally, *Listeria monocytogenes* is a short, gram-positive, nonspore-forming bacillus that can produce neonatal disease or can result in stillbirth. Characteristics that are unique to Listeria include a tumbling motility on hanging drop and an umbrella-shaped motility pattern when a specimen is stabbed into a test tube agar slant.

256–257. The answers are: 256-e, 257-b. (*Damjanov, 10/e, pp 1541–1545. Cotran, 5/e, pp 725–727.*) Pulmonary hamartomas, although infrequent, are still the most common of all benign lung tumors. Hamartomas consist of various tissues normally found in the organ where they develop, but in abnormal amounts and arrangements. In the lung they consist of lobules of connective tissue often containing mature cartilage, fat, or fibrous tissue and separated by clefts lined by entrapped respiratory epithelium. The peak incidence is at age 60, and the tumor is usually found as a well-circumscribed, peripheral, "coin" lesion on routine chest X-ray. Unless the radiographic findings are pathognomonic of hamartoma with "popcorn ball" calcifications, the lesion should be excised or at least carefully followed. Conservative excision is curative.

One type of bronchogenic carcinoma that has unique characteristics is bronchioloalveolar carcinoma (BAC). This tumor is characterized by well-differentiated, mucus-secreting, columnar epithelial cells that infiltrate along the alveolar walls and spread from alveolus to alveolus through the pores of Kohn. This pneumonic spread can be mistaken for pneumonia with a chest X-ray. These tumors, which comprise about 2 to 5 percent of bronchogenic carcinomas, do not arise from the major bronchi. Instead they are thought to arise in terminal bronchioles from Clara cells. Even though these tumors may be multiple, they are well-differentiated and have a good prognosis.

Small-cell carcinomas are undifferentiated malignancies that are of neuroendocrine origin and display neurosecretory granules on electron microscopy. The malignant cells have scant amounts of cytoplasm, and their nuclei are small, round, and rarely have nucleoli. Squamous cell carcinomas histologically reveal keratin pearl formation, intracytoplasmic keratin, or the formation of intercellular bridges. Adenocarcinomas are characterized by the formation of glandular structures. Non-small cell carcinomas of the lung that do have form glands or have squamous differentiation are called undifferentiated large cell carcinomas. Bronchial carcinoids are tumors of low-grade malignancy with neuroendocrine differentiation confirmed by immunostaining for neuron-specific enolase, serotonin, calcitonin, or bombesin. They form intrabronchial polypoid growths but most of the tumor mass lies outside the bronchus. Most arise in central bronchi but 20 percent arise in small bronchi and appear as peripheral lung nodules. Surgical excision is curative in at least 90 percent, but 10 percent of carcinoids are aggressive with local invasion or metastases.

GASTROINTESTINAL SYSTEM

Questions

DIRECTIONS: Each question below contains five suggested responses. Select the **one best** response to each question.

258. A 48-year-old male living in an underdeveloped country presents with pain in the left side of his face. Physical examination reveals a large, indurated area involving the left side of his jaw with multiple sinuses draining pus. This draining material contains a few scattered small yellow granules. This lesion is most likely caused by an infection with

a. *Streptococcus pyogenes*
b. *Borrelia vincentii*
c. *Corynebacterium diphtheriae*
d. *Klebsiella rhinoscleromatis*
e. *Actinomyces israelii*

259. A 24-year-old female presents after having several "attacks" that last for about 24 hours. She states that during these "attacks" she develops nausea, vomiting, vertigo, and ringing in her ears. Physical examination reveals a sensorineural hearing loss. The pathology of her condition involves

a. Acute suppurative inflammation
b. Dilatation of the cochlear duct and saccule
c. A cyst of the middle ear filled with keratin
d. A tumor of the middle ear composed of lobules of cells in a highly vascular stroma
e. New bone formation around the stapes and the oval window

260. Carcinoma of the oral cavity

a. Is predominantly adenocarcinoma in type
b. Is more common in females
c. Is predisposed to by hairy leukoplasia
d. Is predisposed to by erythroplasia
e. Occurs most frequently on the hard palate

261. The lesion shown in the photomicrograph below was removed from a patient's nasal cavity. With no age given and at this low magnification, the most likely diagnosis is

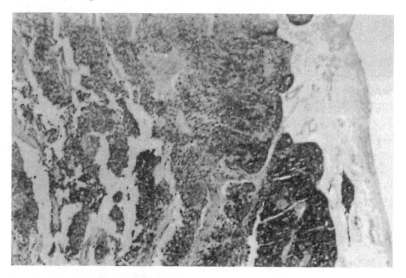

a. Adenocarcinoma
b. Nasal glioma
c. Olfactory neuroblastoma
d. Nasopharyngeal angiofibroma
e. Multiple myeloma

262. A 37-year-old woman presents with a recurrent swelling in her left upper eyelid. The lesion is biopsied by an ophthalmologist, and a section from that specimen, seen in the photomicrograph below, is characteristic of a

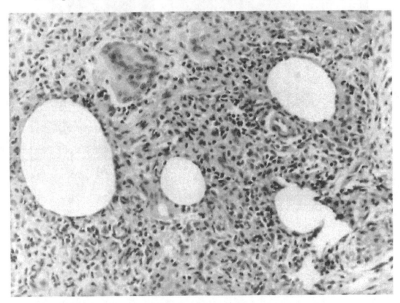

a. Chalazion
b. Hordeolum
c. Xanthelasma
d. Hydrocystoma
e. Sebaceous carcinoma

263. The lesion seen in the photomicrograph below is referred to as

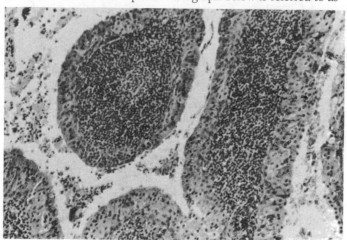

a. Adenoid cystic carcinoma
b. Lymphoepithelioma
c. Thyroglossal duct neoplasm
d. Warthin's tumor
e. Sebaceous lymphadenoma

264. Tumors of the salivary glands are correctly characterized by which of the following statements?

a. They are principally mesenchymal in origin
b. They metastasize early and pursue a rapid course when malignant
c. They tend to have a similar clinical presentation regardless of histologic pattern
d. They are less often malignant in the minor salivary glands than in the parotid
e. They are more common in children than adults

265. A 49-year-old female presents with increasing problems swallowing food (progressive dysphagia). X-ray studies with contrast reveal that she has a markedly dilated esophagus above the level of the lower esophageal sphincter (LES). No lesions are seen within the lumen of the esophagus. This patient's symptoms are most likely caused by

a. Decreased LES resting pressure
b. Absence of myenteric plexus in the body of esophagus
c. Absence of myenteric plexus at the LES
d. Absence of submucosal plexus in the body of esophagus
e. Absence of submucosal plexus at the LES

266. A 45-year-old male alcoholic vomits blood and is hypotensive. The most likely cause of his bleeding episode is related to

a. Achalasia
b. Plummer-Vinson syndrome
c. Sliding hiatal hernia
d. Zenker's diverticula
e. Esophageal varices

267. The photomicrograph below shows an esophageal biopsy taken 10 cm above the lower esophageal sphincter. The condition illustrated

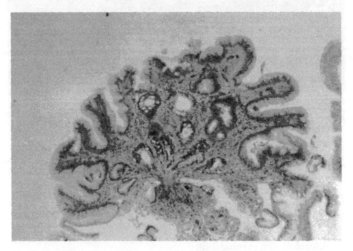

a. Is usually congenital in origin
b. Results from loss of esophageal myenteric ganglion cells
c. Is seen as a white patch at endoscopy
d. Increases the risk of carcinoma by a factor of 30 to 40
e. Is a common precursor of squamous cell carcinoma

268. A 51-year-old male presents with epigastric pain that is lessened whenever he eats. A gastroscopy is performed to evaluate these gastric symptoms and a solitary gastric ulcer is seen. This ulcer is round and has punched-out straight walls. The margins of the ulcer are slightly elevated, and gastric rugae radiate outward from the ulcer. Based on these findings, in order to relieve the epigastric pain this patient should

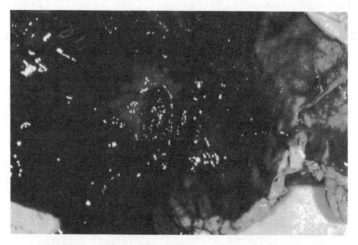

a. Take indomethacin twice a day
b. Abstain from smoking
c. Eat only two meals per day
d. Drink alcohol with evening meal
e. Have surgery to resect the ulcer

269. Gastric tumors with the histologic appearance illustrated in the photomicrograph below

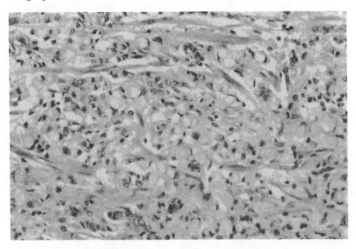

a. Usually fall into the category of early gastric carcinoma
b. Are most commonly located in the cardia
c. Often show a marked desmoplastic response
d. Carry a favorable prognosis
e. Belong to the category of neuroendocrine tumors

270. The abnormality of the ileum illustrated below

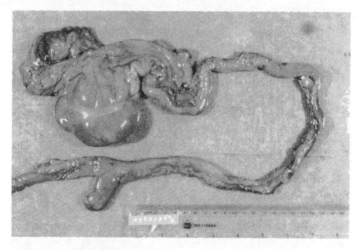

a. Is present in approximately 20 percent of normal persons
b. Is lined by heterotopic gastric mucosa in less than 2 percent of cases
c. Often shows mucosal ulceration
d. Is related to a persistence of the vitello-intestinal duct
e. Usually arises from the mesenteric border of the ileum

271. A 25-year-old schoolteacher was well until she attended a church bazaar where she heartily ate barbecued turkey. The following day she developed bloody diarrhea, crampy pain, and tenesmus. A gastroenterologist who did not take a history took a colon biopsy specimen that showed mucosal edema, congestion, and numerous lymphoid cells in the lamina propria. Which of the following differential diagnoses would apply?

a. Staphylococcal gastroenteritis vs. Crohn's disease
b. Viral gastroenteritis vs. acute diverticulitis
c. Colonic endometriosis vs. amebic dysentery
d. Early ulcerative colitis vs. salmonella colitis
e. Bleeding hemorrhoids vs. Meckel's diverticulitis

272. A 10-month old, previously healthy, male infant develops a severe, watery diarrhea 2 days after visiting the pediatrician for a routine checkup. The most likely diagnosis is

a. Rotavirus infection
b. Enterotoxigenic *E. coli* infection
c. *Entamoeba histolytica* infection
d. Lactase deficiency
e. Ulcerative colitis

273. True statements regarding celiac disease (nontropical sprue) include that

a. There is a strong association with HLA-B8 and HLA-DQw2 antigens
b. Severity of disease often correlates strongly with serum level of antibody to gliadin
c. Malignancy is unassociated
d. Many of the mucosal inflammatory cells express surface IgG antigliadin
e. The distal small bowel shows the most severe involvement

274. The appearance of the small intestinal mucosa illustrated in the photomicrograph below indicates

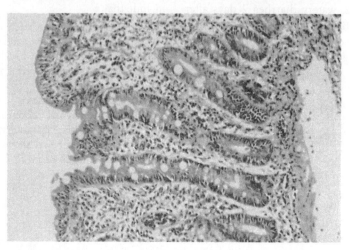

a. Small intestinal lymphoma
b. Whipple's disease
c. Celiac disease
d. Crohn's disease
e. *Giardia lamblia* infestation

275. Two subtotal colectomy specimens are sent to the laboratory with both showing a hemorrhagic cobblestone appearance of the mucosa. One, however, shows longitudinal grooving of the surface, which suggests

a. Ischemic bowel disease
b. Multiple polyposis syndrome
c. Ulcerative colitis
d. Crohn's disease
e. Intestinal tuberculosis

276. A distinguishing feature when comparing ulcerative colitis with Crohn's disease is

a. Colonic involvement
b. Possible malignant transformation
c. Arthritis
d. Fistula formation
e. Absence of granulomas

277. The lesion shown in the colon in the photograph below

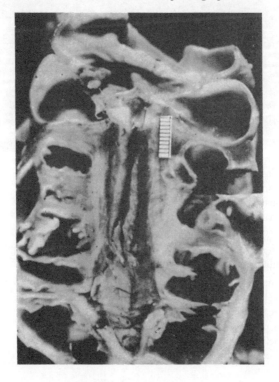

a. Is most prevalent under 50 years of age
b. Occurs most often in the ascending and transverse segments when it occurs in the colon
c. Occurs more often in the small intestine than the colon
d. Is more common in males
e. Is premalignant

278. During routine colonoscopy of a 65-year-old male, a 2mm "dew-drop"-like polyp is found in the sigmoid colon. A biopsy of this lesion is seen in the associated picture. What is the best diagnosis?

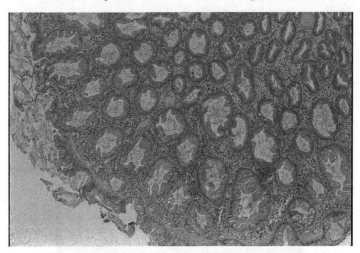

a. Hyperplastic polyp
b. Hamartomatous polyp
c. Inflammatory polyp
d. Adenomatous polyp
e. Lymphoid polyp

279. Familial polyposis coli is characterized by

a. Autosomal recessive pattern of inheritance
b. Multiple hamartomatous polyps throughout the colon
c. 100 percent risk of carcinoma
d. An association with fibromatosis and multiple osteomas
e. An association with tumors of the central nervous system

280. An 18-year-old woman presents with abdominal pain localized to the right lower quadrant, nausea and vomiting, mild fever, and an elevation of the peripheral leukocyte count to 17,000 cells per microliter. Examination of the surgically resected appendix is most likely to reveal

a. An appendix with normal appearance
b. Neutrophils within the muscular wall
c. Lymphoid hyperplasia and multinucleated giant cells within the muscular wall
d. A dilated lumen filled with mucus
e. A yellow tumor nodule at the tip of the appendix

281. A 62-year-old male with hepatic failure secondary to cirrhosis develops a pungent odor in his breath (fetor hepaticus). He is also noted to have marked ascites, gynecomastia, asterixis, and palmar erythema. His serum ammonia levels are found to be elevated. This patient's gynecomastia is the result of

a. Decreased synthesis of albumin
b. Defective metabolism of the urea cycle
c. Deranged bilirubin metabolism
d. Impaired estrogen metabolism
e. The formation of mercaptans in gut

282. Dilated sinusoids and irregular cystic spaces filled with blood within the liver, which may rupture leading to massive intraabdominal hemorrhage, are most commonly associated with

a. Salicylates
b. Estrogens
c. Anabolic steroids
d. Acetaminophen
e. vinyl chloride

283. A 27-year-old female presents with headaches, muscle pain (myalgia), anorexia, nausea, and vomiting. She denies any history of drug or alcohol use, but upon further questioning she states that recently she has lost her taste for coffee and cigarettes. Physical examination reveals a slight yellow discoloration to her sclerae, while laboratory results indicate a serum bilirubin level of 1.8 mg/dL, and the aminotransferases (AST and ALT) levels are increased. These signs and symptoms are most consistent with a diagnosis of

a.   Gilbert's syndrome
b.   Chronic hepatitis
c.   Amebic liver abscess
d.   Acute viral hepatitis
e.   Acute hepatic failure

284. A married second year medical student with two young children is notified by her children's day care center that two other children at the day care center have recently been diagnosed as having viral hepatitis. Without any other information, this second year student correctly assumes that the most likely causative agent for these two cases of hepatitis is

a.   Hepatitis A virus
b.   Hepatitis B virus
c.   Hepatitis C virus
d.   Hepatitis D virus
e.   Cytomegalovirus (CMV)

285. Which one of the following hepatitis profile patterns is most consistent with an asymptomatic hepatitis B carrier?

	HBsAg	HBeAg	anti-HBs	anti-HBc
a.	+	−	−	−
b.	+	+	−	−
c.	+	+	−	+
d.	+	−	−	+
e.	−	−	+	+

286. A mononuclear portal inflammatory infiltrate that disrupts the limiting plate and surrounds individual hepatocytes (piecemeal necrosis), as shown in the photomicrograph below, is characteristic of

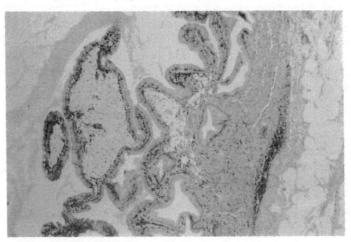

a. Ascending cholangitis
b. Chronic active hepatitis
c. Acute alcoholic hepatitis
d. Cholestatic jaundice
e. Nutritional cirrhosis

287. Chronic hepatitis is most likely to develop in which one of the following clinical situations?

a. Hepatitis A infection
b. Hepatitis B infection
c. Hepatitis C infection
d. Hepatitis D and hepatitis B coinfection
e. Hepatitis E infection

288. A 49-year-old female presents with increasing fatigue and is found to have elevated liver enzymes (AST and ALT). You follow her in your clinical and find over the next nine months that her liver enzymes have remained elevated. All serologic tests for viral markers are within normal limits. A liver biopsy reveals chronic inflammation in the portal triads that focally destroys the limiting plate and "spills over" into the adjacent hepatocytes. There are no granulomas present, and there is no evidence of fibrosis surrounding any of the bile ducts within the portal triads. Antismooth muscle antibodies and antinuclear antibodies are found in her serum. An LE cell test is positive. What is the diagnosis?

a. Autoimmune hepatitis
b. Chronic persistent hepatitis
c. Primary biliary cirrhosis
d. Primary sclerosing cholangitis
e. Systemic lupus erythematosus

289. Which of the following statements regarding alcoholic steatosis and hepatitis is illustrated in the photomicrograph below is true?

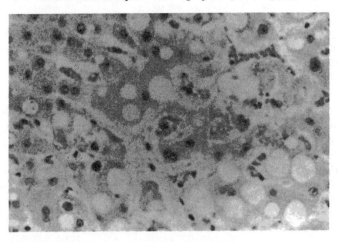

a. Morphological changes of steatosis are irreversible
b. Hepatocyte necrosis is most marked in the periportal area
c. Perivenular and pericellular fibroses are precursors of cirrhosis
d. Mallory's hyaline is pathognomonic of alcoholic liver damage
e. The inflammatory infiltrate is chiefly lymphocytic

290. Which of the following cells found within the liver is the major source of the excess collagen deposited in cirrhosis?

a. Hepatocytes
b. Kupffer cells
c. Ito cells
d. Endothelial cells
e. Bile duct epithelial cells

291. A 38-year-old woman presents with fatigue and pruritus and is found to have high serum alkaline phosphatase and slightly elevated serum bilirubin levels. Serum antimitochondrial antibodies are also present. A liver biopsy reveals a marked lymphocytic infiltrate in the portal tracts along with occasional granulomas. The most likely diagnosis is

a. Impacted gallstone
b. primary biliary cirrhosis
c. Primary sclerosing cholangitis
d. Von Meyenburg's complex
e. Caroli's disease

292. A 51-year-old male alcoholic with a history of chronic liver disease presents with increasing weight loss and ascites. Physical examination reveals a slightly enlarged, soft, nontender prostate. Examination of the scrotum is unremarkable, and fecal occult blood tests are negative. A chest X-ray is unremarkable, but a CT scan of the abdomen reveals a single mass in the left lobe of the liver. Work-up reveals elevated levels of α-fetoprotein in this patient's blood. At this point the most likely diagnosis for the liver mass is

a. Angiosarcoma
b. Cholangiocarcinoma
c. Hepatoblastoma
d. Hepatocellular carcinoma
e. Metastatic colon cancer

293. A 54-year-old male presents with a high fever, jaundice, and colicky abdominal pain in the right upper quadrant. The gallbladder cannot be palpated by physical examination. Work-up reveals hemoglobin level of 15.3 g/dL, unconjugated bilirubin level of 0.9 mg/dL, conjugated bilirubin level of 1.1 mg/dL, and alkaline phosphatase level of 180 IU/L. What is the best diagnosis?

a. Acute cholecystitis
b. Chronic cholecystitis
c. Bile duct obstruction by a stone
d. Carcinoma of the gallbladder
e. Carcinoma of the head of the pancreas

294. The photomicrograph below shows a section through the gallbladder wall. Which of the following statements regarding the condition illustrated is true?

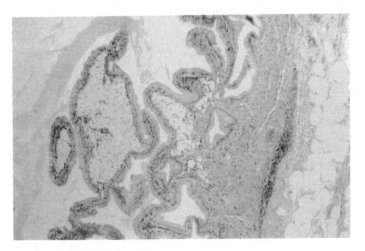

a. It is known as cholesterolosis
b. Changes often extend into the extrahepatic bile ducts
c. It predisposes to acute cholecystitis
d. It is strongly associated with pigment stones
e. None of the above

295. An infant is brought in by his mother, who says that his skin tastes salty. With time this patient's pancreas will be expected to undergo progressive fibrosis with atrophy of the exocrine glands and cystic dilatation of the ducts. The basic abnormality in this infant involves

a.   Decreased synthesis of surface receptor
b.   Decreased intracellular cAMP
c.   Decreased glycosylated chloride channel
d.   Increased phosphorylation of chloride channel
e.   Increased ductal secretion of water

296. A middle-aged male alcoholic has had repeated bouts of pancreatitis following periods of binge drinking. In recent months he has had a low-grade fever, and on examination a mass is palpated in the epigastrium. This mass, removed at celiotomy, is shown in the photograph below. What is the diagnosis?

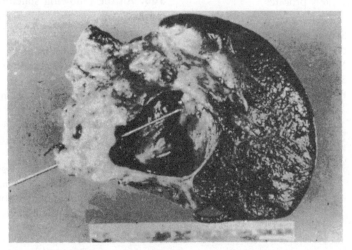

a.   Pancreatic carcinoma
b.   Mucinous cystadenoma
c.   Perforated ulcer
d.   Pancreatic pseudocyst
e.   Cystic hepatoma

297. Which of the following statements regarding carcinoma of the exocrine pancreas is true?

a. It arises from secretory cells of pancreatic acini
b. It is decreasing in frequency
c. It is most often located in the tail of the pancreas
d. It is more common in diabetics than in nondiabetics
e. It carries a 40 percent 5-year survival

298. A pancreatic islet cell tumor of the gastrin-secreting G cells will most likely produce

a. Hypoglycemia
b. Severe peptic ulceration of the duodenum
c. Mild diabetes
d. Steatorrhea
e. Profuse watery diarrhea

299. Retinoblastoma, the most common intraocular tumor of children, is associated with all the following EXCEPT

a. Occurrence in both familial and sporadic patterns
b. Unilateral and unifocal sporadic tumors
c. inactivation of cancer suppressor genes
d. Poor prognosis even with treatment
e. Frequent histologic occurrence of rosettes

300. All the following statements regarding carcinoma of the esophagus are true EXCEPT

a. Most carcinomas arising in the body of the esophagus are squamous
b. Squamous carcinomas begin as lesions in situ
c. Patients with Barrette's esophagus have approximately a 10 percent risk of carcinoma
d. The most common morphological form is a polypoid fungating mass
e. Distant metastases are frequently present at the time of diagnosis

301. All the following statements regarding *Helicobacter pylori* gastritis as illustrated in the photomicrograph below are true EXCEPT

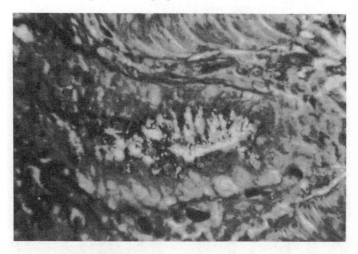

a. It is present in the majority of patients with duodenal ulceration
b. The inflammatory infiltrate is characteristically rich in eosinophils
c. Tissue invasion by microorganisms is inconspicuous
d. Organisms are absent from areas of intestinal metaplasia
e. Urease is an important virulence factor of *H. pylori*

302. All the following statements concerning carcinoma of the stomach are true EXCEPT

a. Diffusely infiltrative carcinoma is associated with a striking desmoplastic reaction
b. Early gastric carcinoma (EGC) is synonymous with carcinoma in situ
c. Over 50 percent of gastric carcinomas are found in the pylorus and antrum
d. There is a striking geographic variation in death rate from gastric carcinoma
e. The death rate from gastric carcinoma has been decreasing for decades

303. The photomicrograph below shows the colonic wall 30 cm from the anal margin in a man with severe bloody diarrhea. All the statements regarding this condition are true EXCEPT

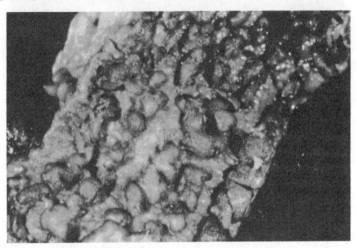

a. Inflammation is usually limited to the lamina propria
b. Multiple crypt abscesses are commonly seen
c. Atypical cytologic changes occur in the mucosa
d. Granulomas occur in the mucosa
e. "skip" lesions are not present

304. A 65-year-old man presents with episodes of facial flushing exacerbated by alcohol and associated with severe diarrhea. All the following findings may be expected on further investigation EXCEPT

a. Increased urinary levels of 5-hydroxyindoleacetic acid (5-HIAA)
b. Increased blood levels of 5-hydroxytryptamine (5-HT)
c. Areas of decreased uptake on liver scintillation scan
d. Right-sided cardiac valvular disease
e. A small yellow nodule in the tip of the appendix

305. All the following statements concerning carcinoma of the colorectum are true EXCEPT

a. 95 percent of all carcinomas of the colorectum are adenocarcinoma
b. Mucin secretion aids extension of the primary malignancy
c. Left-sided lesions tend to grow as polypoid fungating masses
d. Serum levels of carcinoembryonic antigen (CEA) are directly related to tumor size
e. Almost all carcinomas of the colorectum begin within adenomatous polyps

306. All the following produce a predominantly unconjugated hyperbilirubinemia EXCEPT

a. Hemolytic anemias
b. Physiologic jaundice of the newborn
c. Crigler-Najjar syndrome, type I
d. Gilbert's syndrome
e. Dubin-Johnson syndrome

307. Finely nodular (micronodular) cirrhosis, as illustrated in the photomicrograph below, is seen in all the following conditions EXCEPT

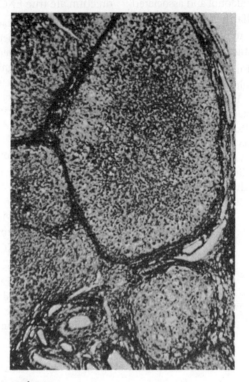

a.   Postnecrotic cirrhosis
b.   Secondary biliary cirrhosis
c.   Primary biliary cirrhosis
d.   Alcoholic cirrhosis
e.   Hemochromatosis

308. The finding of multiple, pale yellow, hard, round stones within the gallbladder is associated with all the following EXCEPT

a. Oral contraceptives
b. Obesity
c. biliary infection
d. Hyperlipidemia syndromes
e. Prevalence within the Native-American population

309. Chronic pancreatitis is associated with all the following EXCEPT

a. Chronic alcoholism
b. Gallstones
c. Pancreatic pseudocyst
d. Pancreatic calcification
e. Fat malabsorption

310. Diseases of the urinary tract occurring with increased frequency in patients with diabetes mellitus include all the following EXCEPT

a. Nodular or intercapillary glomerulosclerosis
b. Nephrotic syndrome
c. Atherosclerosis of the renal artery
d. Renal papillary necrosis
e. Uric acid stones

311. Components of diabetic glomerulopathy include all the following EXCEPT

a. Diffuse glomerulosclerosis
b. Nodular glomerulosclerosis
c. Thickening of capillary basement membranes
d. Mesangial proliferation
e. Fibrin thrombi

DIRECTIONS: Each group of questions below consists of lettered headings followed by a set of numbered items. For each numbered item select the **one** lettered heading with which it is **most** closely associated. Each lettered heading may be used **once, more than once, or not at all**.

Questions 312–313

Match each of the following clinical scenarios with the correct diagnosis from the following list.

a. Congenital aganglionic megacolon
b. Congenital pyloric stenosis
c. Diaphragmatic hernia
d. Esophageal atresia
e. Hiatal hernia
f. Hypertrophic gastropathy
g. Plummer-Vinson syndrome
h. Tracheoesophageal fistula
i. Zenker's diverticuli

312. A newborn infant presents with coughing and cyanosis during feeding. This infant is also noted to have marked gastric dilatation due to "swallowed" air. A chest X-ray does not reveal the presence of bowel gas in the chest cavity. This infant's mother was noted to have had polyhydramnios during this pregnancy.

313. A 2-week-old infant presents with regurgitation and persistent severe vomiting. Physical examination reveals the presence of a mid-epigastric abdominal mass. A chest X-ray does not reveal the presence of bowel gas in the chest cavity. This infant's mother did not have polyhydramnios during this pregnancy. Surgery is performed and the abnormality is easily corrected.

Questions 314–315

Match each of the following clinical scenarios with the correct diagnosis from the following list.

a.   Abetalipoproteinemia
b.   Blind-loop syndrome
c.   Crohn's disease
d.   Disaccharidase deficiency
e.   Hartnup's disease
f.   Intestinal lymphoma
g.   Nontropical sprue
h.   Progressive systemic sclerosis
i.   Tropical sprue
j.   Whipple's disease

314. A patient presents with steatorrhea. Laboratory examination reveals a serum albumin level of 2.9 g/dl and a calcium level of 8.9 mg/dl. Examination of his peripheral smear reveals that many of his peripheral red blood cells have numerous spikes on their surface. A mucosal biopsy of the small intestines reveals the epithelial cells to be filled with lipid.

315. A 45-year-old male presents with fever, chronic diarrhea, and weight loss. He is found to have multiple pain and swelling of his joints (migratory polyarthritis) and generalized lymphadenopathy. Physical examination reveals skin hyperpigmentation. A biopsy from his small intestines reveals the presence of macrophages in the lamina propria that have PAS-positive cytoplasm.

Questions 316–317

Match each of the following clinical scenarios with the correct diagnosis from the following list.

a. Alpha-1-antitrypsin deficiency
b. Dubin-Johnson syndrome
c. Primary hemochromatosis
d. Reye's syndrome
e. Secondary hemochromatosis
f. Viral hepatitis
g. Wilson's disease

316. A 36-year-old male presents because his skin has been darkening recently. You notice that his skin has a dark, somewhat bronze color. Work-up reveals signs of diabetes mellitus. His serum iron is found to be 1,150 μg/dL, and his transferrin saturation is 98 percent. A liver biopsy is performed and reveals extensive deposits of hemosiderin in the hepatocytes and Kupffer cells.

317. A 5-year-old female girl is brought in with severe vomiting that has developed suddenly 5 days after she has had a viral infection. Upon questioning, her parents indicate that she was given aspirin for several days to treat a fever that occurred with this viral illness. She is hospitalized and quickly develops signs of cerebral edema. Liver tissue from this young girl reveals marked steatosis.

GASTROINTESTINAL SYSTEM

Answers

258. The answer is e. (*Cotran, 5/e, p 309. Rubin, 2/e, pp 356–360, 384–385, 391–395, 1258.*) Numerous diseases result from bacterial infections of the oral cavity. *Actinomyces israelii*, a normal inhabitant of the mouth, is a branched, filamentous gram-positive bacteria that may produce an indurated (lumpy) jaw with multiple draining fistulas or abscesses. Small yellow colonies may be seen in the draining material, these being called sulfur granules. Scarlet fever, a disease of children, is caused by several strains of beta-hemolytic group A streptococci (*S. pyogenes*). An erythrogenic toxin damages vascular endothelium and produces a rash on the skin and oral mucosa. The tongue in a patient with scarlet fever may be fiery red with prominent papillae (raspberry tongue) or white-coated with hyperemic papillae (strawberry tongue). Acute necrotizing ulcerative gingivitis (Vincent angina or trench mouth) is caused by two symbiotic organisms, a fusiform bacillus and a spirochete (*Borrelia vincentii*), the combination being termed fusospirochetosis. *Corynebacterium diphtheriae* causes diphtheria, which is characterized by oral and pharyngeal pseudomembranes and a peripheral lymphocytosis. Rhinoscleroma, a chronic inflammation of the nose, is caused by *Klebsiella rhinoscleroma*, and histologically is characterized by numerous foamy macrophages, called Mikulicz cells.

259. The answer is b. (*Cotran, 5/e, pp 746–747. Rubin, 2/e, pp 1266–1271.*) Meniere's disease is an abnormality that is characterized by periodic episodes of vertigo, which are often accompanied by nausea and vomiting, sensorineural hearing loss, and tinnitus (ringing in the ears). These symptoms are related to hydropic dilatation of the endolymphatic system of the cochlea. Inflammation of the middle ear (otitis media), which occurs most often in children, may be acute or chronic. If caused by viruses, there may be a serous exudate, but if produced by bacteria, there may be a suppurative exudate. Acute suppurative otitis media is characterized by acute suppurative inflammation (neutrophils), while chronic otitis media has chronic inflammation with granulation tissue. Chronic otitis media may cause perforation of the eardrum or may lead to the formation of a cyst within the middle ear that is filled with keratin. This cyst is called a cholesteatoma. The name is somewhat of a misnomer as cholesterol deposits are not present. Otosclerosis, a common hereditary cause of bilateral conduction hearing loss, is associated with new spongy bone formation around the stapes and the oval window. Patients present with progressive deafness. Tumors of the middle ear are quite rare, but a neoplasm that arises from the paraganglia of the middle ear (the glomus jugulare or glomus tympanicum) is called a chemodectoma. Other names for this tumor include nonchromaffin paraganglioma and glomus jugulare tumor. This lesion is characterized histologically by lobules of cells in a highly vascular stroma (zellballen). A similar tumor that occurs in the neck is called a carotid body tumor.

260. The answer is d. (*Cotran, 5/e, pp 738–741.*) Carcinoma of the oral cavity accounts for approximately 5 percent of all human malignancies. More than 90 percent are squamous cell type and precursor lesions include leukoplakia (dysplastic leukoplakia) and erythroplasia with transformation rates of approximately 15 and 50 percent, respectively. It is more common in males. Smoking, tobacco chewing, chronic irritation, heat exposure, and irradiation are all thought to contribute to carcinogenesis. The lower lip is the most common site followed by the floor of the mouth, anterior tongue, palate, and posterior tongue. Prognosis varies according to site but is best for lesions of the lip and worst for lesions in the floor of the mouth.

261. The answer is c. (*Damjanov, 10/e, pp 1454–1455, 2758.*) The photomicrograph (at low magnification) shows an intact overlying mucosa with a subjacent highly cellular neoplasm composed of small, dark-staining cells ("tumor of small blue cells"). In the child, small, blue cell tumors comprise lymphoma, neuroblastoma, cerebellar medulloblastoma, undifferentiated nephroblastoma (Wilms' tumor), retinoblastoma, embryonal rhabdomyosarcoma, and Ewing's sarcoma. In the adult, anaplastic, small cell carcinomas of the lung, pancreas, uterine cervix, and anorectum (cloacogenic carcinoma); plasmacytomas; and neuroectodermal tumors of thoracopulmonary origin are also included. In addition to the age of the patient and the organ site, certain structures visible at higher magnification, such as rosettes (retinoblastoma) and pseudorosettes (anaplastic small cell carcinoma, neuroblastoma) aid in the differential diagnosis. In the example given, the lesion is too cellular to be either nasal glioma (large, pale glial cells) or nasopharyngeal angiofibroma (vascular structures). The olfactory neuroblastoma (the tumor depicted in the photomicrograph) arises from the olfactory placode of the stem cell referred to as the esthesioneuroblast. The cells populating the tumor are round or oval neuroepithelial cells occurring in clusters and associated with a fibrillary intercellular matrix.

262. The answer is a. (*Silverberg, 2/e, pp 2047–2050. Rubin, 2/e, p 1458.*) Many lesions of the eyelid are submitted for pathologic examination. One of the most common eyelid lesions is the chalazion, a chronic inflammatory reaction to lipid released into the tissue from the eyelid's sebaceous glands of Meibom or Zeis. Characteristic histologic features of this lesion include a chronic inflammatory reaction with giant cells that surround empty spaces where the lipid vacuoles from the sebaceous glands had been located. Because the major clinical disorder to be differentiated from chalazia is a sebaceous carcinoma, ophthalmologists biopsy recurrent lesions suspected of being chalazia to rule this out. Hordeolums (styes) are acute staphylococcal infections of the eyelash follicles (external hordeolum) or the Meibomian glands (internal hordeolum). Xanthelasma, yellow plaques on the skin, histologically reveal aggregates of foamy macrophages within the dermis. Hydrocystomas are one type of cyst that may affect the eyelid and may be lined by apocrine or eccrine cells.

263. The answer is d. (*Cotran, 5/e, pp 751–752. Rubin, 2/e, pp 1252–1253.*) Warthin's tumors occur mainly in the lower regions of the parotid gland, especially near the angle of the mandible, and on rare occasion may be bilateral. They are completely benign neoplasms although they carry some undesirable synonyms: adenolymphoma, which is a misnomer, and papillary cystadenoma lymphomatosum, a term undesirable both for the lymphomatosum part as well as its length. For these reasons most workers prefer the term Warthin's tumor. The pattern is highly characteristic of an epithelial surface lining of acidophilic cells that overlay benign lymphoid tissue elements, including germinal centers. The epithelial portion probably arises from early duct cells that become entrapped within developing parotid lymph nodes during embryogenesis. Sebaceous lymphadenoma would have sebaceous cells within the lymphoid tissue. Thyroglossal duct cyst is located in the midline of the neck but may be found extending up to the base of the tongue, and there is a similarity between the lymphoid islands seen in thyroglossal duct cysts and in Warthin's tumor; however, thyroid follicles may lead to the correct diagnosis in the former. Lymphoepithelioma is a tumor that is recognized by hyperplastic duct epithelium surrounded by lymphoid tissue. Myoepithelial islands embedded in lymphoid tissue may be seen in the minor and major salivary glands in Sjögren's syndrome.

264. The answer is c. (*Cotran, 5/e, pp 749–753.*) The salivary glands give rise to a wide variety of tumors, the majority of which are of epithelial origin and benign. Most tumors occur in adults and have a slight female predominance. Approximately 75 to 85 percent occur in the parotids, 10 to 20 percent in the submandibular glands, and the remainder in the minor glands. In the parotid the vast majority are benign, whereas in the minor glands 35 to 50 percent are malignant. Mesenchymal tumors are rare. Clinically, most tumors of salivary glands present as palpable masses, regardless of histologic type. They occasionally present with symptoms related to local invasion, such as facial nerve palsy. Masses may be present for years before diagnosis, even when malignant. Carcinomas tend to run an indolent course, invade local structures slowly, recur locally after removal, and metastasize late. Prognosis is usually presented in 10- or 20-year survival rates.

265. The answer is b. (*Cotran, 5/e, pp 757–758.*) Achalasia, which means "unrelaxed," is a term that describes the absence of normal lower esophageal sphincter (LES) relaxation. This disease results from decreased or absent ganglion cells in the myenteric plexus in the body of the esophagus. The etiology of this neuronal loss is unknown in many cases; however, some cases are secondary to other diseases, such as diabetes mellitus, amyloidosis, sarcoidosis, and Chagas disease, which is caused by *Trypanosoma cruzi.* Because of the increased LES pressure and the absence of peristaltic waves in the lower esophagus, the esophagus in these patients is dilated and tortuous above the level of the LES. Barium X-ray studies reveal this dilated esophagus. The distal esophagus has a characteristic "beak-like" appearance. Patients with achalasia have an increased risk of developing aspiration pneumonia and squamous cell carcinoma.

266. The answer is e. *(Cotran, 5/e, pp 756–761.)* Most lesions of the esophagus present with similar symptoms, such as heartburn and dysphagia, but the most serious disease, which carries the risk of exsanguination, is bleeding esophageal varices. Varices occur in about two-thirds of all patients with cirrhosis, and in the majority of patients the etiology is alcoholic cirrhosis. The cirrhosis causes portal hypertension, which shunts blood into connecting channels between the portal and caval systems, such as the subepithelial plexus of veins in the lower esophagus. Varices produce no symptoms until they rupture and cause massive bleeding (hematemesis), which may lead to death. Other diseases may cause hematemesis such as gastritis, esophageal laceration (Mallory-Weiss tears), or peptic ulcer disease. Dysphagia (difficulty swallowing) is another esophageal symptom. It is seen in diseases with abnormal esophageal function, such as achalasia, and diseases that narrow the esophageal lumen, such as webs and rings. The characteristics of achalasia include aperistalsis, incomplete relaxation of the lower esophageal sphincter (LES) with swallowing, and increased resting tone of the LES, all of which lead to esophageal dilatation and symptoms of progressive dysphagia. Plummer-Vinson syndrome is the combination of esophageal webs in the upper esophagus and anemia. Outpouchings in the upper esophagus are called pharyngeal (Zenker's) diverticuli and may result in regurgitation and aspiration. Sliding hiatal hernias are associated with signs and symptoms of reflux esophagitis.

267. The answer is d. *(Cotran, 5/e, pp 762–764.)* The presence of columnar epithelium lining part or all of the distal esophagus is known as Barrette's esophagus. It is considered an acquired change resulting from reflux of acidic gastric contents with ulceration of the esophageal squamous epithelium and replacement by metaplastic, acid-resistant, columnar epithelium. Endoscopically it has a velvety-red appearance. Microscopically, intestinal-type epithelium is most common, but gastric-type epithelium is also seen. Varying degrees of dysplasia may be present. The risk of carcinoma is increased 30- to 40-fold. Virtually all of these tumors are of the adenocarcinoma type and they account for up to 10 percent of all esophageal cancers.

268. The answer is b. *(Cotran, 5/e, pp 773–777. Rubin, 2/e, pp 637–643.)* Gastric ulcers may be either acute gastric ulcers, peptic ulcers, or ulcers from malignant cancers. Acute gastric ulcers are stress ulcers that are really erosions and not true ulcers. Certain gross and microscopic characteristics help to differentiate benign peptic ulcers from malignant ulcers. Benign peptic ulcers tend to be round and regular with punched-out straight walls. The margins are only slightly elevated and rugae radiate outward from the ulcer. Histologically, the surface of the ulcer has acute inflammation and necrotic fibrinoid debris, while the base has active granulation tissue overlying a fibrous scar. Grossly, the floor of the ulcer is smooth. The gastric epithelium adjacent to the ulcer is reactive and is characterized by numerous mitoses and epithelial cells with prominent nucleoli. In contrast, malignant ulcers grossly are irregular with raised irregular margins. *Helicobacter pylori* may be seen with either type of ulcer and its presence is not diagnostic for the type of ulcer. It is also found in 20 percent of the general population. Peptic ulcers are due to the effects of acid and may occur anywhere in the gastrointestinal tract exposed to acid-peptic activity. Over 98 percent of cases occur in the stomach or duodenum with duodenal cases outnumbering gastric by 4:1. Ulcers associated with the Zollinger-Ellison syndrome are typically multiple and frequently involve distal duodenum and jejunum. Duodenal ulceration appears to be related to hypersecretion of acid. Gastric ulceration typically occurs in a setting of normo- or hypochlorhydria with abnormality of mucosal defense mechanisms, back-diffusion of acid, and possibly local ischemia. *Helicobacter pylori* is associated with up to 100 percent of patients with duodenal ulcers, and about 75 percent of patients with gastric ulcers. The treatment of peptic ulcers involves trying to decrease the effects of gastric acid. There are several types of drugs that can be used to treat peptic ulcers, such as cimetidine and omeprazole. Because food neutralizes acid within the stomach and relieves the typical epigastric pain of peptic ulcer disease, patients are advised to eat frequent small meals. Additional therapeutic measures include abstaining from substances or actions that increase gastric acid production, such as coffee, alcohol, and prostaglandin production inhibitors, which include aspirin, indomethacin, ibuprofen, and smoking.

269. The answer is c. (*Cotran, 5/e, pp 779–783.*) "Signet-ring cell" carcinoma is a morphologic variant of adenocarcinoma most often seen in the stomach. In these tumors, intracellular mucin vacuoles coalesce and distend the cytoplasm of tumor cells, which compresses the nucleus toward the edge of the cell and creates a signet-ring appearance. Tumors of this type are usually deeply invasive and fall into the category of advanced gastric carcinoma. There is often a striking desmoplasia with thickening and rigidity of the gastric wall, which may result in the so-called linitis plastica appearance. Advanced gastric carcinoma is usually located in the pyloroantrum and the prognosis is poor with 5-year survival of only 5 to 15 percent.

270. The answer is d. (*Cotran, 5/e, p 786.*) Meckel's diverticulum occurs in the ileum, usually within 30 cm of the ileocecal valve, and is present in approximately 2 percent of normal persons. It represents incomplete involution of the vitello-intestinal duct and always arises from the antimesenteric border of the intestine. Heterotopic gastric or pancreatic tissue may be present in about one-half of cases. Peptic ulceration, which occurs as a result of acid secretion by heterotopic gastric mucosa, is usually located in the adjacent ileum. Complications include perforation, ulceration, intestinal obstruction, intussusception, and neoplasms, including carcinoid tumors.

271. The answer is d. (*Cotran, 5/e, pp 329–334, 790–794, 804–806.*) Early stages of ulcerative colitis (UC) may be indistinguishable from gastroenteritis caused by *Salmonella choleraesuis* and *S. typhimurium*. In early stages, both diseases may show histologically a dense mononuclear inflammatory infiltrate in the lamina propria, occasional crypt abscesses, and mucosal edema and congestion. Even the respective clinical symptoms and colon x-ray changes may be similar, although marked vomiting should point to food poisoning. Salmonellae have been the cause of outbreaks and epidemics of acute gastroenteritis, and the cause has often been found to be contaminated fowl that has been insufficiently cooked to inactivate endotoxins.

272. The answer is a. (*Cotran, 5/e, pp 328–334, 790–794, 800, 804.*) The causes of diarrhea are immense and may be broadly classified into multiple categories including secretory diarrhea, osmotic diarrhea, and exudative diarrhea. Both secretory and exudative diarrhea may have infectious causes. Several viruses may cause secretory diarrhea. Rotavirus is a major cause of diarrhea in children between the ages of 6 and 24 months. Clinical symptoms consisting of vomiting and watery (secretory) diarrhea begin about 2 days after exposure. Bacterial enterocolitis may be related to either the production of preformed toxins, such as with *Vibrio cholerae* and enterotoxigenic *E. coli*, which is a major cause of "traveler's diarrhea," or it may be related to bacterial invasion of the colon, as seen with salmonella and shigella. *Entamoeba histolytica* is a cause of amebiasis and is endemic in underdeveloped countries. It characteristically produces flask-shaped ulcers in the colon and may embolize to the liver, where it produces amebic liver abscesses. Lactase deficiency, a cause of osmotic diarrhea, is very rarely a congenital disorder, but much more commonly is an acquired disorder seen in adults that results in malabsorption of milk and milk products. The onset of symptoms from ulcerative colitis are most commonly apparent between the ages of 20 and 25.

273. The answer is a. (*Cotran, 5/e, pp 797–798. Rubin, 2/e, pp 661–662.*) Celiac disease (gluten-sensitive enteropathy) is a disorder characterized by malabsorption induced by sensitivity to the gluten and gliadin in certain cereals, especially wheat, rye, and barley. Exposure to gluten results in a typical malabsorption syndrome of varying severity. There is a high incidence of HLA-B8 (over 85 percent of cases) and HLA-DQw2 (over 90 percent) antigens. Celiac disease and HLA-B8 are also associated with the skin disease dermatitis herpetiformis. Characteristic morphological changes include villus atrophy, crypt hypertrophy with increased mitotic activity in crypts, and chronic inflammatory infiltrate in the lamina propria of the duodenum and jejunum. The proximal small intestine shows the most severe and extensive involvement. Immunocytes express surface IgA antigliadin antibodies. Antigliadin antibodies are also present in the serum but the level correlates poorly with clinical status. Complications are numerous and, with disease lasting 10 years or more, include a 10 to 15 percent risk of malignancy. Half of these cancers are B-cell lymphomas; the remainder are carcinomas that may arise anywhere in the gastrointestinal tract, but occur frequently in the small bowel.

274. The answer is c. (*Cotran, 5/e, pp 797–799.*) Celiac disease, or gluten-sensitive enteropathy, is an inflammatory condition of the small intestinal mucosa related to dietary gluten. It is more common in females and shows familial clustering. Histologically it is characterized by villus atrophy with hyperplasia of underlying crypts and increased mitotic activity. The surface epithelium shows disarray of the columnar epithelial cells and increased intraepithelial lymphocytes. There is a chronic inflammatory infiltrate in the lamina propria. Definitive diagnosis in patients with these features on biopsy depends on response to a gluten-free diet and subsequent gluten challenge.

275. The answer is d. (*Cotran, 5/e, pp 331–332, 801–806, 813–814.*) Hemorrhagic cobblestone appearance of the colon and small bowel may be seen in multiple states including inflammatory bowel disease, a term that can apply both to ulcerative colitis and regional enteritis (Crohn's disease). Other conditions that resemble cobblestoning of the mucosa of the bowel include multiple polyps such as occur in Gardener's syndrome, Turcot syndrome, familial polyposis, and multiple acquired polyps. Crohn's disease, however, differs from the others in that longitudinal ulcers may be present, yielding a long axis grooving, parallel to the long axis of the bowel. Such ulcers may also be seen in tuberculous enteritis; however, when inflammatory bowel disease is in the differential diagnosis, longitudinal ulcers are indicative of Crohn's disease.

276. The answer is d. (*Cotran, 5/e, pp 800–807.*) The two inflammatory bowel diseases (IBD), Crohn's disease (CD) and ulcerative colitis (UC), are both chronic, relapsing inflammatory disorders of unknown etiology. They both may show very similar morphologic features, such as mucosal inflammation, malignant transformation, and extragastrointestinal manifestations, such as erythema nodosum, arthritis, uveitis, pericholangitis, and ankylosing spondylitis. CD is a granulomatous disease; but granulomas are present in a minority of cases, so that the absence of granulomas does not rule out the diagnosis of CD. CD may involve any portion of the gastrointestinal tract and characteristically has skip lesions. In contrast, UC affects only the colon, and the disease involvement is continuous. Involvement of the intestines by CD is typically transmural, which leads to the formation of fistulas and sinuses. Since UC involves the mucosa and submucosa, fistula formation is absent. Additionally in Crohn's disease, the mesenteric fat wraps around the bowel surface, producing what is called "creeping fat," and the thickened wall narrows the lumen, producing a characteristic "string sign" on x-ray.

277. The answer is d. (*Cotran, 5/e, pp 806–808.*) Diverticula occur most frequently in men over the age of 50 and are most often located in the descending and sigmoid colon. The colon is the most commonly involved segment of the gastrointestinal tract. A majority of these lesions are not true diverticula since the mucosa and muscularis mucosae herniate through defects in the muscularis propria. Complications are not very common but include diverticulitis, hemorrhage, perforation, fistulas, intestinal obstruction, and, more commonly, bowel spasms or abnormal motility (irritable bowel syndrome).

278. The answer is a. (*Cotran, 5/e, pp 809–814.*) Colonic polyps are either non-neoplastic, which have no malignant potential, or neoplastic, which are precursors of cancer. Most colon polyps are non-neoplastic and are the result of abnormal maturation or inflammation. Hyperplastic polyps histologically have a serrated "saw-tooth" appearance, while grossly they tend to be small and have a "dew-drop" appearance. These polyps are thought to be an aging change and are not associated with malignant transformation. Inflammatory polyps or pseudo-polyps may be formed by inflamed regenerating epithelium, as seen with Crohn's disease or ulcerative colitis. Juvenile (retention) polyps contain abundant stroma and dilated glands filled with mucus, while lymphoid polyps contain intramucosal lymphoid tissue. Hamartomatous polyps are similar to juvenile polyps, but they also contain smooth muscle. An interesting fact about juvenile polyps, which are typically found in children or young adults, is that they are prone to self-amputation, and patients may find them floating in the toilet (which can be a disturbing finding for the patient).

Neoplastic polyps arise from proliferative, dysplastic epithelium, which is characterized by stratification of cells having plump, elongated nuclei. As a group these dysplastic polyps are called adenomatous polyps. Based on their architecture they are further classified as either tubular adenomas, villous adenomas, or mixed tubulovillous adenomas. The risk for malignancy is dependent upon the size of the polyp, and the type and the amount of dysplasia present. The risk for developing a malignancy is greater for large villous polyps that have severe dysplasia.

279. The answer is c. (*Cotran, 5/e, pp 813–815.*) Although most colonic polyps occur sporadically, there are several conditions in which colonic polyposis is familial and sometimes associated with extraintestinal abnormalities. Familial polyposis coli is usually transmitted as an autosomal dominant condition and is characterized by multiple adenomatous colonic polyps with a minimum of 100 polyps necessary for diagnosis. As with sporadic adenomatous polyps, there is a risk of malignancy and this increases to 100 percent within 30 years of diagnosis. Panproctocolectomy is, therefore, usually recommended. Gardener's syndrome is the association of colonic polyposis with multiple osteomas, fibromatosis, and cutaneous cysts. The association of colonic polyposis with central nervous system tumors is known as Turcot's syndrome.

280. The answer is b. (*Cotran, 5/e, pp 818–820, 823–825. Rubin, 2/e, pp 343, 696–697.*) Acute appendicitis, a disease found predominantly in adolescents and young adults, is characterized histologically by acute inflammatory cells, neutrophils, within the mucosa and muscular wall. Clinically, acute appendicitis causes right lower quadrant pain, nausea, vomiting, a mild fever, and a leukocytosis in the peripheral blood. These symptoms may not occur in the very young or the elderly. The inflamed appendiceal wall may become gangrenous and perforate in 24 to 48 h. Even with classic symptoms, the appendix may be histologically unremarkable in up to 20 percent of the cases. False positive diagnoses are to be preferred to the possible severe or fatal complications of a false negative diagnosis of acute appendicitis that results in rupture. Lymphoid hyperplasia with multinucleated giant cells (Warthin-Finkeldey giant cells) is characteristic of measles (rubeola). These changes can be found in the appendix, but this is quite rare. Dilatation of the lumen of the appendix is called a mucocele and may be caused by mucosal hyperplasia, a benign cystadenoma, or a malignant mucinous cystadenocarcinoma. If the latter tumor ruptures, it may seed the entire peritoneal cavity, causing the condition called pseudomyxoma peritonei. The most common tumor of the appendix is the carcinoid tumor. Grossly it is yellow in color and is typically located at the tip of the appendix. Histologically, carcinoids are composed of nests or islands of monotonous cells. Appendiceal carcinoids rarely metastasize.

281. The answer is d. (*Cotran, 5/e, pp 841–842. Chandrasoma, 3/e, pp 636–637.*) Despite various underlying causes, the clinical features of all types of liver failure are similar. A defective urea cycle results in hyperammonemia, while a foul-smelling breath (fetor hepaticus) is thought to occur due to volatile, sulfur-containing mercaptans being produced in the gut. If liver cell necrosis is present, serum hepatic enzymes, such as LDH, ALT, and AST, will be increased. Impaired estrogen metabolism in males can result in gynecomastia, testicular atrophy, palmar erythema, and spider angiomas of the skin. Additionally, deranged bilirubin metabolism results in jaundice (mainly conjugated hyperbilirubinemia) and a decreased synthesis of albumin (hypoalbuminemia) results in ascites. Symptoms of hepatic encephalopathy, a metabolic disorder of the neuromuscular system, include stupor, hyperreflexia, and asterixis, which describes a peculiar flapping tremor of the hands.

282. The answer is c. (*Cotran, 5/e, pp 856–857, 865–866, 873.*) Hepatic injury can result from a wide range of drugs, chemicals, and toxins. Peliosis hepatis is an abnormality of the hepatic blood flow that results in sinusoidal dilatation and the formation of irregular blood-filled lakes, which may rupture and produce massive intraabdominal hemorrhage or hepatic failure. It is most often associated with the use of anabolic steroids, but more rarely it may be associated with oral contraceptives. Reye's syndrome, characterized by microvesicular fatty change in the liver and encephalopathy, has been related to the use of salicylates in children with a viral illness. Acetaminophen toxicity results in centrilobular liver necrosis, while estrogens may be related to thrombosis of the hepatic or portal veins. Several hepatic tumors are related to exposure to vinyl chloride, including angiosarcoma and hepatocellular carcinoma.

283. The answer is d. (*Cotran, 5/e, pp 849–856. Chandrasoma, 3/e, pp 643–645.*) Several clinical syndromes may develop after exposure to any of the viruses that cause hepatitis, including asymptomatic hepatitis, acute hepatitis, fulminant hepatitis, chronic hepatitis, and the carrier state. Asymptomatic infection in individuals is documented by serologic abnormalities only. Liver biopsies in patients with acute hepatitis, either the anicteric phase or the icteric phase, will reveal focal necrosis of hepatocytes (forming Councilman bodies) and lobular disarray resulting from ballooning degeneration of the hepatocytes. These changes are nonspecific, but the additional finding of fatty change is suggestive of hepatitis C virus (HCV) infection. Clinically acute viral hepatitis is classified into three phases. During the prodrome phase, patients may develop symptoms that include anorexia, nausea and vomiting, headaches, photophobia, and myalgia. An unusual symptom associated with acute viral hepatitis is altered olfaction and taste, especially the loss of taste for coffee and cigarettes. The next phase, the icteric phase, involves increased bilirubin-producing jaundice. Patients may also develop light stools and dark urine (due to disrupted bile flow), and ecchymoses (due to decreased vitamin K). The final phase is the convalescence phase. Fulminant hepatitis refers to massive necrosis and is seen in about 1 percent of patients with either hepatitis B or C, but very rarely with hepatitis A infection. The biggest risk for fulminant hepatitis is coinfection with both hepatitis B and D. Finally, chronic hepatitis is defined as elevated serum liver enzymes for longer than 6 months. Patients may be either symptomatic or asymptomatic.

284. The answer is a. (*Cotran, 5/e, pp 843–849. Chandrasoma, 3/e, pp 641–643.*) Several types of viruses are implicated as being causative agents of viral hepatitis. Each of these has unique characteristics. Hepatitis A virus, an RNA picornavirus, is transmitted through the fecal-oral route (including shellfish) and is called "infectious hepatitis." It is associated with small outbreaks of hepatitis in the United States, especially in young children at day care centers. Hepatitis B virus, which causes "serum hepatitis," is associated with the development of a serum sickness-like syndrome in about 10 percent of patients. Immune complexes of antibody and HBsAg are present in patients with vasculitis. Hepatitis C virus is characterized by episodic elevations in serum transaminases, and also by fatty change in liver biopsy specimens. Hepatitis D virus is distinct in that it is a defective virus and needs HBsAg to be infective. Finally, hepatitis E virus is characterized by its water-borne transmission. It is found in underdeveloped countries and has an unusually high mortality in pregnant females. It is important to remember that the liver may be infected by other viruses, such as yellow fever virus, Ebstein-Barr virus (EBV, the causative agent of infectious mononucleosis), CMV, and herpes virus. The latter is characterized histologically by intranuclear eosinophilic inclusions (Cowdry bodies) and nuclei that have a "ground-glass" appearance.

285. The answer is d. (*Cotran, 5/e, pp 844–846. Rubin, 2/e, pp 724–726.*) Hepatitis B virus (HBV) is a member of the DNA-containing hepadnaviruses. The mature HBV virion is called the "Dane particle." Products of the HBV genome include the nucleocapsid (hepatitis B core antigen, HBcAg), envelope glycoprotein (hepatitis B surface antigen, HBsAg), and DNA polymerase. After exposure to HBV, there is a relatively long asymptomatic incubation period, averaging 6 to 8 weeks, followed by an acute disease lasting several weeks to months. HBsAg is the first antigen to appear in the blood. It appears before symptoms begin, peaks during overt disease, and declines to undetectable levels in 3 to 6 months. HBeAg, HBV-DNA, and DNA polymerase appear soon after HBsAg. HBeAg peaks during acute disease and disappears before HBsAg is cleared. The presence of either HBsAg or HBeAg without antibodies to either is seen early in hepatitis B infection. Anti-HBsAg appears about the time of the disappearance of HBsAg and indicates complete recovery. Anti-HBc first appears much earlier, shortly after the appearance of HBsAg, and levels remain elevated for life. Its presence indicates previous HBV infection, but not necessarily that the hepatitis infection has been cleared. Persistence of HBeAg is an important indicator of continued viral replication with probable progression to chronic hepatitis. With normal recovery from hepatitis B, both HBsAg and HBeAg are absent from the blood, while anti-HBs and anti-HBc are present. If anti-HBs is never produced, then HBsAg may not be cleared. In this case, the patient may remove the HBeAg and be an asymptomatic carrier, or the HBeAg may persist and the patient could be a chronic carrier who has progressed to chronic active hepatitis. In both of these conditions, anti-HBc is still present.

286. The answer is b. (*Cotran, 5/e, pp 851–852.*) Chronic hepatitis has been defined as an inflammatory process of the liver that lasts longer than 1 year and lacks the nodular regeneration and architectural distortion of cirrhosis. In chronic active hepatitis, an intense inflammatory reaction with numerous plasma cells spreads from portal tracts into periportal areas. The reaction destroys the limiting plate and results in formation of periportal hepatocytic islets. Prognosis is poor, and the majority of patients develop cirrhosis. Chronic persistent hepatitis is usually a sequela of acute viral hepatitis and has a benign course, without progression to chronic active hepatitis or cirrhosis. The portal inflammation does not extend into the periportal areas, and this differentiates it from chronic active hepatitis.

287. The answer is c. (*Cotran, 5/e, pp 843–852.*) The hepatitis viruses are responsible for most cases of chronic hepatitis, but the chance of developing chronic hepatitis varies considerably with the different types of hepatitis viruses. Neither hepatitis A nor hepatitis E virus infection is associated with the development of chronic hepatitis. About 5 percent of adults infected with hepatitis B develop chronic hepatitis, and about one-half of these patients progress to cirrhosis. In contrast to hepatitis B, chronic hepatitis develops in about 50 percent of patients with hepatitis C. In the

United States it is estimated that hepatitis B causes 30,000 new cases of chronic hepatitis each year, but hepatitis C causes about 85,000 new cases annually. Hepatitis D infection occurs in two clinical settings. There might be acute coinfection by hepatitis D and hepatitis B, which results in chronic hepatitis in less than 5 percent of cases. If instead hepatitis D is superinfected upon a chronic carrier of hepatitis B virus, then about 80 percent of cases progress to chronic hepatitis.

288. The answer is a. (*Cotran, 5/e, pp 853, 868–870. Chandrasoma, 3/e, pp 652–653.*) Chronic hepatitis is defined clinically by the presence of elevated serum liver enzymes for longer than 6 months. Liver biopsies in patients with chronic hepatitis may reveal inflammation that is limited to the portal areas (chronic persistent hepatitis), or the inflammation may extend into the adjacent hepatocytes. This inflammation causes necrosis of the hepatocytes (piecemeal necrosis) and is called chronic active hepatitis. These changes are nonspecific and can be seen with hepatitis B virus (HBV) or hepatitis C virus (HCV) infection. The finding of hepatocytes with ground-glass, eosinophilic cytoplasm is highly suggestive of HBV infection, while fatty change (steatosis) is suggestive of HCV. A clinically distinct subtype of chronic hepatitis is called chronic autoimmune ("lupoid") hepatitis. This disease occurs in young females who have no serologic evidence of viral disease. These patients have increased IgG levels and high titers of autoantibodies, such as anti-smooth muscle antibodies and antinuclear antibodies. They also have a positive LE test, which is the basis for the name "lupoid" hepatitis, but there is no relationship of this disease to systemic lupus erythematosus. The prognosis for these patients is poor, as many progress to cirrhosis.

Two diseases classified as primary biliary diseases are primary biliary cirrhosis (PBC) and primary sclerosing cholangitis (PSC). Primary biliary cirrhosis is primarily a disease of middle-aged females and is characterized by pruritus, jaundice, and hypercholesterolemia. More than 90 percent of patients have antimitochondrial autoantibodies, particularly to mitochondrial pyruvate dehydrogenase. A characteristic lesion, called the florid duct lesion, is seen in portal areas and is composed of a marked lymphocytic infiltrate and occasional granulomas. Primary sclerosing cholangitis is characterized by fibrosing cholangitis, which produces concentric "onion-skin fibrosis" in portal areas. It is associated with chronic ulcerative colitis, one type of inflammatory bowel disease.

289. The answer is c. (*Cotran, 5/e, pp 857–860.*) Alcoholic liver disease includes steatosis (fatty liver), hepatitis, and cirrhosis. Steatosis is the earliest hepatic consequence of excess alcohol intake and consists of cytoplasmic accumulation of lipid vacuoles that coalesce and distend the cells with ultrastructural evidence of cell injury. These changes are reversible. Alcoholic hepatitis is usually accompanied by some fatty changes and is characterized by hepatocellular swelling, necrosis, and neutrophil infiltration in the perivenular area, as well as the appearance of Mallory's hyaline-eosinophilic cytoplasmic inclusions composed of cytokeratin proteins. These inclusions may also, however, be seen in liver injury due to other causes. Pericellular fibrosis and fibrosis around the central vein are significant changes considered by some to indicate the possible development of cirrhosis.

290. The answer is c. (*Fawcett, 12/e, pp 657–660. Cotran, 5/e, pp 832, 835.*) Ito cells are fat-containing lipocytes found within the space of Disse of the liver. They participate in the metabolism and storage of vitamin A and also secrete collagen in the normal and the fibrotic (cirrhotic) liver. In normal livers, types I and III collagens (interstitial types) are found in the portal areas and occasionally in the space of Disse or around central veins. In cirrhosis, types I and III collagens are deposited throughout the hepatic lobule. Endothelial cells normally line the sinusoids and demarcate the extrasinusoidal space of Disse. Attached to the endothelial cells are the phagocytic Kupffer cells, which are part of the monocyte-phagocyte system.

291. The answer is b. (*Cotran, 5/e, pp 867–871. Rubin, 2/e, pp 740–744.*) Diseases of the biliary tract may lead to manifestations of jaundice and if prolonged and severe may lead to cirrhosis. These diseases can be classified as either primary or secondary. Causes of secondary biliary cirrhosis include biliary atresia, gallstones, and carcinoma of the head of the pancreas. Histologic examination of the liver may reveal bile stasis in the interlobular bile ducts and bile duct proliferation in the portal areas. Primary biliary cirrhosis (PBC) is primarily a disease of middle-aged women and is characterized by pruritus, jaundice, and hypercholesterolemia. More than 90 percent of patients have antimitochondrial autoantibodies, particularly the "M2" antibody to mitochondrial pyruvate dehydrogenase. A characteristic lesion, called the florid duct lesion, is seen in portal areas and is composed of a marked lymphocytic infiltrate and occasional granulomas. Primary sclerosing cholangitis (PSC) is characterized by fibrosing cholangitis that produces concentric "onion-skin" fibrosis in portal areas. It is highly associated with chronic ulcerative colitis. Abnormal development of the biliary tract may lead to several abnormalities, including von Meyenburg's complex (small bile duct hamartomas near normal portal tracts) and Caroli's disease, which is characterized by segmental dilatation of the larger intrahepatic bile ducts.

292. The answer is d. (*Cotran, 5/e, pp 879–882. Chandrasoma, 3/e, pp 659–662.*) The most common primary malignancy of the liver is the hepatocellular carcinoma (hepatoma). These tumors are associated with certain viral infections (hepatitis B and hepatitis C viruses), aflatoxin (produced by *Aspergillus flavus*), and cirrhosis. Microscopic sections of these tumors reveal pleomorphic tumor cells that form trabecular patterns, which are similar to the normal architecture of the liver. Hepatomas may secrete α-fetoprotein (AFP), but this tumor marker may also be seen in yolk-sac tumors or fetal neural tube defects. Clinically hepatocellular carcinomas have a tendency to grow into the portal vein or the inferior vena cava, and may be associated with several types of paraneoplastic syndromes, such as polycythemia, hypoglycemia, and hypercalcemia. There is a microscopic fibrolamellar variant of hepatocellular carcinoma that is seen more often in females, is not associated with AFP, is grossly encapsulated, and has a better prognosis. It is important to compare the characteristics of hepatocellular carcinomas with another type of primary tumor of the liver, namely cholangiocarcinoma, which is a malignancy of bile ducts. This tumor is associated with Thorotrast and infection with the liver fluke (*Clonorchis sinensis*), but it is not associated with cirrhosis. Histologically, the tumor cells have cytoplasmic mucin, which is not found in hepatomas. Instead these malignant cells may have cytoplasmic bile. Malignant metastatic tumors are the most common tumors found in the liver. Grossly there may be multiple or single nodules, while microscopically they usually resemble the primary tumor. For example, metastatic colon cancer to the liver will histologically reveal adenocarcinoma. Metastatic disease to the liver usually does not cause functional abnormalities of the liver itself, and the liver enzymes and bilirubin levels in the blood are usually normal. Angiosarcomas are highly aggressive malignant tumors that arise from the endothelial cells of the sinusoids of the liver. Their development is associated with certain chemicals, such as vinyl chloride, arsenic, and Thorotrast. A malignant tumor of the liver that is found in children is the hepatoblastoma. Microscopically these tumors consist of ribbons and rosettes of fetal embryonal cells.

293. The answer is c. (*Cotran, 5/e, pp 888–891. Chandrasoma, 3/e, pp 663, 665–667.*) Patients with obstruction of the common bile duct present clinically with Charcot's triad, which consists of biliary colic, high fever (secondary to cholangitis), and jaundice. Jaundice secondary to extra-hepatic obstruction is associated with normal hemoglobin levels, normal serum indirect bilirubin levels, and increased levels of direct bilirubin and alkaline phosphatase. Common causes of obstruction of the common bile duct include cancer in the head of the pancreas and obstruction by a gall-stone. Clinically these two can be differentiated using Courvoisier's law, which states that in a patient with obstructive jaundice, the presence of a palpable gallbladder is indicative of obstruction due to a cancer of the head of the pancreas. This is because the obstruction causes the gallbladder to dilate. In contrast, most patients with gallstones have cholecystitis, which is associated with a thickened gallbladder wall. This will prevent the gall-bladder from dilating. Therefore, if the obstruction is due to a gallstone the gallbladder will not dilate and will not be palpable. Cholecystitis, inflam-mation of the gallbladder, may be either an acute or chronic response. In acute cholecystitis, which may be associated with a stone (calculous) or lack a stone (acalculous), there is an acute inflammatory response which consists mainly of neutrophils. Acute cholecystitis usually presents with right upper quadrant pain and may constitute a surgical emergency. Chronic chole-cystitis, which is associated with stones in more than 90 percent of cases, has a variable histologic appearance, but findings include a thickened muscular wall, scattered chronic inflammatory cells (lymphocytes), and outpouchings of the mucosa (Rokitansky-Aschoff sinuses).

294. The answer is a. (*Cotran, 5/e, p 893.*) Cholesterolosis of the gallblad-der, also known as "strawberry gallbladder," is relatively common and, although associated with cholesterol calculi, is not thought to predispose to acute cholecystitis or malignancy. Lipid-laden macrophages accumulate within the mucosal folds of the gallbladder and result in a yellow-flecked appearance. The pathophysiology is unclear but may be related to the presence of supersaturated bile. Following acute or chronic cholecystitis there may be diffuse calcium deposition in the gallbladder wall (calcified, or "porcelain," gallbladder), which is not associated with cholesterolosis. Pigment stones may occur with increased concentration of unconjugated bilirubin in bile, as in the hemolytic anemias.

295. The answer is c. (*Cotran, 5/e, pp 451–454.*) Cystic fibrosis (CF) is one of the most common lethal genetic diseases that affects white populations (1/2000). The primary abnormality in patients with cystic fibrosis involves the epithelial transport of chloride. Normally, binding of a ligand to a membrane surface receptor activates adenyl cyclase, which leads to increased intracellular cAMP. This in turn activates protein kinase A, which phosphorylates the cystic fibrosis transmembrane conductance regulator (CFTR), causing it to open and release chloride ions. Sodium ions and water then follow the chloride ions to maintain the normal viscosity of mucus. The most common abnormality in patients with CF involves decreased glycosylation of the CFTR, which then does not become incorporated into the cell membrane. A lack of chloride channels then causes decreased chloride, sodium, and water secretion, all of which together results in a very thick mucus (the other name of CF is "mucoviscidosis"). These thick mucus plugs can block the pancreatic ducts, which causes fibrosis and cystic dilatation of the ducts (hence the name "cystic fibrosis"). Decreased excretion of pancreatic lipase leads to malabsorption of fat and steatorrhea, which may lead to deficiency of fat soluble vitamins. Thick mucus may also cause intestinal obstruction in neonates, a condition called meconium ileus. Abnormal mucus in the pulmonary tree leads to atelectasis, fibrosis, bronchiectasis, and recurrent pulmonary infections, especially with *S. aureus* and *Pseudomonas* species. Obstruction of the vas deferens and seminal vesicles in males leads to sterility, while obstruction of the bile duct will produce jaundice. This child's skin tasted salty because of increased sweat electrolytes, the result of decreased reabsorption of electrolytes from the lumens of sweat ducts.

296. The answer is d. (*Cotran, 5/e, pp 904–905.*) Pseudocysts of the pancreas are so named because the cystic structure is essentially unlined by any type of epithelium. True cysts, wherever they are found in the body, are always lined by some type of epithelium, whether columnar cell, glandular, squamous, or flattened cuboidal cell. The pancreatic pseudocyst is most commonly found in a background of repeated episodes of pancreatitis. Eventual mechanical large duct obstruction by either an inflammatory process per se, periductal fibrosis, or an abscess along with inspissated duct fluid from secretions and enzymes leads to the expanding mass. The mass lesion may be located between the stomach and liver, between the stomach and colon or transverse mesocolon, or in the lesser sac. Drainage or excision is necessary for adequate treatment. Acute bacterial infection may complicate the course.

297. The answer is d. *(Cotran, 5/e, pp 905–907.)* Carcinoma of the exocrine pancreas is a highly malignant tumor that accounts for 5 percent of cancer deaths in the U.S. Its occurrence has increased threefold in the past 40 years mainly as a result of smoking and exposure to chemical carcinogens. It is more frequent in diabetics than nondiabetics. Sixty percent of tumors are located in the head of the pancreas, 20 percent in the body, and 5 percent in the tail. The remainder are of indeterminate primary location. Growth is often insidious and presentation is often with jaundice due to compression of the extrahepatic bile ducts. The disease is rarely curable at presentation and prognosis is poor, with median survival from diagnosis of 6 months and 5-year survival of only 1 to 2 percent.

298. The answer is b. *(Cotran, 5/e, pp 922–924.)* Functional islet cell tumors of the pancreas secrete specific substances that result in several syndromes. Pancreatic gastrinomas, tumors of the G cells of the pancreas, secrete gastrin and are a cause of the Zollinger-Ellison syndrome. This syndrome consists of intractable gastric hypersecretion, severe peptic ulceration of the duodenum and jejunum, and high serum levels of gastrin. The majority of gastrinomas are malignant. Insulinomas, tumors of beta cells, are the most common islet cell neoplasm and are usually benign. Symptoms include low blood sugar, hunger, sweating, and nervousness. Glucagonomas, islet cell tumors of the alpha cells, secrete glucagon and are characterized by mild diabetes, anemia, venous thrombosis, severe infections, and a migratory, necrotizing, erythematous skin rash. Delta cell tumors, which secrete somatostatin, produce a syndrome associated with mild diabetes, gallstones, steatorrhea, and hypochlorhydria. The majority of delta cell tumors are malignant. D1 tumors (also called vasoactive intestinal peptide tumors, or VIPomas) produce the Verner-Morrison syndrome, which is characterized by explosive, profuse diarrhea with hypokalemia and hypochlorhydria. This combination of symptoms is referred to as pancreatic cholera.

299. The answer is d. (*Cotran, 5/e, pp 265–268, 461–462.*) Familial cases of retinoblastoma are frequently multiple and bilateral, although like all the sporadic, nonheritable tumors they can also be unifocal and unilateral. Histologically, rosettes of various types are frequent (similar to neuroblastoma and medulloblastoma). There is a good prognosis with early detection and treatment; spontaneous regression occurs rarely. Retinoblastoma belongs to a group of cancers (osteosarcoma, Wilms' tumor, meningioma, rhabdomyosarcoma, uveal melanoma) in which the normal cancer suppressor gene (antioncogene) is inactivated or lost, with resultant malignant change. Retinoblastoma and osteosarcoma arise after loss of the same genetic locus—hereditary mutation in the q14 band of chromosome 13.

300. The answer is e. (*Cotran, 5/e, pp 764–766.*) Carcinoma of the esophagus accounts for about 10 percent of malignancies of the GI tract, but for a disproportionate number of cancer deaths. Predisposing factors include smoking, esophagitis, and achalasia. Sixty to seventy percent are squamous cell carcinomas that characteristically begin as lesions in situ. Adenocarcinoma occurs mainly in the lower esophagus and may arise in up to 10 percent of cases of Barrette's esophagus. Anaplastic and small cell variants also occur. Polypoid lesions are most common, followed by malignant ulceration and diffusely infiltrative forms. Tumors tend to spread by direct invasion of adjacent structures, but lymphatic and hematogenous spread may occur. Distant metastases are, however, a late feature. Five-year survival is less than 10 percent.

301. The answer is b. (*Cotran, 5/e, pp 770–778.*) Helicobacter pylori is a gram-negative, microaerophilic, curved bacillus found only on gastric-type epithelium. It is present in 10 percent of normal persons under 30 years of age with prevalence rising to 60 percent in those over 60 years of age. Virtually all patients with duodenal ulceration and 80 percent of those with gastric ulceration are infected by *H. pylori*. Many virulence factors aid the organism in colonization of the acid environment of the stomach, one of the most important of which is urease, which produces ammonia and buffers gastric acidity. The organism does not invade the tissues but induces surface epithelial cell damage and an inflammatory infiltrate in the lamina propria that is typically superficial and mixed granulocytic and lymphocytic.

302. The answer is b. (*Cotran, 5/e, pp 779–783.*) The death rate from gastric carcinoma has been decreasing for decades but still shows marked variations among countries; Japan, Chile, and Iceland have rates up to six times higher than those of the U.S. and Australia. First-generation migrants carry the risk of their country of origin, but subsequent generations assume the risk of their new country. The decreased rate is due to a decrease in the rate of one type of gastric cancer, the intestinal type. The incidence of the other type, diffuse gastric carcinoma, has not changed recently. Early gastric carcinoma (EGC) refers to a local neoplastic lesion limited to the mucosa and submucosa without penetration of the muscularis propria. Metastasis can occur, however, from EGC to local lymph nodes in up to 5 percent of cases. EGC is usually recognizable on radiographic or endoscopic examination, and so in most cases is potentially curable. It develops very slowly into a frankly invasive lesion and, if detected early and removed, allows a 5-year survival of up to 95 percent compared with 15 percent for gastric carcinoma overall. Of all gastric carcinomas, 50 to 60 percent arise in the pyloroantrum, 10 percent in the cardia, 10 percent in the whole organ, and the remainder in other sites. Diffusely infiltrative carcinoma extends widely through the stomach wall, often without producing an intraluminal mass, and incites a marked desmoplastic reaction that results in a thickened, inelastic stomach wall.

303. The answer is d. (*Cotran, 5/e, pp 804–806. Silverberg, 2/e, pp 1166–1170.*) The condition illustrated is ulcerative colitis, an inflammatory disorder of unknown cause. It involves the distal colon with variable proximal extension; however, skip lesions are not present. Grossly there is ulceration with islands of residual mucosa present, which form pseudopolyps. The inflammation is predominantly superficial with an infiltrate of acute and chronic inflammatory cells in the lamina propria. Cryptitis and crypt abscesses are common. Many lymphoid follicles may be seen but epithelioid cells, giant cells, and granulomas, as may be seen in Crohn's disease, are absent. Cellular atypia is seen in regenerating mucosa. When ulcerative colitis is inactive, morphological abnormalities of glands, goblet cell depletion, and Paneth cell metaplasia indicate underlying disease.

304. The answer is e. (*Cotran, 5/e, pp 818–820. Rubin, 2/e, pp 668–670.*) The patient shows two of the most common clinical manifestations of the carcinoid syndrome, which include flushing, diarrhea, bronchoconstriction, and right-sided cardiac valvular disease. The syndrome results from elaboration of serotonin (5-hydroxytryptamine) by a primary carcinoid tumor in the lungs or ovary, or from hepatic metastases from a primary carcinoid tumor in the gastrointestinal tract. Diagnosis is based on finding increased urinary 5-HIAA excretion from metabolism of excess serotonin and on histologic analysis of tumor tissue. Primary appendiceal carcinoid tumors, the most common gastrointestinal carcinoid tumors, very rarely metastasize and are virtually always asymptomatic.

305. The answer is c. *(Cotran, 5/e, pp 300, 815–817.)* Ninety-five percent of all carcinomas of the colorectum are adenocarcinoma, and almost all begin as in situ lesions within adenomatous polyps. Many of the adenocarcinomas secrete mucin. When this secretion is extracellular, it dissects the gut wall cell planes and so aids extension of the malignancy. The gross pathology of left- and right-sided lesions differs; left-sided lesions tend to grow in an annular, "napkin-ring," encircling fashion, while right-sided lesions tend to be sessile or polypoid fungating masses. Carcinoembryonic antigen is the tumor marker longest used in diagnosis and follow-up of colorectal tumors. Its serum levels are directly related to both size and extent of spread of the primary tumor. Levels fall to zero with complete removal of tumor but rise again with recurrence at primary or secondary sites.

306. The answer is e. *(Henry, 19/e, pp 87–88, 258–260. Cotran, 5/e, pp 837–841.)* Jaundice is caused by increased blood levels of bilirubin, which result from abnormalities of bilirubin metabolism. Bilirubin, the end product of heme breakdown, is taken up by the liver, where it is conjugated with glucuronic acid by the enzyme bilirubin UDP-glucuronosyl transferase (UGT) and then secreted into the bile. Unconjugated bilirubin is not soluble in an aqueous solution, is complexed to albumin, and cannot be excreted in the urine. Unconjugated hyperbilirubinemia may result from excessive production of bilirubin, which occurs in hemolytic anemias. It can also result from reduced hepatic uptake of bilirubin, as occurs in Gilbert's syndrome, a mild disease associated with a subclinical hyperbilirubinemia. Finally, unconjugated hyperbilirubinemia may result from impaired conjugation of bilirubin. Examples of diseases resulting from impaired conjugation include physiologic jaundice of the newborn and the Crigler-Najjar syndrome, which result from either decreased UGT activity (type II) or absent UGT activity (type I). Conjugated bilirubin is water-soluble, nontoxic, and readily excreted in the urine. Conjugated hyperbilirubinemia may result from either decreased hepatic excretion of conjugates of bilirubin, such as in the Dubin-Johnson syndrome, or impaired extrahepatic bile excretion, as occurs with extrahepatic biliary obstruction.

307. The answer is a. *(Cotran, 5/e, pp 834–835. Rubin, 2/e, pp 744–745.)* Cirrhosis is often subdivided into micronodular and macronodular types on the basis of the size of individual nodules within the cirrhotic liver. Although this division is entirely descriptive, most diseases that lead to cirrhosis result in one of these subtypes. Alcoholic liver damage, hemochromatosis, and biliary cirrhosis, both primary and secondary, typically result in a micronodular pattern with nodules < 3 mm in diameter. Postnecrotic cirrhosis is typically macronodular and a mixed or variable pattern may be seen in the cirrhosis of Wilson's disease and a_1-antitrypsin deficiency. It is also apparent that a micronodular pattern may convert over time to a macronodular pattern.

308. The answer is c. *(Cotran, 5/e, pp 884–888.)* Gallstones, which affect 10 to 20 percent of the adult population in developed countries, are divided into two main types. Cholesterol stones are pale yellow, hard, round, radiographically translucent stones that are most often multiple. Their formation is related to multiple factors including female sex hormones (such as with oral contraceptives), obesity, rapid weight reduction, and hyperlipidemic states. Their prevalence approaches 75 percent in some Native-American populations. The other main type of gallstones are pigment stones, which are brown or black in color and composed of bilirubin calcium salts. They are found more commonly in Asian populations and are related to chronic hemolytic states, diseases of the small intestines, and bacterial infections of the biliary tree.

309. The answer is b. *(Cotran, 5/e, pp 899–904.)* Pancreatitis may be either acute or chronic. Acute pancreatitis may be clinically mild or severe. Acute hemorrhagic pancreatitis, which clinically is severe, is associated with alcoholism in men and chronic biliary disease in women. Chronic pancreatitis is characterized histologically by chronic inflammation and irregular fibrosis of the pancreas. The major cause of chronic pancreatitis is chronic alcoholism. Complications of chronic pancreatitis include pancreatic calcifications, pancreatic cysts and pseudocysts, stones within the pancreatic ducts, diabetes, and fat malabsorption, which results in steatorrhea and decreased vitamin K levels. Although gallstones are a common cause of acute pancreatitis, cholelithiasis is not an etiologic factor in chronic pancreatitis.

310. The answer is e. *(Cotran, 5/e, pp 920–921, 961–963, 985.)* Diabetes is a major cause of renal disease. It affects the glomeruli with resultant glomerulosclerosis, fibrin caps, and capsular drops. It also affects the renal vasculature, where it causes atheroma of the major renal arteries and hyaline arteriolosclerosis of both afferent and efferent arterioles. Acute infection of the renal pyramids occurs and in combination with impaired circulation to the papillae may lead to papillary necrosis. Uric acid stones are found in patients with hyperuricemia, such as patients with gout or leukemia.

311. The answer is e. *(Cotran, 5/e, pp 920–921, 961–963.)* Thickening of the capillary basement membrane is a universal finding in diabetic kidney disease and consists of diffuse thickening as is seen in vasculopathy in other organ sites in diabetes. This has to be verified by ultrastructural examination by electron microscopy. Additionally, the mesangium widens and tubular basement membranes also thicken in diabetes. Thickening is produced by hyaline-like material, which reacts with the PAS stain. This may result from glycosylation of the proteins of the basement membrane. Thickening is probably also contributed by an increase in collagen type 4, as well as in the basement membrane glycoprotein laminin; however, the polyanionic proteoglycans are decreased. This may contribute to the increased permeability and consequent leakage of cationic proteins into the urine. Diffuse glomerulosclerosis results from an increase in the mesangial matrix as well as an increase in mesangial cells. This increase in matrix will also react with the PAS stain. Eventually, with continuing disease the glomerular tufts will become obliterated and yield a sclerosed, acidophilic tuft. At this stage the afferent and probably efferent arterioles will also be thickened and appear hyalinized.

Nodular glomerulosclerosis (Kimmelstiel-Wilson disease, intercapillary glomerulosclerosis) appears as laminated hyaline nodules at the peripheries of the glomerulus covered by what appears to be patent capillary loops. They may resemble amyloid and if they are present, amyloid stain should be done. Not always present, but highly characteristic of diabetic glomerulopathy are fibrin caps and capsular drops. The fibrin cap is a deposit that overlies a peripheral capillary within the glomerulus and consists of acidophilic deposits between the basement membrane and the endothelial cells. Capsular drops are PAS-positive proteinaceous foci that compose a thickening of the parietal layer of Bowman's capsule, giving the appearance of being free within the urinary ultrafiltrate.

312–313. The answers are: 312-h, 313-b. (*Cotran, 5/e, pp 756–759, 769–770, 778, 786–787.*) The most common congenital anomaly of the esophagus is trachea-esophageal fistula (TEF). Congenital anomalies of the esophagus are classified into five types, but only four types are associated with esophageal atresia. Type A abnormality consists of atresia of the esophagus without a connection to the trachea (no fistula). Type B consists of atresia of the esophagus with fistula between the trachea and the blind upper segment, while type C (the most common type) is characterized by atresia of the esophagus with fistula between the trachea and the distal esophageal segment. Type D has esophageal atresia with fistula between both segments and the trachea, while type E is characterized by a fistula between a normal esophagus and the trachea. This abnormality has no atresia. To summarize, type A has no fistula, type B connects to the upper segment, type C to the lower segment, and type D to both segments. These defects are dangerous because material that is swallowed may pass into the trachea (aspiration) either directly (types B, D, and E) or indirectly through reflux in that there is a blind upper pouch present (types A and C). Additionally gastric dilatation can occur due to "swallowed" air in those anomalies in which the trachea communicates with the lower esophagus (types C, D, and E). Also important is the fact that any defect that interferes with fetal swallowing in utero will produce polyhydramnios during pregnancy.

Several congenital abnormalities of the gastrointestinal tract present with specific symptoms. Infants with congenital hypertrophic pyloric stenosis present in the second or third week of life with symptoms of regurgitation and persistent severe vomiting. Physical examination reveals a firm mass in the region of the pylorus. Surgical splitting of the muscle in the stenotic region is curative. Diaphragmatic hernias, if large enough, may allow for abdominal contents—including portions of the stomach, intestines, or liver—to herniate into the thoracic cavity and cause respiratory compromise. Congenital aganglionic megacolon, Hirschsprung's disease, is caused by failure of the neural crest cells to migrate all the way to the anus, resulting in a portion of distal colon that lacks ganglion cells and both Meissner's submucosal and Auerbach's myenteric plexuses. This results in a functional obstruction and dilatation proximal to the affected portion of colon. Symptoms of Hirschsprung's disease include failure to pass meconium soon after birth followed by constipation and possible abdominal distention. Hypertrophic gastropathy refers to several diseases, such as Ménétrier's disease, which produce markedly enlarged gastric rugal folds secondary to hyperplasia of the mucosal epithelial cells. This lesion usually presents in older men with symptoms of epigastric pain, weight loss, and bleeding and may be mistaken radiographically for a gastric carcinoma or lymphoma. Dysphagia refers to difficulty swallowing. It may be seen in diseases having abnormal esophageal function, such as achalasia, or diseases that narrow the esophageal lumen, such as webs and rings. Plummer-Vinson syndrome is the combination of esophageal webs in the upper esophagus and anemia. Outpouchings in the upper esophagus are called pharyngeal (Zenker's) diverticuli and may result in regurgitation and aspiration. Sliding hiatal hernias are associated with signs and symptoms of reflux esophagitis.

314–315. The answers are: 76-a, 77-j. (*Cotran, 5/e, pp 799–800. Rubin, 2/e, pp 662–668.*) The malabsorption syndrome refers to the combination of diarrhea, steatorrhea, and the symptoms caused by malabsorption of specific dietary substances. Steatorrhea is defined as excessive fat (>6g/d) in the feces. In these patients, their stools float. Loss of protein in the stool will result in muscle wasting and hypoalbuminemia, which in turn will lead to edema. Loss of calcium will result in hypocalcemia, which in turn will result in tetany (muscle spasms) and secondary hyperparathyroidism. Loss of iron will result in hypochromic microcytic anemia, glossitis, and koilonychia. Loss of either folate or vitamin B12 will result in a megaloblastic anemia. Loss of other B vitamins will result in cheilosis and glossitis. Loss of the fat soluble vitamins will also produce specific symptoms. Loss of vitamin K will result in decreased prothrombin and hemorrhage; loss of vitamin D will result in hypocalcemia and osteomalacia; and loss of vitamin A will result in night blindness.

The causes of malabsorption are vast, but in a few of these cases, small intestinal biopsy specimens may provide clues to a specific diagnosis. Abetalipoproteinemia is a genetic defect in the synthesis of apolipoprotein

B, which leads to an inability to synthesize prebetalipoproteins (VLDL), betalipoproteins (LDL), and chylomicrons. Therefore these individuals have no chylomicrons, VLDL, or LDL in their blood. A biopsy of their small intestine reveals the mucosal absorptive cells to be vacuolated by lipid (triglyceride) inclusions, and their peripheral smear reveals numerous acanthocytes, which are red blood cells that have numerous irregular spikes on their cell surface. Their symptoms of malabsorption may be partially reversed by ingestion of medium-chain triglycerides rather than long-chain triglycerides, because these medium-chain triglycerides are absorbed directly into the portal system and are not incorporated into lipoproteins. Whipple's disease is a systemic disease associated with malabsorption, fever, skin pigmentation, lymphadenopathy, and arthritis. A biopsy of the small intestine will typically reveal the lamina propria to be infiltrated by numerous PAS-positive macrophages, which contain glycoprotein and rod-shaped bacteria. The organism, *Tropheryma whippelii*, is a gram-positive actinomycete. The disease responds promptly to broad-spectrum antibiotic therapy.

Disaccharidases (such as lactase) are located in the brush border of the small intestinal cells and are necessary for the proper absorption of carbohydrates. An acquired deficiency of lactase, quite common in Asian and African adults, results in an osmotic diarrhea due to the excess unbroken-down and unabsorbed lactose. Abdominal distention and flatulence is related to increased hydrogen production from bacterial fermentation of the unabsorbed lactose. Treatment is to restrict milk and dairy products from the diet. Primary intestinal lymphoma usually arises in men under the age of 50 and may present with malabsorption. Malignant lymphoid cells infiltrate the lamina propria of the mucosa. Lymphadenopathy and hepatosplenomegaly are usually absent. Immunoproliferative small intestinal disease (IPSID) is a neoplastic proliferation of small intestinal B lymphocytes that secrete IgA (alpha-chain disease) and is seen in the Mediterranean region (Mediterranean lymphoma). Tropical and nontropical (celiac) sprue are both characterized by shortened to absent villi in the small intestines (atrophy). Celiac sprue is a disease of malabsorption related to a sensitivity to gluten, which is found in wheat, oats, barley, and rye. This disease is related to HLA-B8 and to previous infection with type 12 adenovirus. These patients respond to removal of gluten from their diet. Tropical sprue is an acquired disease found in tropical areas, such as the Caribbean, the Far East, and India. It is the result of a chronic bacterial infection. Granulomas in mucosa and submucosa of an intestinal biopsy, if infectious causes have been excluded, are highly suggestive of Crohn's disease. Fibrosis of lamina propria and submucosa may be seen in patients with systemic sclerosis. Bacterial overgrowth, a result of numerous causes such as the blind-loop syndrome, strictures, achlorhydria, or immune deficiencies, may also cause malabsorption. Treatment is with appropriate antibiotics.

316–317. The answers are: 316-c, 317-d. (*Cotran, 5/e, pp 861–866. Chandrasoma, 3/e, pp 655–658.*) Abnormalities of metabolism are associated with a diverse group of liver disease. Hemochromatosis, excessive accumulation of body iron, may be primary or secondary. Primary hemochromatosis is a genetic disorder of iron metabolism that is inherited as an autosomal recessive disorder. The classic clinical triad for this disease consists of micronodular pigment cirrhosis, diabetes mellitus, and skin pigmentation. The combination of diabetes and skin pigmentation is called "bronze diabetes." In the majority of patients the serum iron is above 250 mg/dL, serum ferritin is above 500 ng/dL, and iron (transferrin) saturation approaches 100 percent. In patients with primary hemochromatosis, the excess iron is deposited in the cytoplasm of parenchymal cells of many organs, including the liver and pancreas. Liver deposition of iron leads to cirrhosis, which in turn increases the risk of hepatocellular carcinoma. Iron deposition in the islets of the pancreas leads to diabetes mellitus. Iron deposition in the heart leads to congestive heart failure, which is the major cause of death in these patients. Iron deposition in the joints leads to arthritis, while deposition in the testes leads to atrophy. Secondary hemochromatosis, also called systemic hemosiderosis, is most common in patients with hemolytic anemias, such as thalassemia. Excess iron may also be due to an excess number of transfusions, or increased absorption of dietary iron. In idiopathic (primary) hemochromatosis iron accumulates in the cytoplasm of parenchymal cells, but in secondary hemochromatosis the iron is deposited in the mononuclear phagocytic system. In both conditions the iron is deposited as hemosiderin, which stains an intense blue color with the Prussian blue stain. Since the iron deposition does not usually occur in the parenchymal cells in secondary hemochromatosis, there usually is no organ dysfunction or injury.

Reyes syndrome (RS) is an acute postviral illness that is seen mainly in children. It is characterized by encephalopathy, microvesicular fatty change of the liver, and widespread mitochondrial injury. Electron microscopy (EM) reveals large budding or branching mitochondria. The mitochondrial injury results in decreased activity of the citric acid cycle and urea cycle and defective beta-oxidation of fats, which then leads to the accumulation of serum fatty acids. The typical patient presents several days after a viral illness with pernicious vomiting. RS is associated with hyperammonemia, elevated serum free fatty acids, and salicylate (aspirin) ingestion.

Wilson's disease, related to excess copper deposition within the liver and basal ganglia of the brain, is characterized by varying liver disease and neurologic symptoms. The liver changes vary from fatty change to jaundice to cirrhosis, while the neurologic symptoms consist of a Parkinson-like movement disorder and behavioral abnormalities. A liver biopsy may reveal steatosis, Mallory bodies, necrotic hepatocytes, or cholestasis. Increased copper can be demonstrated histologically using the rhodamine stain. Alpha-1-antitrypsin deficiency causes both liver disease and lung disease, especially panacinar emphysema. Liver biopsies reveal red blobs within the cytoplasm of hepatocytes that are PAS positive and diastase-resistant.

ENDOCRINE SYSTEM

Questions

DIRECTIONS: Each question below contains five suggested responses. Select the **one best** response to each question.

318. Which of the following is physiologically the most active thyroid hormone?

a. Thyroglobulin
b. Monoiodotyrosine (MIT)
c. Diiodotyrosine (DIT)
d. Triiodothyronine (T$_3$)
e. Thyroxine (T$_4$)

319. An 8-month-old infant is being evaluated for growth and mental retardation. Physical examination reveals a small infant with dry, rough skin, a protuberant abdomen, periorbital edema, a flattened, broad nose, and a large, protuberant tongue. Which one of the listed disorders is the most likely cause of this infant's signs and symptoms?

a. Graves' disease
b. Cretinism
c. Toxic multinodular goiter
d. Toxic adenoma
e. Struma ovarii

320. A perimenopausal woman presents with increasing swallowing difficulty and fatigue. Physical examination reveals that her thyroid is enlarged (palpable goiter). Laboratory examination of her serum reveals T$_4$ of 4.9 µg/dL, free T$_4$ of 2.5 ng/dL, and TSH levels of 5.5 µIU/ml. No thyroid-stimulating immunoglobulins are identified in the serum, but anti-microsomal antibodies are present. Examination of histologic section from her thyroid gland reveals numerous lymphocytes, some forming lymphoid follicles, and atrophy of the thyroid follicles with focal oxyphilic metaplasia. The most likely diagnosis is

a. Hashimoto's thyroiditis
b. DeQuervain's thyroiditis
c. Subacute lymphocytic thyroiditis
d. Riedel's thyroiditis
e. Thyrotoxicosis

321. The section of tissue shown in the photomicrograph below (taken under low power) was probably removed from a patient who has

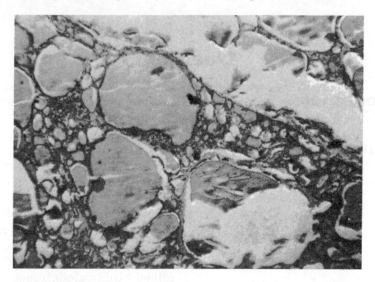

a. A normal thyroid gland
b. Colloid storage goiter
c. Graves' disease
d. Riedel's struma
e. Hashimoto's thyroiditis

322. A 37-year-old man presents with a single, firm mass within the thyroid gland. Histologic examination of this mass reveals organoid nests of tumor cells separated by broad bands of stroma as seen in the photomicrograph below. The stroma stained positively with the Congo red stain and demonstrated yellow-green birefringence. The most likely diagnosis of this lesion is

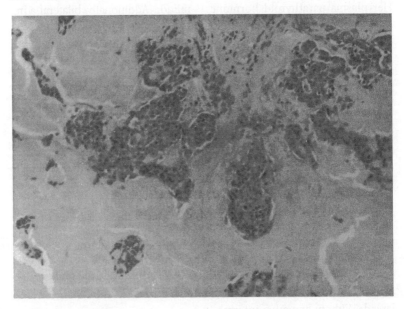

a.   Follicular carcinoma
b.   Papillary carcinoma
c.   Squamous cell carcinoma
d.   Medullary carcinoma
e.   Anaplastic carcinoma

323. A 52-year-old female presents with nausea, fatigue, muscle weakness, and intermittent pain in her left flank. Laboratory examination reveals an increased serum calcium and a decreased serum phosphorus. Her plasma parathyroid hormone levels are increased, but parathyroid hormone-related peptide levels are within normal limits. Urinary calcium is increased, and microhematuria is present. Her abnormality is most likely caused by

a. Primary hyperparathyroidism
b. Primary hypoparathyroidism
c. Pseudohypoparathyroidism
d. Secondary hyperparathyroidism
e. Secondary hypoparathyroidism

324. A 65-year-old male presents with bone pain and is found to have hypocalcemia and increased parathyroid hormone. Surgical exploration of his neck finds all four of his parathyroid glands to be enlarged. Without any other information, which one of the following is most likely the cause of the enlargement of the parathyroid glands?

a. Primary hyperplasia
b. Parathyroid adenoma
c. Chronic renal failure
d. Parathyroid carcinoma
e. Lung carcinoma

325. An XX infant is found to have external male genitalia and internal female genitalia. Physical examination reveals decreased blood pressure, while laboratory examination reveals a serum sodium level of 132 mEq/L. Additionally, bilateral adrenal cortical hyperplasia is present. The findings in this infant are most likely the result of a deficiency of

a. 3 β dehydrogenase
b. 11-hydroxylase
c. 17-hydroxylase
d. 21-hydroxylase
e. 1-α-hydroxylase

326. The most common etiologic factor in Cushing's syndrome is

a. Adrenal adenoma
b. Bilateral adrenal hyperplasia
c. Adrenal carcinoma
d. Ectopic adrenal tissue
e. Hypercorticism secondary to non-endocrine malignant tumors

327. A patient on long-term exogenous glucocorticoid administration is most likely to have which one of the following sets of plasma values?

	ACTH	aldosterone	potassium	sodium
a.	↑	normal	↑	normal
b.	↑	↓	↑	↓
c.	↑	normal	normal	normal
d.	↓	↓	normal	↓
e.	↓	normal	normal	normal

328. In type II polyglandular autoimmune syndrome (Schmidt's syndrome), autoimmune adrenocortical insufficiency may occur along with

a. Hypoparathyroidism
b. Mucocutaneous candidiasis
c. Hashimoto's thyroiditis
d. Islet cell adenoma of the pancreas
e. Medullary carcinoma of the thyroid

329. A 35-year-old male who presents with a neck mass is found to have a serum calcium level of 11.8 mg/dl and periodic elevation of his blood pressure. Extensive work-up reveals the presence of a medullary carcinoma of the thyroid, a pheochromocytoma, and hyperplasia of the parathyroid glands. This patient most likely has

a. Multiple endocrine neoplasia syndrome (MEN) type I
b. MEN syndrome type IIa
c. MEN syndrome type IIb
d. Polyglandular syndrome type I
e. Polyglandular syndrome type II

330. A 2-year-old boy presents with repeated viral and fungal infections and tetany. Work-up reveals hypocalcemia and a marked impairment of cell-mediated immunity resulting from an absence of T cells. Because of these signs and symptoms, the diagnosis of DiGeorge's syndrome is made. Considering this diagnosis, the absence of T cells is a direct consequence of failure of which embryonic structure to develop?

a. Third pharyngeal pouch
b. Fourth pharyngeal pouch
c. Fifth pharyngeal pouch
d. Ultimobranchial body
e. Foramen cecum

331. A 42-year-old man presents because recently he has had to change his shoe size from 9 to 10 1/2. He also says that his hands and jaw are now larger. The disorder is most likely mediated through the actions of excess

a. Prolactin
b. ACTH
c. Somatomedin
d. Antidiuretic hormone
e. Thyrotropin

332. A 25-year-old female presents with the acute onset of cessation of lactation. She delivered her first child several months ago and has been breast feeding since then. She reports that she has not menstruated since the delivery. She also says that lately she has been tired and has been "feeling cold" all of the time. Laboratory work-up reveals a deficiency of ACTH and other anterior pituitary hormones. What is the most likely cause of this patient's signs and symptoms?

a. Craniopharyngioma
b. Cushing's disease
c. Empty sella syndrome
d. Nonsecretory chromophobe adenoma
e. Sheehan's syndrome

333. A 49-year-old man who smokes two packs of cigarettes a day presents with a lung mass on x-ray and recent weight gain. Laboratory examination shows hyponatremia with hyperosmolar urine. The patient probably has

a. Renal failure
b. Pituitary failure
c. Conn's syndrome
d. Cardiac failure
e. Inappropriate ADH

334. A lesion that originates within and selectively destroys the ventromedial nucleus of the hypothalamus would most likely result in

a. Decreased appetite
b. Increased appetite
c. Increased urination
d. Paralysis of the extraocular muscles
e. Tunnel vision

335. Graves' disease is associated with all the following EXCEPT

a. Tachycardia
b. Anti-TSH receptor antibodies
c. Localized myxedema
d. Toxic nodular goiter
e. Exophthalmos

336. Follicular carcinoma of the thyroid may show all the following features EXCEPT

a. Vascular invasion and hematogenous metastasis
b. Multiple foci within the gland
c. A clear cell variant that resembles
   renal carcinoma
d. An insular type that is an aggressive
   form
e. Absence of ground-glass nuclei

337. Signs and symptoms seen in
patients with defects in parathyroid
hormone interaction with G protein (Albright's hereditary osteodystrophy) include all the following
EXCEPT

a. Short stature
b. Short fourth and fifth metacarpal
   bones
c. Mental retardation
d. Hypocalcemia
e. Decreased secretion of parathyroid
   hormone

338. Primary hyperaldosteronism
is associated with all the following
features EXCEPT

a. Carcinoma
b. Adenoma
c. Muscle weakness
d. Expansion of intravascular volume
e. Edema

339. Components of the normal
thymus gland include all the following EXCEPT

a. Thymocytes
b. Epithelial cells

c. Neuroendocrine cells
d. Myoid cells
e. Germinal centers

340. All the following statements
concerning thymomas are true
EXCEPT

a. They originate from epithelial cells
b. They are most common in the anterosuperior mediastinum
c. They are asymptomatic or cause
   local pressure effects
d. Neoplastic lymphocytes are a component
e. Most thymomas are benign

DIRECTIONS: Each group of questions below consists of lettered headings followed by a set of numbered items. For each numbered item select the **one** lettered heading with which it is **most** closely associated. Each lettered heading may be used **once, more than once, or not at all**.

Questions 341–342

Match each of the following clinical scenarios with the correct diagnosis from the following list.

a. Cortical carcinoma
b. Corticotrophic adenoma
c. Gonadotrope adenoma
d. Nephroblastoma
e. Neuroblastoma
f. Null cell adenoma
g. Paraganglioma
h. Pheochromocytoma
i. Prolactinoma
j. Somatotrope adenoma

341. A 34-year-old female presents with recurrent episodes of severe headaches, palpitations, tachycardia, and sweating. A physical examination reveals her blood pressure to be within normal limits, however, during one of these episodes of headaches, palpitations, and tachycardia, her blood pressure is found to be markedly elevated. What tumor is most likely to be present in this individual?

342. A 25-year-old female presents because she thinks that she may be pregnant. She states that she has had menstrual cycles since the age of 13, but now they have stopped completely. She preformed an "at-home" pregnancy test that she had bought at a local drugstore, but this was negative. A repeat pregnancy test done by the laboratory is also negative. Physical examination reveals the presence of a bilateral "milky" discharge from both nipples. Additional laboratory tests reveal decreased serum LH and estradiol levels. A CT scan reveals enlargement of the pituitary gland. What tumor is most likely to be present in this individual?

Questions 343–344

Match each of the following clinical scenarios with the labeled box in the associated graph that depicts the correct serum levels of calcium and parathyroid hormone.

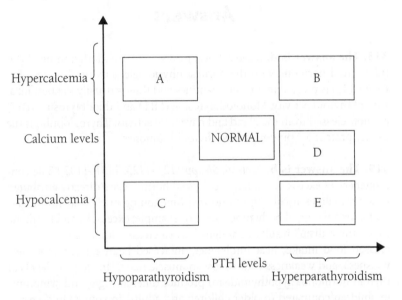

343. A 65-year-old female presents with numbness and tingling of her hands, feet, and lips. Physical examination reveals hyperactivity of her muscles, which is illustrated by a positive Chvostek's sign.

344. A 23-year-old female has a familial deficiency of α-1-hydroxylase. Resultant parathyroid hyperplasia brings the calcium and phosphorous serum levels to within normal limits.

ENDOCRINE SYSTEM

Answers

318. The answer is d. *(Henry, 19/e, pp 333–335.)* Triiodothyronine (T_3) is the thyroid hormone with the greatest physiologic activity, although thyroxine (T_4) is present in greater quantities and thus is usually the best measure of thyroid activity. Monoiodotyrosine (MIT) and diiodotyrosine (DIT) are not released from the gland and have little activity. Thyroglobulin is the carrier protein for binding stored thyroid hormones.

319. The answer is b. *(Cotran, 5/e, pp 1124–1125, 1131–1133.)* The consequences of excess or inadequate thyroid hormone are directly attributed to abnormalities involving the normal functioning of thyroid hormones, such as regulation of body processes. For example, excess thyroid hormone (hyperthyroidism) results in weight loss (increased lipolysis) despite increased food intake, heat intolerance, increased heart rate, tremor, nervousness, and weakness (due to loss in muscle mass). Inadequate levels of thyroid hormone (hypothyroidism) produce different signs and symptoms in children compared to older children and adults. In young children hypothyroidism produces cretinism, a disease that is characterized by marked retardation of physical and mental growth (severe mental retardation). Patients develop dry, rough skin and a protuberant abdomen. Characteristic facial features include periorbital edema, a flattened broad nose, and a large, protuberant tongue. In contrast, hypothyroidism in older children and adults produces myxedema. This disease is characterized by a decrease in the metabolic rate, which can result in multiple different signs and symptoms, such as cold intolerance and weight gain. Neurologic features of this abnormality include slowing of intellectual and motor function (fatigue, lethargy, and slow speech), apathy, sleepiness, depression, paranoia, and prolonged relaxation phase in deep tendon reflexes ("hung-up" reflexes). Other signs and symptoms of hypothyroidism include dry skin and brittle hair, which can produce hair loss, decreased erythropoiesis, which produces a normochromic normocytic anemia; increased cholesterol, which increases the risk of atherosclerosis; and myxedema, which is the increased interstitial deposition of mucopolysaccharides. The latter abnormality can result in diffuse non-pitting edema of the skin, hoarseness, and enlargement of the heart. Other systems affected by hypothyroidism include the heart, the GI tract, and the GU tract. Patients may develop a slowed heart rate and decrease stroke volume (resulting in cool, pale skin), constipation, and impotence in men, and menorrhagia and anovulatory cycles in women.

Graves' disease (diffuse toxic hyperplasia) is an autoimmune disorder that clinically produces hyperthyroidism. Other common causes of primary diseases of the thyroid that cause hyperthyroidism include toxic multinodular goiter and toxic adenoma. These three diseases have in common the word "toxic," which refers to the symptoms of hyperthyroidism. Goiters and adenomas are not necessarily "toxic," and these patients may instead be euthyroid, e.g., diffuse nontoxic (simple) goiter, multinodular nontoxic goiter, and nontoxic adenoma. Uncommon causes of hyperthyroidism include choriocarcinomas, hydatidiform moles (both of which may produce TSH-like substances in addition to chorionic gonadotropins), struma ovarii (a monodermal teratoma of the ovary that is composed of thyroid), and TSH-secreting pituitary tumors.

320. The answer is a. (*Cotran, 5/e, pp 1125–1128.*) Four types of thyroiditis may be associated with hypothyroidism. Hashimoto's thyroiditis, one of the autoimmune thyroid diseases, is associated with the HLA-B8 haplotype and high titers of circulating autoantibodies, including anti-microsomal, anti-thyroglobulin, and anti-TSH receptors antibodies. This abnormality is not that uncommon in the United States.

Histologically there is infiltration of the thyroid stroma by an intense lymphoplasmacytic infiltrate with the formation of lymphoid follicles with germinal centers. This produces destruction and atrophy of the follicles and transforms the thyroid follicular cells into acidophilic cells. There are many different names for these cells, including oxyphilic cells, oncocytes, Hurthle cells, and Askanazy cells. Not uncommonly, patients develop hypothyroidism as a result of follicle disruption, and the manifestations consist of fatigue, myxedema, cold intolerance, hair coarsening, and constipation. Rarely cases of Hashimoto's thyroiditis may develop hyperthyroidism (Hashitoxicosis), while the combination of Hashimoto's disease, pernicious anemia, and type I diabetes mellitus is called Schmidt's syndrome. This is one type of the multiglandular syndromes.

Whereas subacute thyroiditis, Riedel's thyroiditis, and psychosomatic complaints may cause common symptoms, biopsy findings of these disorders are distinctly different from those of Hashimoto's disease. Subacute (DeQuaervain's, granulomatous, or giant cell) thyroiditis is a self-limited viral infection of the thyroid. It typically follows an upper respiratory tract infection. Patients develop the acute onset of fever, painful thyroid enlargement, and may develop a transient hypothyroidism. Histologically there is destruction of the follicles with a granulomatous reaction and multinucleated giant cells that surround fragments of colloid. One-half of the patients with Riedel's thyroiditis are hypothyroid, but in contrast to the other types of thyroiditis, microscopic examination reveals dense fibrosis of the thyroid gland, often extending into extrathyroidal soft tissue. This fibrosis produces a rock-hard enlarged thyroid gland that may produce the feeling of suffocation. This combination of signs and symptoms may be mistaken clinically for a malignant process. Additionally these patients may develop similar fibrosis in the mediastinum or retroperitoneum. Finally, subacute lymphocytic thyroiditis is also a self-limited, painless enlargement of the thyroid that is associated with hypothyroidism, but lacks antithyroid antibodies or lymphoid germinal centers within the thyroid.

321. The answer is b. (*Cotran, 5/e, pp 1131–1133.*) The histologic appearance of colloid storage goiter generally includes abnormally large, colloid-filled follicles compressing the intervening small or normal-sized follicles that contain very little colloid. The epithelium of the follicles is predominantly flat cuboidal, with occasional epithelial papillary structures protruding into the follicles. In primary hyperplasia with Graves' disease, the follicular epithelium is tall, with papillary infoldings and peripheral vacuolation of the colloid. Riedel's struma appears histologically as a marked fibrous tissue replacement of the normal thyroid tissue. In Hashimoto's thyroiditis, only remnants of thyroid follicles and epithelial cells are found in sheets of lymphocytes with germinal centers.

322. The answer is d. (*Cotran, 5/e, pp 1136–1142.*) The four major histologic subtypes of thyroid carcinoma are papillary, follicular, medullary, and undifferentiated (anaplastic). Medullary carcinoma, which originates from the parafollicular C cells, is characterized by its amyloid stroma, which classically has a yellow-green birefringence staining pattern with the Congo red stain; by its genetic (familial) associations with pheochromocytomas and parathyroid hyperplasia or adenomas (Sipple's syndrome, multiple endocrine neoplasia IIa); and by its elaboration of calcitonin and other substances. In contrast, papillary carcinomas are composed of papillary structures with fibrovascular cores, while follicular carcinomas typically have a microfollicular pattern. It is important prognostically to differentiate papillary carcinomas from follicular carcinomas, as papillary carcinomas tend to be indolent (up to 80 percent survival at 10 years), while follicular carcinomas are much more aggressive (5-year mortality up to 70 percent). Follicular areas may be present within a papillary carcinoma and in fact may be quite extensive. If present, these changes can make the diagnosis difficult. It is important to recognize this follicular variant of papillary carcinoma as its behavior remains similar to that of indolent papillary carcinoma. Features consistent with papillary carcinoma, even in predominantly follicular areas, include optically clear nuclei ("ground glass," "Orphan Annie eyes"), nuclear grooves, calcospherites (psammoma bodies), and intranuclear cytoplasmic pseudoinclusions.

323. The answer is a. (*Cotran, 5/e, pp 1144–1147. Chandrasoma, 3/e, pp 857–863.*) Hyperparathyroidism is caused by excess production of parathyroid hormone (PTH). In patients with hyperparathyroidism it is important to distinguish primary hyperparathyroidism from secondary hyperparathyroidism. Both forms may be associated with the development of bone lesions, but excess PTH production in primary hyperparathyroidism leads to different laboratory values than those seen with secondary hyperparathyroidism. Increased levels of PTH in primary hyperparathyroidism result in the following laboratory results: increased serum calcium (hypercalcemia) and decreased serum phosphorus. The serum calcium levels are elevated because of increased bone resorption and increased intestinal calcium absorption, the result of increased activity of vitamin D. PTH also increases calcium reabsorption in the distal renal tubule, but because the filtered load of calcium exceeds the ability for reabsorption, calcium is increased in the urine (hypercalciuria). PTH also increases the urinary excretion of phosphate. The excess calcium in the urine predisposes to renal stone formation, especially calcium oxalate or calcium phosphate stones. Urinary stones can produce flank pain and hematuria. This is the most common presentation for patients with hyperparathyroidism. The hypercalcemia of hyperparathyroidism may also cause peptic ulcer disease, which is due to the stimulation of gastrin release and increased acid secretion from the parietal cells. The hypercalcemia also results in muscle weakness, fatigue, and hypomotility of the GI tract, which can lead to constipation and nausea. Alterations of mental status are also common.

In contrast to primary hyperparathyroidism, secondary hyperparathyroidism results from hypocalcemia. This causes secondary hypersecretion of PTH and produces the combination of hypocalcemia and increased PTH production. It is primarily found in patients with chronic renal failure. Patients with hypoparathyroidism develop hypocalcemia, hyperphosphatemia, but have normal serum creatinine levels. Primary hypoparathyroidism and pseudohypoparathyroidism also result in decreased 24-hour excretion of calcium and phosphate.

324. The answer is c. *(Cotran, 5/e, pp 1144–1147. Rubin, 2/e, pp 1126–1128.)* Parathyroid hyperplasia may be associated with either primary or secondary hyperparathyroidism. In contrast to primary hyperparathyroidism, secondary hyperparathyroidism results from hypocalcemia and causes secondary hypersecretion of parathyroid hormone (PTH). This results in the combination of hypocalcemia and increased PTH. This abnormality is principally found in patients with chronic renal failure where phosphate retention is thought to cause hypocalcemia. Since the failing kidney is not able to synthesize 1,25-dihydroxycholecalciferol, the most active form of vitamin D, this deficiency leads to poor absorption of calcium from the gut and relative hypocalcemia, which stimulates excess PTH secretion. Chronic renal failure is the most important cause, but secondary hyperparathyroidism also occurs in vitamin D deficiency, malabsorption syndromes, and pseudohypoparathyroidism. In any of the causes of parathyroid hyperplasia all four parathyroid glands are typically enlarged. Parathyroid hyperplasia can be differentiated from parathyroid adenomas by the fact that parathyroid hyperplasia, either primary or secondary, results in enlargement of all four glands, while a parathyroid adenoma or parathyroid carcinoma will produce enlargement of only one gland. In most cases the other three glands are smaller than normal.

325. The answer is d. *(Cotran, 5/e, pp 1154–1157. Rubin, 2/e, pp 1129–1131.)* In the adrenal cortex, cholesterol is converted into either mineralocorticoids (aldosterone) in the zona glomerulosa, glucocorticoids (cortisol) in the zona fasciculata, or sex steroid precursors in the zona reticularis. Congenital adrenal hyperplasia (CAH) is a syndrome that results from a defect in the synthesis of cortisol. This leads to excess ACTH secretion by the anterior pituitary and resultant adrenal hyperplasia. The defect in the synthesis of cortisol is the result of a deficiency in one of the enzymes in the normal pathway of cortisol synthesis, such as 21-hydroxylase or 11-hydroxylase. Most cases of CAH result from a deficiency of 21-hydroxylase. Two forms of this deficiency include salt-wasting adrenogenitalism and simple virilizing adrenogenitalism. The salt-wasting syndrome results from a complete lack of the hydroxylase. There is no synthesis of mineralocorticoids or glucocorticoids in the adrenal cortex. Decreased mineralocorticoids causes marked sodium loss in the urine, hyponatremia, hyperkalemia, acidosis, and hypotension. Because of the enzyme block there is increased formation of 17-hydroxyprogesterone, which is then shunted into the production of testosterone. This may cause virilism (pseudohermaphroditism) in female infants. That is, XX females with CAH develop ovaries, female ductal structures, and external male genitalia. Much more often there is only a partial deficiency of 21-hydroxylase, and this leads to decreased production of both aldosterone and cortisol. The decreased cortisol levels cause increased production of ACTH by the pituitary, which results in adrenal hyperplasia, enough to maintain adequate serum levels of aldosterone and cortisol. In contrast to a complete deficiency of 21-hydroxylase, there is no sodium loss with a partial deficiency of 21-hydroxylase. The excess stimulation by ACTH, however, again leads to increased production of androgens, which may cause virilism in female infants.

A deficiency of 11-hydroxylase, which is rare, also leads to decreased cortisol production and increased ACTH secretion. This in turn leads to the accumulation of DOC (deoxycorticosterone) and 11-deoxycortisol, both of which are strong mineralocorticoids. This results in increased sodium retention by the kidneys and hypertension. Patients also develop hypokalemia and virilization due to androgen excess. Patients with a deficiency of 17-hydroxylase also have impaired cortisol production, increased ACTH, and secondary increased DOC. These patients, however, cannot synthesize normal amounts of androgens and estrogens. This is because the gene that codes for 17-α hydroxylase is the same for the enzyme in the adrenal cortex and the gonads, and the deficiency is the same in both organs. Because of decreased sex hormones, genotypic females develop primary amenorrhea and fail to develop secondary sex characteristics, while genotypic males will present as pseudohermaphrodites.

Additionally, the plasma LH levels will be increased due to decreased feedback inhibition.

326. The answer is b. (*Henry, 19/e, pp 353–355. Rubin, 2/e, pp 1133–1138.*) Cushing's syndrome may be the result of bilateral adrenal hyperplasia, adrenal neoplasia, or excessive use of adrenocorticotropic hormone or glucocorticoids. However, bilateral adrenal hyperplasia is the most common etiologic factor. The clinical manifestations of the syndrome—whether it is induced by ectopic ACTH (small cell carcinoma of the lung), or exogenously, or endogenously by the adrenal—are similar. Levels of plasma and urinary cortisol and urinary 17-hydroxycorticoid are usually elevated.

327. The answer is e. (*Cotran, 5/e, pp 1157–1160. Rubin, 2/e, pp 1131–1133.*) Hypofunctioning of the cortex of the adrenal gland (adrenocortical insufficiency) may be the result of abnormalities involving either the adrenal gland itself (primary adrenocortical insufficiency) or the pituitary gland, which controls the adrenal (secondary adrenocortical insufficiency). Primary insufficiency may arise from either an acute process or a chronic process. Causes of primary acute adrenocortical insufficiency include acute hemorrhagic necrosis of the adrenals, as seen in children as Waterhouse-Friderichsen syndrome. This syndrome is most commonly due to Neisseria meningitidis septicemia, which is characterized by meningitis, septicemia, DIC, and hypovolemic shock. Acute adrenocortical insufficiency may also occur with too rapid a withdrawal of steroid therapy if a patient has additional stress. Causes of primary chronic adrenocortical insufficiency (Addison's disease) include autoimmune adrenalitis, infections, amyloidosis, and metastatic cancer. Previously the most common cause of Addison's disease was tuberculosis of the adrenal gland, but now the majority of patients have adrenal autoantibodies and are thought to have autoimmune adrenalitis. Half of these cases have other autoimmune endocrine diseases, the resulting syndromes being called polyglandular syndromes.

Secondary adrenocortical insufficiency, such as caused by decreased functioning of the pituitary or in prolonged suppression of the pituitary by exogenous glucocorticoid therapy, results in decreased ACTH and hypofunctioning of the adrenal. This produces symptoms that are similar to Addison's disease, such as weakness and weight loss. In contrast to Addison's disease, patients with secondary adrenocortical insufficiency have normal secretion of aldosterone, because aldosterone production is not controlled by the pituitary gland. Therefore these patients do not develop symptoms of aldosterone deficiency such as volume depletion, hypotension, hyperkalemia, or hyponatremia. Additionally, since ACTH levels are not elevated there is no hyperpigmentation.

328. The answer is c. *(Cotran, 5/e, pp 1158–1160. Rubin, 2/e, pp 1131–1133.)* In 1855, when Addison first described primary adrenal insufficiency, the most common cause was tuberculosis of the adrenal gland. Now the majority of patients have adrenal autoantibodies and are thought to have autoimmune Addison's disease. Half of these patients have other autoimmune endocrine diseases. Patients with type I polyglandular autoimmune syndrome have at least two of the following three diseases or abnormalities: Addison's disease, hypoparathyroidism, and mucocutaneous candidiasis. Type II polyglandular autoimmune syndrome, also called Schmidt's syndrome, lacks hypoparathyroidism and mucocutaneous candidiasis, and instead is associated with autoimmune thyroid disease (Hashimoto's thyroiditis) and insulin-dependent diabetes. Islet cell adenomas of the pancreas may be found in multiple endocrine neoplasia type 1 (MEN 1) syndrome along with pituitary adenomas and parathyroid hyperplasia or adenomas. Medullary carcinoma of the thyroid along with pheochromocytomas of the adrenal gland and parathyroid hyperplasia is seen in MEN 2A (Sipple's syndrome).

329. The answer is b. *(Cotran, 5/e, pp 1159, 1169–1170. Rubin, 2/e, pp 1132, 1140.)* Combinations of neoplasms affecting different endocrine organs in the same patient are referred to as multiple endocrine neoplasia (MEN) syndromes. There are several types of MEN syndromes. Patients with type I MEN syndrome (Wermer syndrome) have pituitary adenomas, parathyroid hyperplasia (or adenomas), and neoplasms of the pancreatic islets. The latter most commonly are gastrinomas, which secrete gastrin and produce the Zollinger-Ellison syndrome. Type IIa MEN syndrome (Sipple syndrome) is characterized by the combination of medullary carcinoma of the thyroid, pheochromocytoma of the adrenal medulla, and hyperparathyroidism. MEN type IIb syndrome (also known as type III) is associated with medullary carcinoma of the thyroid, pheochromocytoma of the adrenal medulla, and multiple mucocutaneous neuromas.

In contrast to the MEN syndromes, combinations of autoimmune diseases affecting different endocrine organs is called polyglandular syndromes. There are several types of polyglandular syndromes. Patients with type I polyglandular autoimmune syndrome have at least two of the triad of Addison's disease, hypoparathyroidism, and mucocutaneous candidiasis. Type II polyglandular syndrome (Schmidt's syndrome) is not associated with either hypoparathyroidism or mucocutaneous candidiasis, but instead is associated with autoimmune thyroid disease (Hashimoto's thyroiditis) and insulin-dependent diabetes mellitus.

330. The answer is b. (*Cotran, 5/e, pp 217–218, 1166.*) The branchial apparatus consists of the branchial clefts (ectoderm), the branchial arches (mesoderm and neural crest), and the branchial (pharyngeal) pouches (endoderm). The third pouch (dorsal wings) develops into the inferior parathyroid glands; the third pouch (ventral wings) develop into the thymus; the fourth pouch develops into the superior parathyroids; while the fifth pouch develops into the ultimobranchial bodies, which in turn gives rise to the C cells of the thyroid. DiGeorge's syndrome results from a failure of the development of the third and fourth pharyngeal pouches. This abnormality is associated with tetany and an absence of T cells. The tetany results from the hypocalcemia caused by the lack of the parathyroid glands, while the absence of T cells is caused by the lack of the thymus gland.

331. The answer is c. (*Henry, 19/e, pp 323–324. Cotran, 5/e, p 1117.*) The constellation of cartilaginous-periosteal soft tissue growth of the distal extremities (acromegaly) and growth of the skull and face bones is characteristic of hypersecretion of growth hormone (GH) from an anterior pituitary adenoma. GH modulates the production of hepatic somatomedin (sulfation factor). Somatomedins are small peptides that act on the target organs after being synthesized under the influence of growth hormone. They have insulin-like properties but are immunologically distinct from insulin. In addition to acral-skeletal expansion, patients with hyperpituitarism of the adult-onset variety (occurring after epiphyseal plate closure) have organomegaly, including increased size of the heart, kidneys, liver, and spleen. Cardiac failure is usually the mechanism of death.

332. The answer is e. (*Cotran, 5/e, pp 1118–1121.*) Hypopituitarism results from destructive processes that involve the adenohypophysis (anterior pituitary). These processes may be acute (sudden) or chronic. Sheehan's syndrome, also known as post-partum pituitary necrosis, results from the sudden infarction of the anterior lobe of the pituitary. This can occur with obstetric complications, such as hemorrhage or shock. The pituitary gland normally doubles in size during pregnancy; hypovolemia during delivery decreases blood flow and may result in infarction of the anterior pituitary. Sheehan's syndrome will produce symptoms of hypopituitarism, the initial sign being cessation of lactation, which may be followed by secondary amenorrhea due to the loss of gonadotropins. Other signs of hypopituitarism include hypothyroidism and decreased functioning of the adrenal gland. Acute destruction of the pituitary is also associated with DIC and thrombosis of the cavernous sinus. Chronic causes of hypopituitarism include nonsecretory chromophobe pituitary adenomas, empty sella syndrome, and suprasellar (hypothalamic) tumors. Nonsecretory chromophobe adenomas present as space-occupying lesions that cause decreased hormone production. The gonadotropins are lost first, which results in signs of hypogonadism. Types of chromophobe adenomas include null cell adenomas (no cytoplasmic granules), chromophobes (sparse granules), and oncocytic adenomas (increased cytoplasmic mitochondria). The term pituitary apoplexy refers to spontaneous hemorrhage into a pituitary tumor, while the empty sella syndrome is caused by a defective diaphragma sella, which permits CSF from the third ventricle to enter the sella. It may also be secondary to infarction or necrosis. A CT scan reveals the sella to be enlarged or appear to be empty.

The metyrapone test can be used to evaluate patients with possible hypopituitarism. Metyrapone blocks the enzyme 11-hydroxylase in the adrenal cortex. This produces decreased production of cortisol with resultant increased production of ACTH and increased production of 11-deoxycortisol. Decreased production of the latter during the performance of this test indicates a problem with either the pituitary or the adrenal gland. Although this test does not differentiate these two, with the former, ACTH levels are decreased, while with the latter, ACTH levels are increased.

A craniopharyngioma (adamantinoma or ameloblastoma) is a tumor that is derived from vestigial remnants of Rathke's pouch, an ectodermal outpouching of the floor of the mouth. These tumors grossly are multiloculated (multicystic) and contain a thick brown oily fluid ("motor oil"). They also contain calcifications that can be seen radiographically. Histologically these tumors recapitulate the enamel of the tooth and form nests of squamous epithelial cells in a fibrous stroma.

333. The answer is e. *(Cotran, 5/e, p 1121.)* The syndrome of inappropriate antidiuretic hormone (SIADH) is an important cause of dilutional hyponatremia that has been identified in tumors of the thymus gland, malignant lymphoma, and pancreatic neoplasms. It occurs predominantly, however, as a result of ectopic secretion of ADH by oat cell carcinomas of the lung. Since the tumor cells per se are autonomously producing ADH, there is no feedback inhibition from the hypothalamic osmoreceptors, and the persistent ADH effect on the renal tubules causes water retention even with concentrated urine. Hence the term inappropriate ADH arises. Laboratory findings of the syndrome include low plasma sodium levels (dilutional hyponatremia), low plasma osmolality, and high urine osmolality caused by disproportionate solute excretion without water.

334. The answer is b. *(Ganong, 17/e, pp 215–217. Cotran, 5/e, pp 1116–1118.)* Lesions that selectively destroy portions of the hypothalamus will produce characteristic signs and symptoms that depend upon the normal functions controlled by that area. For example, destruction of the hypothalamic ventromedial nucleus will lead to rage, obesity, and hyperphagia, which is due to increased appetite. These same symptoms can result from stimulation rather than destruction of the dorsomedial nucleus. In contrast to obesity, starvation due to decreased appetite will result from lesions that destroy the lateral hypothalamus (lateral nuclei). Destruction of the supraoptic nucleus will lead to decreased production of antidiuretic hormone (ADH) and will lead to the development of diabetes insipidus, one symptom of which is polyuria. Destruction of the posterior hypothalamus (posterior nucleus) will result in the inability to produce heat when cold. Such an affected person would become "cold-blooded" (poikilotherm), like a reptile. In contrast, destruction of the anterior hypothalamus (anterior nucleus) would result in excess heat production (hyperthermia).

Vision loss, such as tunnel vision, can result from large pituitary tumors impinging upon the optic chiasm, while hyperglycemia can result from pituitary tumors that secrete growth hormone. A deficiency of thiamine can produce the Wernicke-Korsakoff syndrome. Wernicke encephalopathy consists mainly of foci of hemorrhage and necrosis in the mammillary bodies. Symptoms of Wernicke syndrome include progressive dementia, ataxia, and paralysis of the extraocular muscles (ophthalmoplegia). Korsakoff psychosis is a thought disorder that produces memory failure and confabulation.

335. The answer is d. (*Cotran, 5/e, pp 1129–1131.*) Graves' disease, or diffuse toxic goiter, is one of the three most common disorders associated with thyrotoxicosis or hyperthyroidism (the other two are toxic multinodular goiter and toxic adenoma). This hyperfunctioning and hyperplastic diffuse goiter is accompanied by infiltrative ophthalmopathy, including exophthalmos or proptosis—only seen in Graves' disease. Dermopathy or pretibial "myxedema" is present in up to 15 percent of cases. Graves' disease is an autoimmune form of goiter caused by thyroid-stimulating immunoglobulins or thyroid-stimulating hormone receptor antibodies. Autoantibodies to TSH receptor antigens are produced because of a defect in antigen-specific suppressor T cells. The antibodies bind to TSH receptors on thyroid follicular cells and function as TSH, with resultant thyroid growth and hyperfunction. Such antibodies can be identified in almost all cases of Graves' disease. Cardiac manifestations include tachycardia, cardiomegaly, and occasional arrhythmias (atrial fibrillation), and these are often early features. Diffuse toxic goiter is associated with HLA-DR3 genotype.

336. The answer is b. (*Cotran, 5/e, pp 1136–1142.*) The four major histologic subtypes of thyroid carcinoma, in decreasing order of frequency, are papillary, follicular, medullary, and undifferentiated (anaplastic). Follicular carcinoma has a frequency of approximately 10 to 20 percent compared with papillary cancer at 60 to 70 percent. There are, of course, follicular variants of both papillary and medullary carcinoma, but these behave as papillary and medullary cancer, not as the follicular type. Other, much rarer variants of follicular cancer include the type resembling renal clear cell carcinoma and the insular type of thyroid cancer, which is an aggressive form of follicular carcinoma with a solid growth pattern. Vascular invasion and hematogenous metastasis are usual with follicular cancer, so that intrathyroidal foci from lymphatic spread would not occur, although they are very common with papillary cancer. Absence of ground-glass nuclei or well-formed papillae or psammoma bodies differentiates follicular from papillary carcinoma.

337. The answer is e. (*Cotran, 5/e, pp 1147–1148. Rubin, 2/e, pp 1125–1126.*) Hypoparathyroidism may be caused by either decreased secretion of parathyroid hormone (PTH) or end-organ insensitivity to PTH (pseudohypoparathyroidism), both of which are associated with hypocalcemia and hyperphosphatemia. Many patients with pseudohypoparathyroidism have a defect in binding of many hormones to guanine nucleotide-binding protein (G protein). These hormones include PTH, thyroid-stimulating hormone, glucagon, and the gonadotropins follicle-stimulating hormone and luteinizing hormone. These patients have characteristic signs and symptoms including short stature, round face, short neck, reduced intelligence, and abnormally short metacarpal and metatarsal bones. In contrast to patients with hypothyroidism caused by decreased levels of PTH, patients with pseudohypoparathyroidism (Albright's hereditary osteodystrophy) have normal or increased levels of circulating PTH and in fact have hyperparathyroidism.

338. The answer is e. (*Cotran, 5/e, pp 1153–1154.*) Edema is not a feature of primary hyperaldosteronism (Conn's syndrome), which is characterized by weakness, hypertension, polydipsia, and polyuria. The underlying physiologic abnormalities include alkaline urine, an elevated level of serum sodium, hypokalemic alkalosis, and excessive potassium loss by the kidneys. The level of serum aldosterone is elevated; that of plasma renin is suppressed. The elevated level of serum sodium causes expansion of the intravascular volume. A single adenoma has been described as the causative factor of primary hyperaldosteronism in the majority of patients, and carcinoma, multiple adenomas, and cortical hyperplasia have been cited occasionally as causes of this syndrome.

339. The answer is e. (*Cotran, 5/e, pp 1166–1167. Rubin, 2/e, pp 1144–1145.*) The thymus, derived from the third pair of pharyngeal pouches and inconsistently from the fourth pair, is divided into an outer cortex and an inner medulla and is composed of lymphocytes and epithelial cells. The lymphocytes are mainly T cells, which in the cortex are immature (thymocytes) and in the medulla are mature (having phenotypic characteristics of peripheral blood T lymphocytes). The epithelial cells are mainly located in the medulla, where they form Hassall's corpuscles. The thymus normally has a few neuroendocrine cells, which can give rise to carcinoid tumors or small cell carcinoma, and a few myoid cells, which are similar to striated muscle cells and may play a role in the autoimmune pathogenesis of myasthenia gravis. The appearance of lymphoid follicles with germinal centers is diagnostic of thymic hyperplasia and is not a normal component of the thymus gland.

340. The answer is d. (*Cotran, 5/e, pp 1167–1168.*) Thymomas are tumors arising from thymic epithelial cells and form one of the most common mediastinal neoplasms, especially in the anterosuperior mediastinum. There is a scant or rich lymphocytic infiltrate of T cells, which are not neoplastic, although their size and prominent nucleoli may cause histologic confusion with lymphoma. About 90 percent of thymomas are benign and occur at a mean age of 50 years. They are very rare in children. They may be asymptomatic or cause pressure effects of dysphagia, dyspnea, or vena cava compression. Associated systemic disorders include myasthenia gravis, hematologic cytopenias, collagen vascular disease (lupus), and hypogammaglobulinemia. Malignant thymomas show infiltration and capsular invasion plus pleural implants or distant metastasis.

341–342. The answers are: 341-h, 342-i. (*Cotran, 5/e, pp 459–461, 464–465, 1114–1118, 1162–1165.*) Tumors of the adrenal medulla include pheochromocytomas, ganglioneuromas, and neuroblastomas. Pheochromocytomas are composed of cells that contain membrane-bound, dense-core neurosecretory granules and have high cytoplasmic levels of catecholamines. Secretion of these catecholamines produces the characteristic symptoms associated with pheochromocytomas, such as hypertension, palpitations, tachycardia, sweating, and glucose intolerance (diabetes mellitus). Pheochromocytomas are associated with the urinary excretion of catecholamines or their metabolic breakdown products. The catecholamines include dopamine, norepinephrine, and epinephrine. These catecholamines are broken down by two enzymes, catecholamine orthomethyltransferase (COMT) and monoamine oxidase (MAO) into homovanillic acid, normetanephrine, metanephrine, or vanillylmandelic acid (VMA). Any of these metabolic products may be found in the urine of patients with pheochromocytomas; however, VMA is most common. The best screening test are 24-hour urinary metanephrine and VMA levels. Pheochromocytomas have been called the "10 percent tumor" as 10 percent are malignant, 10 percent are multiple (bilateral), 10 percent are extra-adrenal, 10 percent calcify, and 10 percent are familial. These familial tumors are associated with neurofibromatosis, MEN IIa or MEN IIb.

Neuroblastomas are malignant tumors of the adrenal medulla that occur in very young patients. Histologically these tumors are composed of small cells, which may form Homer-Wright rosettes. Electron microscopy reveals the presence of neurosecretory granules, while immunohistochemical stains are positive for neuron-specific enolase (NSE). These highly aggressive tumors are special because some will spontaneously regress and some will de-differentiate into benign tumors, such as ganglioneuromas. Malignant tumors of the kidney in children are called nephroblastomas (Wilms' tumor), and histologically reveal a combination of metanephric blastema, undifferentiated mesenchymal cells, and immature tubule or glomerular formation. Cortical carcinomas are found in the adrenal cortex, while paragangliomas are found in paraganglia outside of the adrenal gland. None of these tumors, except for neuroblastomas, occur in the adrenal medulla.

Pituitary adenomas are the most common neoplasms of the pituitary gland. These benign neoplasms are classified according to the hormone or hormones that are produced by the neoplastic cells. The cell types, in order of decreasing frequency, are the following: lactotrope adenomas (which secrete prolactin), null cell adenomas (which do not secrete hormones), somatotrope adenomas (which secrete growth hormone), corticotrophic adenomas (which secrete ACTH), gonadotrope adenomas (which secrete FSH and LH), and thyrotrope cell adenoma (which secrete TSH). Prolactin secreting tumors (lactotrope adenomas or prolactinomas) produce symptoms of hypogonadism and galactorrhea, which is milk secretion that is not associated with pregnancy. In females this hypogonadism produces amenorrhea and infertility, while in males it produces impotence and decreased libido. The same symptoms that are seen with a prolactin-secreting pituitary adenoma can also be produced by certain drugs, such as methyldopa and reserpine. A somatotropic adenoma that secretes growth hormone may produce gigantism if it occurs in children prior to the closure of the epiphyseal plates or acromegaly if it occurs in adults after the closure of the epiphyseal plates. Additional findings in patients with excess growth hormone production include enlargement of the viscera, thickening of the skin, and diabetes mellitus. A functioning thyrotroph adenoma may produce hyperthyroidism, while a functioning gonadotroph cell adenoma usually present with hypogonadism. Excess production of adrenocorticotropin (ACTH) by a corticotrophic adenoma will produce Cushing's disease.

343–344. The answers are: 343-c, 344-d. (*Cotran, 5/e, pp 1144–1148. Chandrasoma, 3/e, pp 857–863.*) To summarize the diseases of the parathyroid glands, since serum calcium levels are affected by serum PTH levels, plotting serum calcium levels and serum PTH on a graph will separate the different abnormalities of PTH functioning into different areas of the graph.

Increased levels of PTH (hyperparathyroidism) may be either primary or secondary. Primary hyperparathyroidism is associated with increased PTH and increased calcium (area B), while secondary hyperparathyroidism is associated with increased PTH and decreased or normal calcium levels (areas E and D, respectively). This can be seen in patients with a deficiency of α-1-hydroxylase, because decreased active vitamin D levels will produce decreased absorption of calcium, hypocalcemia, and resultant hyperparathyroidism.

Hypoparathyroidism may be caused by either decreased secretion of parathyroid hormones (primary hypoparathyroidism) or end organ insensitivity to parathyroid hormone (pseudohypoparathyroidism). Both of these are associated with hypocalcemia and hyperphosphatemia, which is due to decreased urinary phosphate excretion. The signs of hypoparathyroidism are mainly due to the effects of hypocalcemia. The hypocalcemia may produce numbness and tingling of the hands, feet, and lips, or tetany, which refers to spontaneous tonic muscular contractions. Two clinical tests that can be used to demonstrate tetany are Chvostek's sign and Trousseau's sign. Chvostek's sign refers to the finding that tapping on the facial nerve produces twitching of the ipsilateral facial muscles, while Trousseau's sign refers to inflating a blood pressure cuff for several minutes to produce painful carpal muscle contractions. Primary hypoparathyroidism refers to decreased levels of PTH and decreased levels of calcium (area C). Causes of primary hypoparathyroidism include iatrogenic, such as surgical accident during thyroidectomy, congenital abnormalities (DiGeorge's syndrome), and type I polyglandular autoimmune syndrome. Patients with the latter abnormality have at least two of the triad of Addison's disease, hypoparathyroidism, and mucocutaneous candidiasis. Pseudohypoparathyroidism refers to decreased levels of calcium and increased levels of PTH (area E, which is the same as hyperparathyroidism). Pseudohyperparathyroidism would theoretically refer to decreased levels of PTH and increased levels of calcium (area A). This combination does not occur with diseases of the parathyroid glands, but instead can be seen in patients with hypercalcemia, the result of production of a substance with parathyroid hormone-like function (paraneoplastic syndrome). This substance is called parathyroid-hormone-related protein. In these patients, serum levels of PTH are decreased because of the high levels of calcium.

GENITOURINARY SYSTEM

Questions

DIRECTIONS: Each question below contains five suggested responses. Select the **one best** response to each question.

345. A major role in the exclusion of albumin from the ultrafiltrate in the normal human glomerulus is played by

a. Sodium-potassium ATPase
b. Parietal epithelium
c. Endothelial fenestrations
d. Proteoglycans
e. Podocytes

346. A significant role in vascular permeability, particularly in the renal glomerulus, is played by

a. Collagen type IV
b. Desmin
c. Fibronectin
d. Podocytes
e. Polyanions

347. An 8-month-old infant presents with progressive renal and hepatic failure. Despite intensive medical therapy, this young infant dies. At the time of autopsy the external surface of his kidneys were found to be smooth, but the cut section revealed numerous cysts that were lined up in a row. What is the mode of inheritance of this renal abnormality?

a. Autosomal dominant
b. Autosomal recessive
c. X-linked dominant
d. X-linked recessive
e. Mitochondrial

348. An 18-month-old infant is evaluated for generalized tissue edema and ascites. Urinalysis shows numerous hyaline casts and lipid droplets. Total plasma protein and albumin are markedly decreased, whereas total lipids are increased. A light micrograph of a renal biopsy glomerulus is shown below. Statements applicable to this disorder include that

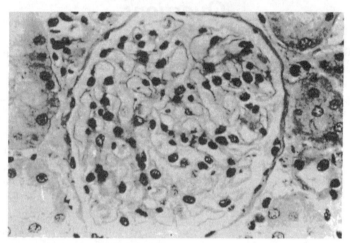

a. The problem is hepatic, not renal
b. Electron microscopy is diagnostic
c. Light microscopy is diagnostic
d. Exacerbations are uncommon
e. Response to steroid therapy is poor

349. An adult medical laboratory technician recovering from hepatitis B develops hematuria, proteinuria, and red cell casts in the urine. Which of the following would best describe the changes within the kidney in this patient?

a. Plasma cell interstitial nephritis
b. IgG linear fluorescence along the glomerular basement membrane
c. Granular deposits of antibodies in the glomerular basement membrane
d. Diffuse thickening of the glomerular basement membrane by subepithelial immune deposits
e. Nodular hyaline glomerulosclerosis

350. A 7-year-old boy presents with bilateral swelling around his eyes. His parents state that this child's eyes have become "puffy" over the past several weeks, and his urine has become cocoa-colored. Physical examination reveals bilateral periorbital edema, but peripheral edema is not found. He is afebrile, and his blood pressure is slightly elevated. A urinary dipstick reveals mild proteinuria, while microscopic examination of his urine reveals hematuria with red blood cell casts. Laboratory tests reveal increased ASO titers and decreased serum C3 levels, but C2 and C4 levels are normal. A throat swab for *streptococcus* is negative. A microscopic section from his kidney reveals increased numbers of cells within the glomeruli. An electron microscopic section of his kidney reveals large electron-dense deposits in the glomeruli that are located between the basement membrane and the podocytes. The foot processes of the podocytes are otherwise unremarkable. Which one of the following renal diseases most likely produced the abnormalities in this young boy?

a. Acute post-streptococcal glomerulonephritis
b. Focal segmental glomerulonephritis
c. Focal segmental glomerulosclerosis
d. Membranous glomerulonephritis
e. Minimal change disease

351. Immune complexes located within the glomerular basement membrane would most likely be found in a patient with

a. Acute glomerulonephritis (GN)
b. Membranous GN
c. Type I membranoproliferative glomerulonephritis (MPGN)
d. Type II MPGN
e. IgA nephropathy

352. A 21-year-old female presents because her urine has turned a brown color. She states that about two months ago her urine turned brown two days after a cold and stayed brown for about three days. At the current time a urinalysis reveals 2+ blood with red cells and red cell casts. Further laboratory tests include a complete blood count (CBC), serum electrolytes, BUN, creatinine, glucose, antinuclear antibodies (ANA), and serum complement levels (C3 and C4). All of these tests are within normal limits. Immunofluorescence examination of a renal biopsy from this patient reveals the presence of large, irregular deposits of IgA/C3 in the mesangium. A linear staining pattern is not found. What is the most likely diagnosis for this patient?

a. Berger's disease
b. Focal segmental glomerulosclerosis
c. Goodpasture's disease
d. Lipoid nephrosis
e. Membranoproliferative glomerulonephritis

353. A linear pattern of immunoglobulin deposition along the glomerular basement membrane that can be demonstrated by immunofluorescence is typical of

a. Lupus nephritis
b. Diabetic glomerulopathy
c. Goodpasture's syndrome
d. Goldblatt's kidney
e. Renal vein thrombosis

354. Marked thickening of the glomerular basement membrane, as shown in the photomicrograph below, may be seen in

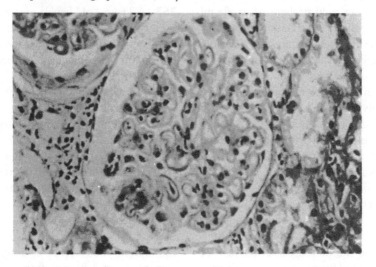

a. Lipoid nephrosis
b. Membranous glomerulonephritis
c. Goodpasture's syndrome
d. Acute pyelonephritis
e. Chronic glomerulonephritis

355. The gross appearance of the kidney shown is most compatible with which of the following conditions?

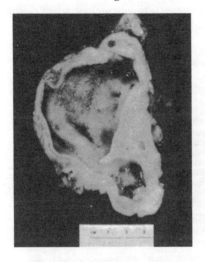

a. Cystic renal dysplasia
b. Acute pyelonephritis
c. Chronic pyelonephritis
d. Acute glomerulonephritis
e. Chronic glomerulonephritis

356. A 42-year-old female during a routine physical examination is found to have an elevated blood pressure of 150/100 mmHg. Workup reveals a small left kidney and a normal-sized right kidney. Laboratory examination reveals elevated serum renin levels. Further workup reveals that renal vein renin levels are increased on the left, but decreased on the right. This patient's hypertension is most likely the result of

a. Atherosclerotic narrowing of the left renal artery
b. Atherosclerotic narrowing of the right renal artery
c. Fibromuscular hyperplasia of the left renal artery
d. Fibromuscular hyperplasia of the right renal artery
e. Hyaline arteriolosclerosis

357. The photomicrograph below shows evidence of glomerular fibrin deposition. This histopathology is a supplemental finding in a 2-year-old child who has a history of abdominal pain and bloody diarrhea, followed by acute glomerulonephritis, Coombs'-negative severe hemolytic anemia, and renal failure. The likely diagnoses might include

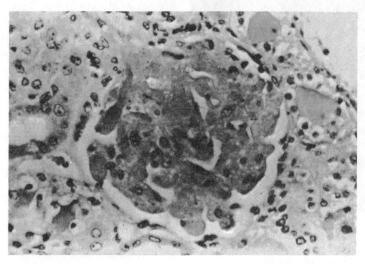

a. Lupus erythematosus
b. Acute poststreptococcal glomerulonephritis
c. Lipoid nephrosis
d. Hemolytic-uremic syndrome
e. Bacterial endocarditis

358. A middle-aged man comes to you with the single presenting symptom of occasional hematuria of very recent onset. The most probable cause is

a. Acute pyelonephritis
b. Nephroblastoma
c. Renal cell carcinoma
d. Mesoblastic nephroma
e. Renal pelvic urothelial tumor

359. A sexually active man who has had a negative evaluation for gonococcal infection and who complains of persistent dysuria but no other symptoms should be considered to have

a. Prostatic hypertrophy
b. Epididymitis
c. Orchitis
d. Nonspecific urethritis
e. Renal stones

360. The condition shown in the photomicrograph, malacoplakia of the urinary bladder, is considered to be associated with

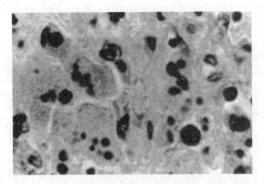

a. Tuberculosis
b. Urothelial carcinoma
c. Schistosomiasis
d. Staphylococcal infections
e. Defects in phagocytosis

361. Which of the following is sufficiently different from the others to be discriminated by histologic examination only?

a. Bowen's disease
b. Squamous cell carcinoma in situ
c. Erythroplasia of Queyrat
d. Bowenoid papulosis
e. Human papillomavirus (HPV) condyloma

362. Histologic examination of an excision specimen from a lesion on the dorsal surface of the penis reveals a papillary lesion with clear vacuolization of epithelial cells on the surface and extension of the hyperplastic epithelium into the underlying tissue along a broad front. The most likely diagnosis of this lesion is

a. Condyloma acuminatum
b. Bowen's disease
c. Erythroplasia of Queyrat
d. Verrucous carcinoma
e. Squamous cell carcinoma

363. The photomicrograph below is of a section from a testis removed from the inguinal region of a man aged 25. Which of the following statements is true regarding the condition illustrated?

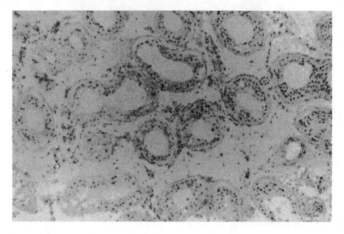

a. It is bilateral in the majority of cases
b. Teratoma is the most common malignancy to arise
c. Risk of associated malignancy is reduced by orchiopexy
d. There is increased risk of malignancy in the contralateral testis
e. Both Leydig and Sertoli cells are reduced in number

364. The photomicrograph below shows a section through a testis removed from a 30-year-old man with acute scrotal pain. True statements regarding this condition include that

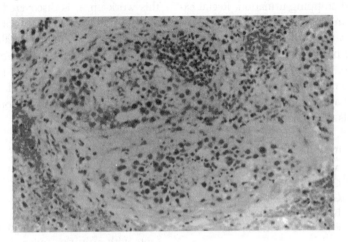

a. Infection is usually by the hematogenous route
b. Sterility is a rare condition
c. The epididymis is usually spared
d. Chlamydia trachomatis is a common pathogen
e. Interstitial cells of Leydig are destroyed

365. A small, palpable, well-circumscribed nodule in the epididymis is most likely to be

a. Androblastoma
b. Tuberculous granuloma
c. Carcinoma
d. Adenomatoid tumor
e. Adrenocortical rest

366. Which of the following testicular tumors is most radiosensitive?

a. Seminoma
b. Embryonal carcinoma
c. Choriocarcinoma
d. Yolk sac tumor
e. Immature teratoma

367. A 69-year-old male presents with urinary frequency, nocturia, dribbling, and difficulty in starting and stopping urination. Rectal examination reveals the prostate to be enlarged, firm, and rubbery. A needle biopsy reveals increased numbers of glandular elements and stromal tissue. The glands are found to have a double layer of epithelial cells. Prominent nuclei or back-to-back glands are not seen. What is the most likely diagnosis?

a.   Acute prostatitis
b.   Chronic bacterial prostatitis
c.   Granulomatous prostatitis
d.   Benign prostatic hyperplasia
e.   Prostatic adenocarcinoma

368. A newborn female is being worked up clinically for several congenital abnormalities. During this work-up, it is discovered that the normal development of the vagina and uterus in this female infant had not occurred. Failure of the uterus to develop (agenesis) is directly related to the failure of what embryonic structure to develop?

a.   Urogenital ridge
b.   Mesonephric duct
c.   Paramesonephric duct
d.   Metanephric duct
e.   Epoophoron

369. A 75-year-old woman presents with a pruritic vulvar lesion. Physical examination reveals an irregular white rough area involving her vulva. If this area of leukoplakia was due to lichen sclerosis, then biopsies from this area would most likely reveal

a.   Atrophy of epidermis with dermal fibrosis
b.   Epidermal atypia with dysplasia
c.   Epithelial hyperplasia and hyperkeratosis
d.   Individual malignant cells invading the epidermis
e.   Loss of pigment in the epidermis

370. Vaginal adenosis precedes the development of which of the following?

a. Condyloma acuminatum
b. Cervical carcinoma
c. Clear cell carcinoma
d. Carcinoma of the endometrium
e. Squamous carcinoma of the vagina

371. The photomicrograph below depicts a biopsy of the uterine cervix that was done following an abnormal Pap smear report. This histologic section shows

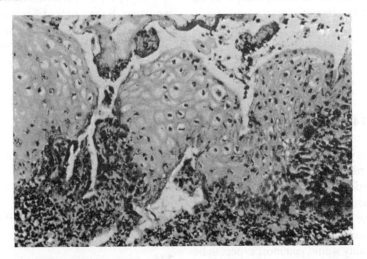

a. Condyloma acuminatum
b. Carcinoma in situ
c. Dysplasia
d. Cervical intraepithelial neoplasia
e. Squamous metaplasia

372. A major risk factor for squamous carcinoma of the cervix is now considered to be

a. Early sexual activity
b. Multiple sexual partners
c. Human papillomavirus types 16/18
d. Herpes simplex virus type 2
e. *Chlamydia trachomatis*

373. A 29-year-old female presents with severe pain during menstruation (dysmenorrhea). During work-up an endometrial biopsy is obtained. The pathology report from this specimen makes the diagnosis of chronic endometritis. Based on this pathology report, which one of the following was present in the biopsy sample of the endometrium?

a. Neutrophils
b. Lymphocytes
c. Lymphoid follicles
d. Plasma cells
e. Decidualized stromal cells

374. A 25-year-old female presents to your office for work-up of infertility. In taking a history she describes severe pain during menses, and she also tells you that in the past another doctor told her that she had "chocolate in her cysts." Based on this history, what abnormality would you most expect to be present in this patient?

a. Metastatic ovarian cancer
b. Endometriosis
c. Acute pelvic inflammatory disease
d. Adenomyosis
e. A posteriorly located subserosal uterine leiomyoma

375. A 25-year-old female presents with a three year history of infertility. Obtaining a history you find out that her cycles have averaged consistently about 33 days in length, and the length of menstruation has also been a constant 4 days in length. You decide to take an endometrial biopsy approximately 2 to 3 days after the predicted time of ovulation. If the cause of her infertility relates to inadequate functioning of the corpus luteum, then biopsies of her endometrium would most likely reveal

a. Non-secretory endometrium with mild hyperplasia
b. Chronologic day and histologic appearance asynchrony
c. Inactive glands within predecidualized stroma
d. Atrophic endometrium (glands and stroma)
e. Secretory glands mixed with proliferative glands

376. A woman harboring endometrial adenocarcinoma nearly always has antecedent

a. Obesity
b. Diabetes mellitus
c. Endometrial polyps
d. Endometrial hyperplasia
e. Systemic hypertension

377. A 46-year-old woman undergoes an abdominal hysterectomy
for a "fibroid" uterus. The surgeon
requests a frozen section on the
tumor, which is deferred because of
the lesion's degree of cellularity.
Which of the following criteria will
be used by the pathologist in determining benignancy versus malignancy in permanent sections?

a. Mitotic rate
b. Cell pleomorphism
c. Cell necrosis
d. Nucleocytoplasmic (NC) ratio
e. Tumor size

378. A female patient is being
treated with penicillin for acute
salpingitis and pelvic inflammatory
disease without benefit. Which of
the following organisms should
now be considered in the differential diagnosis?

a. *Treponema pallidum*
b. *Neisseria gonorrhoeae*
c. *Chlamydia trachomatis*
d. Adenoviruses
e. Herpesviruses

379. A 19-year-old female presents with oligomenorrhea. Physical examination reveals an obese
young female with acne and increased facial hair. A pelvic examination is essentially within normal
limits, excluding the adnexal regions which could not be palpated
secondary to obesity. Work-up reveals increased serum levels of
luteinizing hormones (LH), androgens, and estrogens, normal
amounts of thyroid stimulating
hormone (TSH) and prolactin, and
decreased levels of follicle stimulating hormone (FSH). Exploration of
this individual's abdomen would
most likely reveal

a. A benign ovarian neoplasm
b. A malignant ovarian neoplasm
c. Bilateral atrophy of the ovaries
   (streak ovaries)
d. Bilateral enlargement of the ovaries
   with multiple subcortical cysts
e. Endometriosis of the ovaries and
   the fallopian tubes

380. A 23-year-old female presents with pelvic pain and is found to have an ovarian mass of the left ovary that measures 3 cm in diameter. Grossly the mass consisted of multiple cystic spaces. Histologically these cysts were lined by tall columnar epithelium, some of which were ciliated. What is your diagnosis for this ovarian tumor, which histologically recapitulates the histology of the fallopian tubes?

a.   Serous tumor
b.   Mucinous tumor
c.   Endometrioid tumor
d.   Clear cell tumor
e.   Brenner tumor

381. The ovarian lesion in the photomicrograph below is

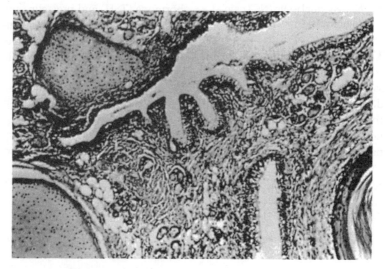

a.   Chronic salpingitis
b.   An ectopic pregnancy
c.   A granulosa cell tumor
d.   A cystic teratoma
e.   Metastatic squamous cell carcinoma

382. A 32-year-old female presents with the recent onset of oligomenorrhea followed by amenorrhea, and then the loss of female secondary characteristics. She has also developed acne, deepening' of her voice, and temporal balding. Which one of the following ovarian tumors would most likely produce these symptoms?

a. Epithelial tumor
b. Stromal tumor
c. Germ cell tumor
d. Surface tumor
e. Metastasis

383. A 24-year-old female delivers a normal 8 pound baby boy at 40 weeks of gestation. She has no history of drug abuse, and her pregnancy was unremarkable. Examination had revealed the placenta to be located normally, but following delivery she fails to deliver the placenta and subsequently develops massive postpartum hemorrhage and shock. Emergency surgery is performed to stop the bleeding. Her post-partum bleeding was most likely caused by

a. An abruptio placenta
b. A placenta previa
c. A placenta accreta
d. A hydatidiform mole
e. An invasive mole

384. A young woman with lower pelvic pain, menometrorrhagia, and a negative β-hCG test undergoes uterine dilatation and curettage. The pathology report on the endometrial sample states, "Compatible with decidualized gestational hyperplasia, no chorionic villi present." The next step would be to

a. Repeat the β-hCG test
b. discharge the patient
c. Consider ectopic pregnancy
d. Consider appendicitis
e. Consider pelvic inflammatory disease

385. A 26-year-old female in the third trimester of her first pregnancy develops persistent headaches and swelling of her legs and face. Early during her pregnancy a physical examination was unremarkable, however, now her blood pressure is 170/105 mm Hg, and a urinalysis reveals slight proteinuria. What is the diagnosis?

a. Eclampsia
b. Gestational trophoblastic disease
c. Nephritic syndrome
d. Nephrotic syndrome
e. Preeclampsia

386. A 25-year-old woman in her 15th week of pregnancy presented with uterine bleeding and passage of a small amount of watery fluid and tissue. She is found to have a uterus that is much larger than estimated by her gestational dates. Her uterus is found to be filled with cystic, avascular, grapelike structures that do not penetrate the uterine wall. No fetal parts are found. The most likely diagnosis for this abnormality is

a. Partial hydatidiform mole
b. Complete hydatidiform mole
c. Invasive mole
d. Placental site trophoblastic tumor
e. Choriocarcinoma

387. All the following renal disorders are associated with the nephrotic syndrome EXCEPT

a. Membranous glomerulonephritis
b. Lipoid nephrosis
c. Membranoproliferative glomerulonephritis
d. Acute tubular necrosis
e. Focal segmental glomerulosclerosis

388. A patient being investigated for hematuria and proteinuria has a renal biopsy that shows changes in the glomeruli as depicted below. All the following diseases can be associated with changes seen in this biopsy EXCEPT

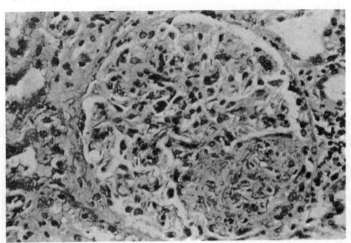

a. Bacterial endocarditis
b. Anaphylactoid purpura
c. Systemic lupus erythematosus
d. Hereditary nephritis (Alport's syndrome)
e. Diabetes mellitus

389. Acute tubular necrosis (ATN) is a fairly common renal lesion and is associated with all the following EXCEPT

a. Red cell casts in the urine
b. Proteinuria
c. Proximal tubular damage in toxic ATN
d. Oliguria
e. Acute renal failure

390. All the following renal diseases cause hypertension EXCEPT

a. Small, bilateral renal infarcts
b. Renal artery arteriosclerosis
c. Fibromuscular dysplasia of the renal artery
d. Hydronephrosis
e. Pyelonephritis

391. All the following statements are true of urinary calculi EXCEPT that

a. They are more common in males
b. They are bilateral in 40 percent of cases
c. They are radiopaque in about 90 percent of cases
d. They may be associated with Pseudomonas infections
e. The incidence is increased in leukemia

392. The kidney shown in the photomicrograph below exhibits a tumor that has originated in the upper pole. Correct statements about this tumor include all the following EXCEPT that

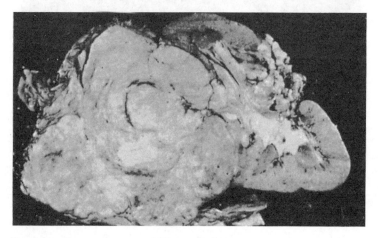

a. It is sometimes associated with polycythemia
b. It is sometimes associated with tuberous sclerosis
c. It may produce glucocorticoids
d. It originates from proximal convoluted tubular cells
e. It occurs predominantly in the sixth decade

393. All the following abnormalities are associated with an increased incidence of Wilms' tumor EXCEPT

a. Aniridia
b. Male pseudohermaphroditism
c. Hemihypertrophy
d. Renal medullary cysts
e. Hypoplasia of radii

394. The photomicrograph below shows an abnormal renal tubular epithelial cell with a large, intranuclear inclusion surrounded by a clear halo. It was found in a urinary specimen from a very ill renal transplant patient. The disease diagnosed is associated with all the following EXCEPT

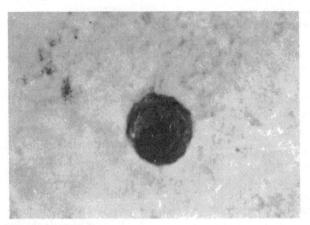

a. Interstitial pneumonitis
b. Hepatitis
c. A herpesvirus
d. Gastrointestinal ulcers
e. Detection of antigen in 1 to 3 weeks

395. All the following statements are true regarding transitional cell carcinoma of the bladder EXCEPT that

a. It is more common in men than in women
b. It is associated with infection by *Schistosoma haematobium*
c. It is associated with cigarette smoking
d. It shows increased incidence in aniline dye workers
e. It tends to recur after excision, regardless of grade

396. Primary germ cell tumors of the testis occur predominantly in the younger male with the exception of

a. Embryonal carcinoma
b. Spermatocytic seminoma
c. Polyembryoma
d. Choriocarcinoma
e. Teratocarcinoma

397. Within prostatic glands, features consistent with prostatic intraepithelial neoplasia (PIN) include all the following EXCEPT

a. Cellular crowding
b. Absence of a basal cell layer
c. Variation in nuclear size
d. Nucleoli
e. Hyperchromatism

398. Carcinoma of the prostate tends to do all the following EXCEPT

a. Be adenocarcinoma
b. Arise in the posterior lobe
c. Cause elevation of serum acid phosphatase
d. Be estrogen-dependent
e. Form osteoblastic metastases

399. Primary malignant neoplasms of the vagina include all the following EXCEPT

a. Sarcoma botryoides
b. Clear cell carcinoma
c. Squamous carcinoma
d. Vaginal adenosis
e. Rhabdomyosarcoma

400. All the following endometrial changes are consistent with secretory endometrium EXCEPT

a. Basal cytoplasmic vacuoles
b. Secretions within glandular lumen
c. Predecidual reaction within stroma
d. Neutrophil infiltrate
e. Plasma cell infiltrate

401. Cystic hyperplasia of the endometrium is associated with all the following EXCEPT

a. Occurrence at or just before menopause
b. Increased estrogen administration or production
c. Excessive uterine bleeding
d. Secretory cells lining the cystically dilated glands
e. functioning granulosa-theca cell tumors

402. True statements about endometrial adenocarcinoma include all the following EXCEPT

a. It is more common than invasive squamous cervical cancer
b. It causes fewer deaths than invasive cervical cancer
c. The peak incidence is at age 55 to 65 years
d. The major symptom is pain
e. Abnormal glucose tolerance is a risk factor

403. Common outcomes of the uterine abnormality illustrated below include all the following EXCEPT

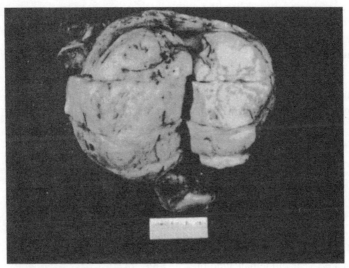

a. Malignant change
b. Cystic degeneration
c. Calcification
d. Rapid enlargement during pregnancy
e. Atrophy after menopause

DIRECTIONS: Each group of questions below consists of lettered headings followed by a set of numbered items. For each numbered item select the **one** lettered heading with which it is **most** closely associated. Each lettered heading may be used **once, more than once, or not at all.**

Questions 404–405

Match each of the following clinical scenarios with the correct diagnosis from the following list.

a. Acute pyelonephritis
b. Chronic pyelonephritis
c. Xanthogranulomatous pyelonephritis
d. Benign nephrosclerosis
e. Malignant nephrosclerosis
f. Renal artery stenosis

404. Examination of a renal biopsy from a 48-year-old female who presented with a blood pressure of 150/105 and decreased kidney function revealed hyaline changes within the wall of the smaller blood vessels.

405. A 53-year-old male presents with severe headaches, nausea, and vomiting. He states that he sees "spots" before his eyes. Physical examination reveals a diastolic blood pressure of 140 mm Hg and a microscopic section from his kidney reveals hyperplastic arteriolitis.

Questions 406–407

Match each disease with the pathologic finding that is most characteristic.

a. Malignant nephrosclerosis
b. Benign nephrosclerosis
c. Preeclampsia
d. Analgesic abuse nephropathy
e. Systemic lupus erythematosus

406. Swollen glomerular endothelial cells.

407. Papillary necrosis.

Questions 408–409

Match each of the following clinical scenarios with the correct diagnosis from the following list.

a. Balanoposthitis
b. Bladder exstrophy
c. Epispadia
d. Hypospadia
e. Meckel's cyst
f. Omphalocele
g. Paraphimosis
h. Phimosis
i. Urachal fistula

408. Physical examination of a 3-day-old male infant reveals urine leaking from the area of the umbilicus.

409. An uncircumcised 49-year-old male presents with the sudden onset on severe pain in the distal portion of his penis. The emergency room physician examines the patient and finds that the foreskin is retracted but cannot be rolled back over the glans penis. The ER physician calls the urologist who performs an emergency resection of this patient's foreskin.

GENITOURINARY SYSTEM

Answers

345. The answer is d. *(Cotran, 5/e, pp 929–931. Rubin, 2/e, pp 806–809.)* The unique structure and composition of the glomerular basement membrane and associated cells account for the formation of the plasma ultrafiltrate referred to as urine. The glomerular basement membrane is approximately 320 nm wide in the normal human with a central electron-dense lamina densa and electron-lucent lamina rara interna and externa with fenestrated endothelial cells immediately adjacent to the capillaries and the visceral epithelial cells (podocytes). Glomerular basement membrane is made up of collagen type 4, with laminin especially concentrated on both laminae rarae. Clustered also on both laminae rarae are polyanionic proteoglycans (especially heparan sulfate), which are thought to play a major role in the exclusion of albumin in the urinary filtrate by a mechanism of charge dependence restriction. This is based on the electronegative charge of the proteoglycans and the anionic charges of albumin. The mechanism is based on different isoelectric points. Thus it is felt that the glomerulus, because of these proteoglycans, may be able to discriminate materials passing through it according to electronegative charge. Glomerular basement membrane does function by exclusion of materials based on size. Mesangial cells, by nature of their contractility, are thought to control intraglomerular blood flow under neurohormonal stimulation. Mesangial cells are not thought to function in filtration per se. The parietal cells lining the Bowman's membrane may function as a barrier but do not participate in the ultrafiltration. The fenestrated endothelial cells and podocytes are part of the filtering membranes but probably play a minor role compared with the glomerular polyanion barrier.

346. The answer is e. *(Cotran, 5/e, pp 929–931. Rubin, 2/e, pp 806–809.)* It has been recently shown that polyanionic molecules at sites on the luminal endothelial cells retard anions by electronegativity forces, which aids the transport of cationic proteins. They may greatly increase vascular permeability, especially in the renal glomerulus. The glomerular basement membrane contains the glycoprotein entactin, fibronectin, collagen type IV, laminin, and polyanionic proteoglycans (heparan sulfate) found at sites on both laminae rarae. The glomerular filtration barrier is made possible by these polyanions. The podocyte is attached to the lamina rara externa on the epithelial (urine filtrate) side of the glomerular basement membrane. Desmin is an intermediate filament protein found in fibroblasts and muscle cells. Bowman's capsule epithelial cells line the inner side of the glomerulus and are bathed in urinary ultrafiltrate. Fibronectin—a connective tissue protein formed by endothelial cells, fibroblasts, and macrophages—stabilizes endothelial cell attachments and functions in wound healing.

347. The answer is b. (*Cotran, 5/e, pp 934–938.*) Cystic diseases of the kidney, which may be congenital, acquired, or inherited diseases, have characteristic gross appearances. In two types of cystic renal disease, the numerous cysts are found in both the cortex and medulla. These two types of polycystic disease of the kidney are the infantile type and the adult type. Adult polycystic kidney disease typically presents in adulthood and has an autosomal dominant inheritance pattern. Histologically the cysts are lined by tubular epithelium, while the stroma between the cysts is normal. Adult polycystic renal disease is associated with liver cysts and berry aneurysms, which may rupture and cause a subarachnoid hemorrhage. About one-half of patients with adult polycystic renal disease eventually develop uremia. Infantile polycystic kidney disease typically presents in newborns, has an autosomal recessive pattern of inheritance, and is associated with hepatic cysts (microhamartomas) and congenital hepatic fibrosis. Grossly these renal cysts have a radial spoke arrangement.

In two types of cystic renal disease, the cysts are limited to the medulla. Medullary sponge kidney is usually asymptomatic, is not familial, and has normal sized kidneys with small cysts in the renal papillae. Medullary cystic disease complex (nephronophthisis) has small sclerotic kidneys with multiple cysts at the corticomedullary junction. Individuals with this abnormality present in the first two decades of life with salt wasting polyuria and progressive renal failure. Most cases are familial and display both recessive and dominant inheritance patterns. Two other types of cysts that are not limited to the medulla are simple cysts and acquired cysts. Simple cortical cysts are single, unilateral cysts found in adults that are benign. Patients are usually asymptomatic, but they may present with microscopic hematuria. Acquired polycystic renal disease is associated with chronic renal dialysis. These kidneys are shrunken and have multiple cysts and an irregular surface.

348. The answer is b. *(Damjanov, 10/e, pp 2089–2090. Cotran, 5/e, pp 950–952.)* There are numerous causes of nephrotic syndrome (NS), including immune complex diseases, diabetes, amyloidosis, toxemia of pregnancy, and such circulating disturbances as bilateral renal vein thrombosis, but NS in small children (under 3 years of age) should suggest the possibility of the renal disease known as minimal change nephropathy, which is synonymous with foot process disease, or nil disease. This peculiar entity presents clinically as insidious nephrotic syndrome, characteristically occurring in younger children, but also seen in adults (rarely), with hypoalbuminemia, edema, hyperlipidemia, massive proteinuria, and lipiduria. The glomeruli are known for their rather normal appearance on light microscopy—at worst, there is mild and focal sclerosis. Electron microscopy is necessary for demonstrating characteristic attenuation and flattening of the foot processes of the podocytes attached to the Bowman's space side of the glomerular basement membrane. The podocytes may revert to normal (with steroid immunosuppressive therapy), or the foot-process attenuation may persist to some extent, in which case the proteinuria also persists. To date, no immune complex deposits or abnormalities of the glomerular basement membrane or mesangium have been demonstrated ultrastructurally.

349. The answer is c. *(Cotran, 5/e, pp 939–945, 949–950.)* Glomerular injury caused by circulating antigen-antibody complexes is a secondary effect from a nonprimary renal source. Numerous clinical examples exist of a serum sickness-like nephritis as a consequence of systemic infection, with classic clinical models such as syphilis, hepatitis B, malaria, and bacterial endocarditis leading to renal disease. Immune complexes to antigens from any of these sources are circulating within the vascular system and become entrapped within the filtration system of the glomerular basement membranes. This can be seen as granular, bumpy deposits by immunofluorescence within the basement membranes of the glomeruli. Linear fluorescence, on the other hand, is seen in primary antiglomerular basement membrane disease, wherein antibodies are directed against the glomerular basement membrane itself. Plasma cell interstitial nephritis is seen in immunologic rejection of transplanted kidneys. Nodular glomerulosclerosis is an effect of diabetes mellitus. The presence of red blood cell casts in the urine nearly always indicates that there has been glomerular injury but is not specific for any given cause. Thickening of the glomerular basement membrane caused by subepithelial immune deposits is seen in membranous glomerulonephritis. While the morphology of membranous glomerulonephritis is different from that of nephritis caused by circulating antigen-antibody complexes (immune complexes), there are similarities in the pathogenesis in that both disorders may be a consequence of or in association with infections such as hepatitis B, syphilis, and malaria. Other causes for membranous glomerulonephritis include reactions to penicillamine, gold, and certain malignancies such as malignant melanoma.

350. The answer is a. *(Cotran, 5/e, pp 945–947. Rubin, 2/e, pp 828–831.)* In a young patient who presents with signs of edema, three renal diseases are in the differential diagnosis. These diseases have similar names and findings, which makes them easily confused with each other. For example, minimal change disease (MCD), focal segmental glomerulosclerosis (FSGS), and post-streptococcal glomerulonephritis may all produce the nephrotic syndrome, characterized by marked proteinuria. This finding can be documented by the presence of protein in a dipstick examination of the urine. MCD characteristically is associated with a selective proteinuria in which albumin is found in the urine rather than immunoglobulins. In contrast, FSGS is associated with a nonselective proteinuria. MCD is a selective proteinuria because it results from decreased amounts of polyanions (mainly heparan sulfate) in the glomerular basement membrane. These polyanions normally block the filtration of the small, but negatively charged albumin molecules. The glomeruli in patients with MCD lack electron dense deposits, and immunofluorescence (IF) tests are negative. These patients have no tendency to develop chronic renal failure, and they respond to steroid therapy. In contrast, FSGS has granular IgM and C3 deposits seen by IF, and patients do not respond to steroids. It is important to realize that FSGS, with no cellular proliferation, is different from focal segmental glomerulonephritis (FSGN), which has cellular proliferation, the main cause of FSGN being IgA (Berger's) nephropathy. Both MCD and FSGN have fusion of the foot processes of the podocytes that can be seen with electron microscopy, but since FSGS is focal and segmental, the biopsy specimen may not demonstrate other findings of FSGS that are not seen with MCD, such as thickening of the basement membrane with hyalinosis (the focal deposition of PAS positive material).

Although signs of the nephritic syndrome, such as hematuria, may be seen with FSGS, young children are more often found with acute post-strep-tococcal glomerulonephritis. This illness typically occurs 1 to 3 weeks after a group A, β-hemolytic streptococcal infection of the pharynx or skin, such as impetigo or scarlet fever. Patients develop hematuria, red cell casts, mild periorbital edema, and increased blood pressure. Laboratory tests reveal increased ASO titers and decreased C3. Cultures taken at the time of presentation with renal symptoms are negative. Light microscopy reveals diffuse endothelial and mesangial cell proliferation with neutrophil infil-tration, so that narrowing of capillary lumens and enlargement of the glomerular tuft to fill Bowman's space occur. Electron microscopy reveals the mesangial deposits and large, hump-shaped subepithelial deposits in peripheral capillary loops that are characteristic. Immunofluorescence shows granular deposits containing IgG, C3, and often fibrin in glomerular capillary walls and mesangium. Children with post-streptococcal glomeru-lonephritis usually recover, and therapy is supportive only.

351. The answer is d. (*Cotran, 5/e, pp 942, 954–957, 960.*) Electron dense deposits composed of immunoglobulin and complement are deposited in characteristic locations of the glomerulus in different renal diseases. De-posits within the basement membrane are seen in type II membranoprolif-erative glomerulonephritis (MPGN or "dense deposit disease"), while subendothelial deposits are seen in type I MPGN. Note that membra-noproliferative glomerulonephritis occurs in two types. Type I, which is as-sociated with nephrotic syndrome, is driven by immune complexes; type II is associated with hematuria and chronic renal failure, and in addition to immune complexes, involves alternate complement activation. In either type there is mesangial proliferation accompanied by thickening of the glomerular basement membranes, and a special finding that often supports the diagnosis of membranoproliferative glomerulonephritis is the presence of actual splitting of the glomerular basement membranes. In type I there are subendothelial deposits of IgG, C3, C1, and C4. In type II there are dense deposits of C3 with or without IgG, and no C1.

Subepithelial deposits are seen in acute glomerulonephritis (GN), such as post-streptococcal glomerulonephritis. Epimembranous deposits (similar to subepithelial deposits) are found in patients with membranous

GN or in the experimental disease Heymann's GN. Note that the deposits in MGN are relatively small and are deposited in a very uniform fashion, while the deposits in post-strep GN are comparably large (subepithelial humps) and are not uniformly distributed. Subendothelial deposits are also seen with systemic lupus erythematosus. Deposits within the mesangial matrix are found in IgA nephropathy (Berger's disease) and Henoch-Schonlein glomerulonephritis. Electron dense deposits are not usually found within Bowman's space, nor are they usually found in patients with Goodpasture's disease or lipoid nephrosis.

352. The answer is a. (*Cotran, 5/e, pp 956–957, 960.*) Many diseases involve hematuria, and a few diseases occur in the setting of an upper respiratory infection or of upper respiratory signs and symptoms. When the hematuria follows within 2 days of the onset of an upper respiratory infection without skin lesions in a young patient, IgA nephropathy (Berger's disease) should be considered. This disease involves the deposition of IgA in the mesangium of the glomeruli. Light microscopic examination may suggest the disease, but renal biopsy immunofluorescence (IF) must be performed to confirm it. This disorder may be the most common cause of the nephritic syndrome worldwide. The hematuria may become recurrent, with proteinuria that may approach nephrotic syndrome proportions. Serum levels of IgA may be elevated. A small percentage of patients may progress to renal failure over a period of years. In contrast to Berger's disease, a linear IF pattern suggests a type II hypersensitivity reaction, such as Goodpasture's disease, while a granular pattern is seen with post-streptococcal glomerulonephritis (GN), membranous GN, focal segmental glomerulosclerosis, and membranoproliferative GN. Most positive immunofluorescence patterns involve IgG and C3, except that a granular IgM pattern is present in focal segmental glomerulosclerosis, while mesangial IgA is seen in IgA nephropathy (Berger's disease). Lipoid nephrosis would have a negative IF pattern; that is, there would be no staining present.

353. The answer is c. (*Cotran, 5/e, pp 717–718, 940.*) In Goodpasture's syndrome, circulating antibodies reactive with the glomerular basement membrane will bind in a linear pattern along the entire length of the glomerular basement membrane, which is their specific antigen. IgG is deposited in the basement membrane, along with complement. There are focal interruptions of the glomerular basement membrane as well, along with deposits of fibrin, as seen with electron microscopy.

354. The answer is b. *(Cotran, 5/e, pp 949–950, 954–956, 958–960.)* The thickening of the basement membrane in systemic lupus erythematosus and membranous glomerulonephritis is thought to result from deposition of immune complexes. The pathogenesis of this same lesion in diabetes mellitus and renal vein thrombosis is unknown. Electron-dense deposits are classically seen in a subendothelial position on the glomerular basement membrane but may be subepithelial as well in some cases.

355. The answer is c. *(Cotran, 5/e, pp 934–935, 958–959, 971–972.)* The kidney shown is typical of chronic pyelonephritis with dilatation of the renal pelvis, clubbing of the calyces, and irregular reduction in parenchymal mass. Chronic pyelonephritis is an asymmetric, irregularly scarring process that may be unilateral or bilateral. Microscopically, there is atrophy and dilatation of tubules with colloid in some tubules. Chronic inflammation and fibrosis occur in the cortex and medulla. Chronic glomerulonephritis causes bilateral, symmetrically shrunken and scarred kidneys. Histologic changes depend on the stage of the disease. Cystic dysplasia is characterized by undifferentiated mesenchyme and immature cartilage and collecting ductules.

356. The answer is c. *(Cotran, 5/e, pp 978–979.)* A much rarer cause of hypertension is renal artery stenosis, which may occur secondary to either an atheromatous plaque at the orifice of the renal artery or fibromuscular dysplasia of the renal artery. The former is more common in elderly men, while the latter is more common in young women. The decrease in blood flow to the kidney with the renal artery obstruction (the Goldblatt kidney) causes hyperplasia of the juxtaglomerular apparatus and increased renin production. This will produce increased secretion of angiotensin and aldosterone, which will lead to retention of sodium and water and produce hypertension. Increased levels of aldosterone will also produce a hyperkalemic alkalosis. The kidney with the stenosis of the renal artery will become small and shrunken due to the effects of chronic ischemia, but the stenosis protects this kidney from the effects of the increased blood pressure. The other kidney, however, is not protected and may develop microscopic changes of benign nephrosclerosis (hyaline arteriolosclerosis).

357. The answer is d. (*Cotran, 5/e, pp 979–981.*) The group of renal diseases associated with microangiopathic hemolytic anemia includes both childhood and adult hemolytic-uremic syndrome (HUS), thrombotic thrombocytopenic purpura, and scleroderma. Endothelial injury and intravascular coagulation occur in all. HUS is characterized by acute renal failure, microangiopathic hemolytic anemia, and thrombocytopenia and is one of the main causes of acute renal failure in children. Prodromal features in children include a gastrointestinal or respiratory tract infection. Lupus erythematosus does not occur in very young children. Acute poststreptococcal glomerulonephritis occurs in older children, is a proliferative lesion, and is not usually associated with hemolytic anemia or fibrin deposition. Lipoid nephrosis shows no glomerular changes with light microscopy.

358. The answer is e. (*Cotran, 5/e, pp 462–465, 986–988.*) A middle-aged patient is highly unlikely to have either of the predominantly childhood tumors nephroblastoma (Wilms' tumor) or mesoblastic nephroma (benign hamartoma). Mesoblastic nephroma, which may be seen in the first year of life, has caused difficulty in differential diagnosis from Wilms' tumor in children. Acute pyelonephritis features signs of acute infection with flank pain, pyuria, fever, and a high bacterial colony count in urine. Renal cell carcinoma is unlikely to cause hematuria until far advanced with invasion of the collecting system. Urothelial renal pelvis tumors cause hematuria early, even when quite small. They form 5 to 10 percent of primary renal tumors and range from apparently benign papillomas to papillary or anaplastic carcinomas. There may be multicentric involvement of ureters or bladder. Diagnosis is by x-ray and cytologic examination of at least three voided urine specimens; malignant cells are not found if the ureter is obstructed by tumor, or if the cells are degenerate or mildly atypical, as in papilloma. Prognosis is not very good for high-grade infiltrating tumors and is very poor for the squamous cell variant (about 15 percent of pelvic tumors); therefore, early diagnosis is paramount.

359. The answer is d. (*Cotran, 5/e, p 1004.*) Nonspecific urethritis may actually be the most common cause of dysuria in sexually active males, although gonorrhea should always be excluded by laboratory examination. Causes of nonspecific urethritis include some bacteria, such as *Escherichia coli* and streptococci, but recent evidence implicates chlamydiae of the TRIC group as being perhaps the most common offending agents. The organism may take up residence in the prostate, producing chronic and active prostatitis. Prostatic hypertrophy, epididymitis, orchitis, and renal stones may cause urinary symptoms but also produce other signs and symptoms that distinguish them from nonspecific urethritis.

360. The answer is e. (*Damjanov, 10/e, pp 2151–2152. Cotran, 5/e, pp 996–997.*) Malacoplakia is an uncommon chronic inflammatory disease of unknown cause, characterized by soft yellow mucosal plaques, infiltration of large histiocytes containing phagolysosomes, and intracytoplasmic and extracellular laminated calcospherules, Michaelis-Gutmann (MG) bodies. While malacoplakia usually involves the mucosa of the urinary bladder, it occurs also in extravesical sites such as the colon, lungs, kidneys, prostate, and brain. It occurs with greater frequency in the immunosuppressed. Histologically, the plaques contain numerous, large, foamy or granular macrophages that are PAS-positive and often include bacterial debris. Laminated, mineralized MG bodies are also numerous in and between macrophages. The cause of malacoplakia is not clear, but it has been associated with *E. coli* infections and is thought to be due to defective removal by macrophages of phagocytosed bacteria with overloaded phagosomes and MG bodies resulting from calcium deposition on the phagosomes. In recent reports, however, cerebral malacoplakia was not associated with bacterial infection.

361. The answer is e. (*Cotran, 5/e, pp 1008–1010, 1045–1052.*) Of all the choices given, human papillomavirus (HPV) condyloma without dysplasia is the only lesion that can be histologically discriminated from the others. The typical HPV condyloma has hyperplastic squamous mucosa that shows progressive maturation from the stratum germinativum to the surface that is often parakeratotic, without cells of dysplasia or malignancy. There often are vacuolated squamous cells in several layers of the mucosa. However, condylomas, whether arising in the female or the male genital areas, may have atypia or dysplasia or even be associated histologically with carcinoma. If present, these features must be commented upon in a pathology report. Condyloma not otherwise specified indicates that none of these disorders of growth are present along with it. Bowen's disease and erythroplasia of Queyrat are different clinical forms of squamous cell carcinoma in situ. Erythroplasia of Queyrat is a specialized form of squamous carcinoma in situ or severe dysplasia occurring on the glans penis mainly.

It is characterized by a moist, macular, spreading red surface. It usually occurs in males of advanced age. Bowen's disease is also squamous carcinoma in situ but may have an association with malignancies of the viscera. Bowenoid papulosis refers to multiple, small, banal-appearing clinical papules on the vulvar or penile surfaces; it histologically shows features of Bowen's disease, and for all practical purposes cannot be distinguished from that disease on histologic grounds only. It is a rather new entity, histologically similar to carcinoma in situ, and it behaves as a self-healing and reversible lesion. Bowenoid papulosis usually occurs in young patients and is often associated with condylomas.

362. The answer is d. (*Cotran, 5/e, pp 1008–1010.*) Clear vacuolization of the superficial layers of the epithelial cells, koilocytosis, is characteristic of infection by human papillomavirus (HPV). These changes are found in both condyloma acuminatum and verrucous carcinoma, but condyloma is a benign papillary lesion that does not grow into the underlying tissue, while verrucous carcinoma, also known as giant condyloma or Buschke-Löwenstein tumor, invades into the underlying tissue along a broad front. This type of invasion is in contrast to squamous cell carcinomas, which invade tissue as fingerlike projections of atypical squamous epithelial cells. Three dysplastic, precancerous intraepithelial lesions of the penis that do not invade into the underlying tissue are Bowen's disease, erythroplasia of Queyrat, and bowenoid papulosis.

363. The answer is d. (*Cotran, 5/e, pp 1011–1013.*) The condition illustrated is cryptorchidism, failure of the testis to descend into the scrotum. It is present in up to 1 percent of males after puberty and is unilateral in the majority of cases. The testis is small, brown, and atrophic grossly. Microscopically, the tubules are atrophic with thickened basement membranes. The interstitial cells are usually prominent and occasional focal proliferations of Sertoli cells may be seen. The incidence of malignancy is increased 7- to 11-fold, and this risk is greater for abdominal than for inguinal location. Seminoma is the most common malignancy. The risk of malignancy is not reduced by orchiopexy. There is a smaller but definite risk of malignancy in the contralateral, correctly placed testis.

364. The answer is d. (*Cotran, 5/e, p 1013.*) The condition illustrated is acute orchitis. There is hemorrhage and inflammation in and between tubules with disruption of spermatogenesis. Bacteria are present in the tubules. Orchitis is somewhat less common than epididymitis and, when present, is usually due to extension of infection from the urinary tract via epididymal lymphatics or the vas deferens. Infection is rarely blood-borne. *E. coli* and *C. trachomatis* are the most common pathogens. Sequelae include tubular atrophy and excretory duct obstruction, both of which may cause sterility. Chronic infection may occur. Interstitial cells are more likely to survive or regenerate, so sexual function is often retained.

365. The answer is d. (*Damjanov, 10/e, pp 2189, 2275, 2277.*) The adenomatoid tumor is benign and is the most common tumor of the epididymis. Its origin is probably the mesothelium. It presents as a small, firm, gray-white nodule less than 5 cm in diameter; similar tumors occur in the fallopian tube, ovary, and posterior uterus. Histology reveals glandlike, mesothelium-lined, spaced and fibrous connective tissue stroma with smooth muscle fibers. Androblastoma, or Sertoli cell tumor, is a sex cord testicular tumor, often benign; tuberculous epididymitis presents multiple confluent tubercles with caseation. Carcinomas of the epididymis and adjacent structures occur but are very rare. Adrenocortical rests are common but usually too small for clinical detection.

366. The answer is a. (*Cotran, 5/e, pp 1015–1022.*) Germ cell tumors of the testis are clinically divided into two categories, seminomas and nonseminomatous germ cell tumors (NSGCTs), because of their differences in presentation, metastasis, prognosis, and therapy. The NSGCTs include embryonal carcinoma, yolk sac tumor (also called infantile embryonal carcinoma or endodermal sinus tumor), choriocarcinoma, and immature teratoma. When compared with NSGCTs, seminomas are extremely radiosensitive, and they are more commonly present with stage I disease. NSGCTs are relatively radioresistant, are more aggressive, and have a worse prognosis. Seminomas typically spread by lymphatics after having remained localized for a long time. Embryonal carcinoma, choriocarcinoma, and mixed tumors with an element of choriocarcinoma tend to metastasize early via the blood. Choriocarcinomas are the most aggressive variant.

367. The answer is d. (*Cotran, 5/e, pp 1023–1029.*) Benign enlargement of the prostate is caused by benign prostatic hyperplasia (BPH) and produces clinical symptoms of urinary frequency, nocturia, difficulty in starting and stopping urination, dribbling, and dysuria. Histologically the hyperplastic nodules are composed of a variable mixture of hyperplastic glands and hyperplastic stromal cells. Histologic signs of malignancy are not present. The development of BPH is associated with increased age and higher testosterone levels. BPH results from androgen-induced glandular proliferation, but estrogen also sensitizes the tissue to androgens. Urinary obstruction results as the inner, periurethral portions of the prostate (the middle and lateral lobes) are affected most commonly. BPH does not predispose the individual to cancer. In contrast to the benign histology of BPH, the histologic signs characteristic of prostatic adenocarcinoma include small glands that appear "back-to-back" without intervening stroma, or they appear to be infiltrating beyond the normal prostate lobules. Histologically these malignant glands are composed of a single layer of cuboidal epithelial cells, as the outer basal layer of epithelial cells, seen in normal and hyperplastic glands, is not present. These malignant cells often contain one or more enlarged nucleoli.

Inflammation of the prostate (prostatitis) is characterized by finding at least fifteen leukocytes per high power field in prostatic secretions. Prostatitis is classified as being either acute or chronic prostatitis. Patients with acute prostatitis present with fever, chills, and dysuria. It is usually caused by bacteria that cause urinary tract infections, such as *E. coli*. Chronic prostatitis presents clinically as low back pain, dysuria, and suprapubic discomfort. It is divided into chronic bacterial prostatitis, which is associated with recurrent urinary tract infections (UTI) with the same organism, and chronic abacterial prostatitis, which is not associated with recurrent UTI's. Instead chronic abacterial prostatitis is associated with infections with either *Chlamydia trachomatis* or *ureaplasma urealyticum*. Granulomatous prostatitis causes vague symptoms and has an unknown etiology. This diagnosis is made histologically.

368. The answer is c. (*Cotran, 5/e, pp 1033–1034. Larsen, 1/e, pp 247–253.*) The paired genital ducts consist of the mesonephric (Wolffian) duct, which extends from the mesonephros to the cloaca, and the paramesonephric (Müllerian) duct, which runs parallel and lateral to the wolffian duct. The mesonephric ducts in males, if stimulated by testosterone secreted by the Leydig cells, develop into the vas deferens, epididymis, and seminal vesicles. In contrast because normal females do not secrete testosterone, the wolffian ducts regress and form vestigial structures. They may, however, form mesonephric cysts in the cervix or vulva, or they may form Gartner duct cysts in the vagina. The cranial group of mesonephric tubules, the epoöphoron, remain as vestige structures in the broad ligament above the ovary, while the caudal group of mesonephric tubules, the paroöphoron, form vestigial structures in the broad ligament beside the ovary. The paramesonephric (Müllerian) ducts in the female form the fallopian tubes, the uterus, the uppermost vaginal wall, and the hydatid of Morgagni. The lower portion of the vagina and the vestibule develop from the urogenital sinus. Males secrete Müllerian inhibiting factor (MIF) from the Sertoli cells of the testes, which causes regression of the Müllerian ducts. This results in the formation of the vestigial appendix testis. The metanephric duct in both sexes will form the ureter, renal pelvis, calyces, and renal collecting tubules. Several abnormalities result from abnormal embryonic development of the Müllerian ducts. Uterine agenesis may result from abnormal development of fusion of these paired paramesonephric ducts. Developmental failure of the inferior portions of the Müllerian ducts results in a double uterus, while failure of the superior portions to fuse (incomplete fusion) may form a bicornuate uterus. Retarded growth of one of the paramesonephric ducts along with incomplete fusion to the other paramesonephric ducts will result in the formation of a bicornuate uterus with a rudimentary horn.

369. The answer is a. (*Cotran, 5/e, pp 1039–1043.*) Several pathologic conditions are associated with the formation of white plaques on the vulva, which clinically are referred to as leukoplakia. Lichen sclerosus is seen histologically as atrophy of the epidermis with underlying dermal fibrosis. This abnormality is seen in post-menopausal women who develop pruritic white plaques of the vulva. This abnormality is not thought to be premalignant. Loss of pigment in the epidermis, called vitiligo, can also produce leukoplakia. Inflammatory skin diseases, such as chronic dermal inflammation, squamous hyperplasia (characterized by epithelial hyperplasia and hyperkeratosis), and vulvar intraepithelial neoplasia (characterized by epithelial atypia or dysplasia) can also present with leukoplakia. A term related to leukoplakia is vulvar dystrophy, but this term refers specifically to either lichen sclerosis or squamous hyperplasia. Because the latter is sometimes associated with epithelial dysplasia, it is also referred to as hyperplastic dystrophy. It is most commonly seen in postmenopausal women. The male counterpart for lichen sclerosis, which is found on the penis, is called balanitis xerotica obliterans.

Paget's disease is a malignant tumor that can be found in the breast or the vulva. The latter is seen clinically as pruritic red crusted, sharply demarcated map-like areas. Histologically these malignant lesions reveal single anaplastic tumor cells surrounded by clear spaces ("halos") infiltrating the epidermis. These malignant cells stain positively with PAS and mucicarmine stains.

370. The answer is c. (*Cotran, 5/e, pp 1044–1045. Rubin, 2/e, pp 920–921.*) Adenocarcinomas of the vagina and cervix have existed for years but increased in young women whose mothers received diethylstilbestrol (DES) while they were pregnant. DES was used in the past to terminate an attack of threatened abortion and thereby stabilize the pregnancy. However, a side effect of this therapy proved to be a particular form of adenocarcinoma, clear cell carcinoma. This phenomenon was elucidated by Herpses and Scully in 1970. This unique adenocarcinoma was discovered in daughters between the ages of 15 and 20 of those women who had received DES. The tumor, which carries a poor prognosis, has at least three histologic patterns. One is a tubulopapillary configuration, followed by sheets of clear cells and glands lined by clear cells, and solid areas of relatively undifferentiated cells. Many of the cells have cytoplasm that protrudes into the lumen and produces a "hobnail" (nodular) appearance. Prior to the development of adenocarcinoma, a form of adenosis consisting of glands with clear cytoplasm that resembles that of the endocervix can be seen. This has been termed vaginal adenosis and may be a precursor of clear cell carcinoma. Clinically adenosis of the vagina is manifested by red, moist granules superimposed on the pink-white vaginal mucosa.

371. The answer is a. (*Cotran, 5/e, pp 1041–1043, 1047–1053.*) Cervical condylomata, particularly flat condylomata, although benign are considered to be precursors of cervical intraepithelial neoplasia (CIN), which comprises both dysplasia and carcinoma in situ (CIS). Histologically, these condylomata consist of connective tissue stroma covered by hyperplastic epithelium with prominent perinuclear cytoplasmic vacuolization (koilocytosis). Koilocytotic cells are characteristic of human papillomavirus (HPV) infection. More than 50 genotypes of HPV are known at present, and condylomata acuminata are associated with types 6/11 while HPV types 16/18 are usually present in CIN. Following an abnormal Pap smear report suggesting condyloma, CIN, or possible invasive carcinoma, workup of the patient should include colposcopy, multiple cervical punch biopsies, and endocervical curettage to distinguish patients who have invasive cancer, CIN, or flat condylomata.

372. The answer is c. *(Cotran, 5/e, pp 1047–1053. Rubin, 2/e, pp 926–931.)* Cervical squamous cell cancer and its precursors (dysplasia) are considered to be sexually transmitted diseases. Women having sexual intercourse at an early age or with multiple male partners, particularly those with penile condylomas, are at risk for development of genital tract squamous neoplasms. Herpes simplex virus (HSV) type 2 was considered an important cause, but now the major risk factor is human papillomavirus (HPV) types 16/18. Existence of the genome of HPV types 6, 11, 16, 18, 31, and 33 has been documented by DNA hybridization methods in several genital lesions including condylomas, cervical intraepithelial neoplasia (CIN) carcinoma in situ, and invasive cervical cancer. In most studies HPV 6 and 11 were confined to lesions with a good prognosis such as condylomas and mild dysplasia (CIN I), whereas HPV 16 and 18 were found predominantly in CIN III (severe dysplasia and carcinoma in situ) and in invasive carcinoma.

373. The answer is d. *(Cotran, 5/e, pp 1035–1037, 1053–1054.)* The endometrium and myometrium are relatively resistant to infections. Therefore, inflammation of the endometrium (endometritis) is rare. The diagnosis of endometritis depends on finding inflammatory cells within the endometrium that are not present during the normal menstrual cycle. Polymorphonuclear leukocytes (neutrophils) are normally present during menstruation, while a stromal lymphocytic infiltrate can be seen at other times during the menstrual cycle. Lymphoid aggregates and lymphoid follicles may also be seen in normal endometrium. Therefore the presence of any of these types of leukocytes is not diagnostic of endometritis. Acute endometritis is usually caused by bacterial infections following delivery or a miscarriage and is characterized by the presence of neutrophils in endometrial tissue that is not menstrual endometrium. The histologic diagnosis of chronic endometritis depends on finding plasma cells within the endometrium. All it takes is one plasma cell to make the diagnosis. Chronic endometritis may be seen in patients with intrauterine devices (IUD's), pelvic inflammatory disease (PID), retained products of conception (postpartum), or tuberculosis. The latter is characterized histologically by the presence of caseating granulomas with Langhans giant cells. These are secondary causes of chronic endometritis. In a significant number of cases, no underlying cause is found. Decidualized stromal cells are the result of the effects of progesterone and are seen normally in the late secretory phase or in patients who are pregnant. Histologically these stromal cells have abundant eosinophilic cytoplasm.

374. The answer is b. (*Cotran, 5/e, pp 1054–1055.*) Endometrial tissue located in abnormal locations is still under the cyclic influence of hormones and may produce menorrhagia, dysmenorrhea, and cyclic pelvic pain. Menorrhagia refers to an increased amount of regular bleeding, while dysmenorrhea refers to severe pain during menstruation. The ectopic endometrial tissue may be located within the myometrium or it may be found outside of the uterus. The former, nests of endometrial stroma within the myometrium, is called adenomyosis. It is thought to result from the abnormal downgrowth of the endometrium into the myometrium. Ectopic endometrial tissue outside of the uterus is called endometriosis and histologically reveals endometrial glands, stroma, and hemosiderin pigment (from the cyclic bleeding). Repeated cyclic bleeding in patients with endometriosis can lead to the formation of cysts that contain areas of new and old hemorrhages. Because they grossly contain blood clots, these cysts have been called "chocolate cysts." Endometriosis is thought to possibly arise from metaplasia of coelomic epithelium into endometrial tissue, or implantation of normal fragments of menstrual endometrium either via the fallopian tubes or via the blood vessels. Other sites of endometriosis include the uterine ligaments (associated with dyspareunia), rectovaginal pouch (associated with pain on defecation and low back pain), fallopian tubes (associated with peritubular adhesions, infertility, and ectopic pregnancies), urinary bladder (associated with hematuria), GI tract (associated with pain, adhesions, bleeding, and obstruction), and vagina (associated with bleeding).

375. The answer is b. (*Cotran, 5/e, pp 1055–1057.*) Dysfunctional uterine bleeding (DUB) is defined as abnormal uterine bleeding that is due to a functional abnormality rather than an organic lesion of the uterus. In contrast, secondary dysmenorrhea refers to painful menses associated with an organic cause, such as endometriosis, which is the most common cause. Most cases of DUB are related to an endocrine abnormality affecting the hypothalamic-pituitary-ovarian axis. The three main categories of DUB are anovulatory cycles (most common form), inadequate luteal phase, and irregular shedding. Anovulatory cycles consist of persistence of the graafian follicle without ovulation. This results in continued and excess estrogen production without the normal postovulatory rise in progesterone levels. With no progesterone production, no secretory endometrium is formed. Instead biopsies will reveal non-secretory (proliferative) endometrium with mild hyperplasia. The mucosa becomes too thick and is sloughed off, and this results in the abnormal bleeding. Anovulatory cycles characteristically occur at menarche and menopause. They are also associated with the polycystic ovary (Stein-Leventhal) syndrome. It is important to note that other causes of unopposed estrogen effect can lead to this appearance of a proliferative endometrium with mild hyperplasia. These causes include exogenous estrogen administration or estrogen-secreting neoplasms, such as a granulosa cell tumor of the ovary or an adrenal cortical neoplasm. If there is ovulation but the functioning of the corpus luteum is inadequate, then the levels of progesterone will be decreased. This will result in asynchrony between the chronologic dates and the histologic appearance of the secretory endometrium. This is referred to as an inadequate luteal phase (luteal phase defect) and is an important cause of infertility. Biopsies are usually performed several days after the predicted time of ovulation. If the histologic dating of the endometrium lags 4 of more days behind the chronologic date predicted by the menstrual history, the diagnosis of luteal phase defect can be made. Clinically these patients have low serum progesterone, FSH, and LH levels. In contrast to the above, prolonged functioning of the corpus luteum (persistent luteal phase with continued progesterone production) will result in prolonged heavy bleeding at the time of menses. Histologically there will be a combination of secretory glands mixed with proliferative glands (irregular shedding). Clinically these patients have regular periods, but the menstrual bleeding is excessive and prolonged (lasting 10 to 14 days). Current oral contraceptives, being a combination of estrogen and progesterone, will cause the endometrium to have inactive glands with predecidualized stroma. The endometrium from women who are postmenopausal will reveal an atrophic pattern with atrophic or inactive glands.

376. The answer is d. (*Cotran, 5/e, pp 1060–1062.*) Endometrial adenocarcinoma appears to be increasing in frequency in the United States, especially in younger women. It is now accepted that a high estrogen-to-progestin ratio predisposes to the development of this tumor. At menopause, estrogen in the form of estrone continues to be produced in the adrenal glands, and the amounts are directly proportional to body fat. This continues in a milieu in which progesterone is at a minimum because of noncycling. These factors explain why obese women are at an increased risk during and after menopause. Diabetes and hypertension are also associated factors, but they are more likely to be effects of obesity than isolated risk factors for developing cancer. Endometrial adenocarcinoma is nearly always preceded by endometrial hyperplasia in some form. This, of course, is not documented in every case because not every patient has had a diagnostic dilatation and curettage of the endometrium prior to development of the carcinoma. Furthermore, endometrial hyperplasia does not always lead to adenocarcinoma.

377. The answer is a. (*Damjanov, 10/e, pp 2273–2275. Rubin, 2/e, p 946.*) "Fibroids" of the uterus are among the most common abnormalities seen in uteri surgically removed in the United States in women of reproductive age. They arise in the myometrium, submucosally, subserosally, and midwall, both singly and several at a time. Sharply circumscribed, they are benign, smooth muscle tumors that are firm, gray-white, and whorled on cut section. Their malignant counterpart, leiomyosarcoma of the uterus, is quite rare in the de novo state and arises even more rarely from an antecedent leiomyoma. Whereas cell pleomorphism, tissue necrosis, and cytologic atypia per se are established criteria in assessing malignancy in tumors generally, they are important to the pathologist in uterine fibroids only if mitoses are also present. Regardless of cellularity or atypicality, if 10 or more mitoses are present in 10 separate high-power microscopic fields, the lesion is leiomyosarcoma. If 5 or fewer mitoses are present in 10 fields with bland morphology, the leiomyoma will behave in a benign fashion. Problems arise when the mitotic counts range between 3 and 7 per 10 fields with varying degrees of cell and tissue atypicality. These equivocal lesions should be regarded by both pathologist and clinician as "gray-area" smooth muscle tumors of unpredictable biologic behavior. Fortunately, the "gray-area" leiomyoma of the uterus is rarely seen. Thus mitoses are the most important criteria in assessing malignancy in smooth muscle tumors of the uterus.

378. The answer is c. (*Damjanov, 10/e, pp 1115–1116, 1325–1326. Cotran, 5/e, pp 1038–1039, 1063.*) Neisseria gonorrhoeae is a very common bacterium in this country that causes acute pelvic inflammatory disease with salpingitis as a result of venereal infection. Tuboovarian abscesses may develop from this bacterium, as well as other bacteria, but these organisms are susceptible to penicillin therapy. In the presence of unresponsiveness to penicillin, consideration should be given to Bacteroides species, which are important anaerobic gram-negative bacilli and are generally refractory to penicillin. These anaerobic bacteria may produce serious infections if uncontrolled. Chlamydiae, while considered to be nongonococcal in origin, are nevertheless important agents in venereal transmission and often are contracted at the same time as Neisseria species. When the gonococcus is adequately treated with penicillin, and symptoms continue, there may have been concurrent infection with chlamydia that is not responsive to penicillin but is sensitive to tetracycline. Adenoviruses are responsible for keratoconjunctivitis, tracheobronchitis, pneumonia in children, acute gastroenteritis, and occasionally hemorrhagic cystitis, but are not ordinarily causative in pelvic inflammatory disease.

379. The answer is d. (*Cotran, 5/e, pp 1064–1065. Chandrasoma, 3/e, pp 764–767.*) Infertility affects close to 20 percent of married couples in the United States, and in many of these cases, the infertility is related to polycystic ovary (Stein-Leventhal) syndrome in the female. The symptoms of patients with this syndrome are related to increased androgen production, which causes hirsutism, and decreased ovarian follicle maturation, which can lead to amenorrhea. These patients typically have excess androgens (androstenedione), increased estrogen levels, increased LH levels, increased GnRH levels, and decreased FSH levels. The cause of this syndrome is thought to be the abnormal secretion of gonadotropins by the pituitary. Increased secretion of LH stimulates the thecal cells to secrete excess amounts of androgens, which are converted to estrone by the peripheral aromatization of androgens by the adrenal gland. Excess estrogens in turn increase the levels of gonadotropin-releasing hormone (GnRH), but decrease the levels of FSH. The GnRH increases the levels of LH, which then stimulate the theca cells of the ovary to secrete more androgens, and this hormonal cycle begins again. The ovaries in these patients are enlarged and have thick capsules, hyperplastic ovarian stroma, and numerous follicular cysts, which are lined by a hyperplastic theca interna. Since these patients do not ovulate there is a marked decreased number of corpora lutea, which in turn results in decreased progesterone levels. These patients also have an increased risk of developing endometrial hyperplasia and endometrial carcinoma because of the excess estrogen production. Treatment for these patients in the past involved surgical wedge resection of the ovary, but now treatment is with clomiphene, which stimulates ovulation.

380. The answer is a. (*Cotran, 5/e, pp 1067–1077.*) The surface epithelial tumors of the ovary are derived from the surface coelomic epithelium, which embryonically gives rise to the Müllerian epithelium. Therefore these ovarian epithelial may recapitulate the histology of organs derived from the Müllerian epithelium. For example, serous ovarian tumors are composed of ciliated columnar serous epithelial cells, which are similar to the lining cells of the fallopian tubes. Endometrioid ovarian tumors are composed of nonciliated, columnar cells, which are similar to the lining cells of the endometrium. Mucinous ovarian tumors are composed of mucinous nonciliated columnar cells, which are similar to the epithelial cells of the endocervical glands. Spread of mucinous tumors, either from metastasis or rupture of an ovarian mucinous cyst, can result in the formation of multiple mucinous masses within the peritoneum. This condition is called pseudomyxomatous peritonei. Other epithelial ovarian tumors are similar histologically to other organs of the urogenital tract, such as the clear cell ovarian carcinoma and the Brenner tumor. The clear cell carcinoma of the ovary is similar histologically to clear cell carcinoma of the kidney, or more accurately, the clear cell variant of endometrial adenocarcinoma or the glycogen-rich cells associated with pregnancy. The Brenner tumor is similar to the transitional lining of the renal pelvis or bladder. This ovarian tumor is associated with benign mucinous cystadenomas of the ovary.

381. The answer is d. (*Damjanov, 10/e, pp 2293–2294. Cotran, 5/e, pp 1072–1073.*) Benign cystic teratomas constitute about 10 percent of cystic ovarian tumors. The cysts contain greasy sebaceous material mixed with a variable amount of hair. The cysts' walls contain skin and skin appendages, including sebaceous glands and hair follicles. A variety of other tissues—such as cartilage, bone, tooth, thyroid, respiratory tract epithelium, and intestinal tissue—may be found. The presence of skin and skin appendages gives the tumor its other name, "dermoid cyst." Dermoid cysts are benign, but in less than 2 percent, one element may become malignant, most frequently the squamous epithelium.

382. The answer is b. (*Cotran, 5/e, pp 1071–1077. Chandrasoma, 3/e, pp 775–776.*) Ovarian neoplasms are divided into four main categories:

epithelial tumors, sex cord-stromal tumors, germ cell tumors, and metas-tases. Examples of ovarian stromal tumors include thecomas, fibromas, granulosa cell tumors, and Sertoli-Leydig cell tumors. Histologically the-comas are composed of spindle-shaped cells with vacuolated cytoplasm. They are vacuolate because of steroid hormone (estrogen) production, which can be stained with an oil red O stain. Fibromas are also composed of spindle-shaped cells, but they do not produce steroid hormones and are oil red O negative. Fibromas are associated with Meig's syndrome, which consists of an ovarian fibroma, ascites, and hydrothorax. Granulosa cell tumors vary in the clinical behavior, but they are considered to be poten-tially malignant. The stromal cells of the ovary are the precursors of en-docrine active cells, so it is easy to understand that neoplasms derived from these stromal cells are often associated with hormone production. For example, granulosa cells normally secrete estrogens, thecal cells nor-mally secrete androgens, and hilar cells (Leydig cells) may secrete andro-gens. Excess androgen production in females may lead to masculinization and produce symptoms such as amenorrhea, loss of secondary female sex characteristics, and the development of secondary male characteristics, such as hirsutism, temporal balding, and deepening of the voice. Ovarian tumors associated with excess androgen production include androblas-tomas (Sertoli-Leydig cell tumors). Other ovarian diseases associated with excess androgen production include polycystic ovarian disease and hy-perthecosis. Excess estrogen production is associated with precocious puberty in the young, or endometrial hyperplasia and cancer in older women. Ovarian tumors that may secrete estrogens include granulosa cell tumors and thecomas.

383. The answer is c. (*Cotran, 5/e, pp 1077–1078. Chandrasoma, 3/e, pp 809–811.*) Abruptio placenta refers to premature separation of a normal-ly located placenta. This abnormality produces marked hemorrhage, pre-mature labor, and fetal demise. Factors that predispose an individual to abruptio placenta include certain drug use (cocaine, alcohol, smoking), maternal hypertension, preeclampsia, multiparity, and increasing mater-nal age. Placenta previa occurs when the placenta implants in the lower uterine segment. This may also result in severe bleeding problems at the time of delivery. Vaginal examination of a patient with this condition could also be dangerous. Placenta accreta refers to the absence of the de-cidua and the direct attachment of the placenta to the myometrium. There is no plane of separation between the placental villi and the myometrium. It is an important cause of post-partum hemorrhage because the placenta fails to separate from the myometrium at the time of labor. The hemorrhage can be life threatening, and a total hysterectomy is the treatment of choice. In both placenta accreta and placenta previa the villi are histologically normal, and there is no trophoblastic proliferation.

Gestational trophoblastic disease refers to abnormal proliferation of trophoblastic tissue and includes hydatidiform mole, the invasive mole, and the malignant choriocarcinoma. These neoplasms all secrete β human chorionic gonadotropin (β HCG) and should be suspected clinically whenever the uterus is too large for the estimated gestational age and no fetal movement or heart sounds are present.

384. The answer is a. (*Cotran, 5/e, p 1079.*) Ectopic pregnancy is a potentially life-threatening condition if it is not treated by removal before rupture and hemorrhage with fatal exsanguination. The most common location for extrauterine implantation is the fallopian tube (more than 85 percent of cases), with rare implantation in the ovary or abdomen. If the tubal implantation has existed from 1 to 4 weeks, the β-hCG test result is likely to be negative; thus a negative result does not exclude pregnancy. It is always worthwhile to repeat a laboratory test when the result is unexpected. Tubal pregnancy is not uncommon and should always be considered if endometrial samples suggest gestational change without chorionic villi.

385. The answer is e. (*Cotran, 5/e, pp 1079–1084. Chandrasoma, 3/e, pp 811–814.*) Toxemia of pregnancy refers to the combination of hypertension, proteinuria, and pitting edema. This combination of signs is also called preeclampsia. When convulsions develop in an individual with preeclampsia the condition is then referred to as eclampsia. These signs and symptoms result from abnormal placental implantation with incomplete conversion of the blood vessels of the decidua. Both of these result in placental ischemia. Normally the blood vessels of the uterine wall at the site of implantation increase in diameter and lose their muscular components. These changes increase the blood flow to the placenta and are the result of increased production of prostacyclin (a strong vasodilator) and decreased production of thromboxane (a potent vasoconstrictor). These changes do not take place at the implantation site of patients who develop preeclampsia. This causes placental ischemia and damages the endothelial cells of the blood vessels of the placenta. This endothelial damage disrupts the normal balance between vasodilation and vasoconstriction. As a result, there are increased levels of vasoconstrictors, such as thromboxane, angiotensin, and endothelin, and decreased levels of vasodilators, such as PGI_2, PGE_2, and nitric oxide. This results in arterial vasoconstriction, which produces systemic hypertension, and can lead to activation of intravascular coagulation (DIC). Risk factors for the development of preeclampsia include nulliparity, twin gestation, and hydatidiform mole. Other complications associated with preeclampsia include renal disease and liver disease, such as the HELLP syndrome, which refers to hemolytic anemia, elevated liver enzymes, and low platelets.

386. The answer is b. (*Cotran, 5/e, pp 1081–1086.*) Gestational trophoblastic diseases include the benign hydatidiform mole (partial and complete), the invasive mole (chorioadenoma destruens), placental site trophoblastic tumor, and choriocarcinoma. Hydatidiform moles are composed of avascular, grapelike structures that do not invade the myometrium. In complete (classic) moles, all the chorionic villi are abnormal and fetal parts are not found. They have a 46,XX diploid pattern and arise from the paternal chromosomes of a single sperm by a process called androgenesis. In partial moles, only some of the villi are abnormal and fetal parts may be seen. These moles have a triploid or a tetraploid karyotype and arise from the fertilization of a single egg by two sperm. About 2 percent of complete moles may develop into choriocarcinoma, but partial moles are rarely followed by malignancy. The invasive mole penetrates the myometrium and may even embolize to distant sites. A similar lesion is the placental site trophoblastic tumor, which is characterized by invasion of the myometrium by intermediate trophoblasts. Gestational choriocarcinomas, composed of malignant proliferations of both cytotrophoblasts and syncytiotrophoblasts without the formation of villi, can arise from either normal or abnormal pregnancies; 50 percent arise in hydatidiform moles, 25 percent in previous abortions, 22 percent in normal pregnancies, and the rest in ectopic pregnancies or teratomas. Both hydatidiform moles and choriocarcinomas have high levels of human chorionic gonadotropin (hCG); the levels are extremely high in choriocarcinoma unless considerable tumor necrosis is present.

387. The answer is d. (*Cotran, 5/e, pp 948–958.*) While many varieties of glomerulonephritis can produce the nephrotic syndrome, a few disorders will virtually always produce it. Included in the latter group are focal (segmental) glomerulosclerosis, membranous glomerulonephritis (GN), lipoid nephrosis, membranoproliferative glomerulonephritis, systemic diseases (such as amyloidosis and systemic lupus erythematosus), some tumors, hep-atitis B, syphilis, drugs such as penicillamine, and certain allergies. Light microscopy shows very little change in glomeruli in lipoid nephrosis, and a diffuse absence of glomerular epithelial foot processes is noted with electron microscopy. Membranoproliferative GN is characterized by an increase in mesangial cellularity accompanied by splitting of the glomerular basement membranes ("double contour"). Membranous GN shows electron-dense deposits of immunoglobulin in the subepithelial portion of the basement membrane. The nephrotic syndrome includes massive albuminuria with significant loss of protein (more than 3 to 5 g of protein) in 24 h, consequent reduced plasma albumin (less than 3 g/dL), hyperlipidemia, and anasarca (generalized edema).

388. The answer is e. (*Cotran, 5/e, pp 947–948, 952–954, 956–958.*) The photomicrograph shows focal glomerulonephritis with crescent formation and focal hypercellularity involving only one portion of the glomerulus. Focal glomerulonephritis involves some glomeruli, but not all, and may involve the entire glomerulus (global) or only parts of the glomerulus (segmental). The photomicrograph demonstrates focal segmental glomerulonephritis, which may be seen in systemic diseases as well as disorders affecting only the kidney. Hypercellularity involved several mesangia with proliferation of epithelial cells lining Bowman's capsule near the damaged capillary loops. This process is referred to as crescent formation. The disease may be seen in bacterial endocarditis and other systemic infections. Immunologic disorders causing focal segmental glomerulonephritis may include IgA focal glomerulonephritis, systemic lupus erythematosus, polyarteritis nodosa, and Schönlein-Henoch purpura (anaphylactoid purpura). IgA focal glomerulonephritis, also known as Berger's disease, has deposits of IgA and some IgG in the involved mesangium as demonstrated by immunofluorescence. Alport's syndrome is a hereditary form of chronic renal disease that may be associated with neural deafness and death at an early age, usually less than 30. Large collections of foam cells are also seen in the renal cortex in these patients. Electron microscopy shows splitting of the glomerular basements accompanied by small, electron-dense granules. Diabetes mellitus is associated with nodular glomerulosclerosis (Kimmelstiel-Wilson disease).

389. The answer is a. (*Cotran, 5/e, pp 964–967.*) In ATN, renal tubular damage follows toxic or ischemic injury and is the commonest cause of acute renal failure (ARF). Red blood cells and proteinaceous casts are usually present, but red cell casts are not associated and would suggest nephritis. Toxic ATN is caused by drugs, toxins, heavy metals (Hg), and organic solvents, and the tubular injury is predominant in proximal convoluted tubules, probably because this is the major site of nephrotoxin reabsorption. Ischemic ATN occurs after shock caused by severe infections, burns, or crush injuries with peripheral circulatory collapse. In ischemic ATN there is multiple focal tubular necrosis along the nephron often with rupture of basement membranes. Although urinary output in ATN often decreases to less than 400 mL per day (oliguria), up to 50 percent of patients with ATN may not have oliguria but may have increased urinary volumes.

390. The answer is a. (*Cotran, 5/e, pp 484–489, 976–978, 982.*) Many pathologic processes affecting the kidney can lead to hypertension. The three main categories are renovascular, renal parenchymal, and urinary tract obstruction. The renin-angiotensin system has been implicated in renovascular hypertension but has not been proved to be of etiologic importance in the other two categories. The most common parenchymal diseases leading to hypertension are pyelonephritis and hydronephrosis. Large infarcts of one kidney can cause hypertension, but many small infarcts are clinically silent.

391. The answer is b. (*Cotran, 5/e, pp 984–985.*) Urinary calculi are a common problem and may arise at any level of the urinary tract, but mainly in the kidney. They are more common in males and most patients are over 30 years of age. Urinary calculi are unilateral in 80 percent of cases, and 90 percent are radiopaque since most contain calcium oxalate or calcium phosphate. Other constituents include magnesium ammonium phosphate, cystine, and uric acid. Urate stones are radiolucent and are increased in hyperuricemia due to gout and in conditions with rapid cell turnover such as leukemia. Urea-splitting organisms such as Pseudomonas predispose to calculi.

392. The answer is b. (*Cotran, 5/e, pp 986–987.*) Renal cell carcinoma (renal adenocarcinoma) accounts for 85 percent of primary renal tumors and usually occurs in the sixth decade, although sometimes at a much younger age. These tumors may produce hormones or hormonelike substances, for example, renin (hypertension), glucocorticoids (Cushing's syndrome), and gonadotropins (feminization and masculinization). More frequently, though in only 5 to 10 percent of patients, polycythemia or erythrocytosis occurs owing to production of erythropoietin. Renal cell carcinoma is not associated with tuberous sclerosis in which the common renal lesion is angiomyolipoma (hamartoma). It is associated with the von Hippel-Lindau syndrome in which many patients develop bilateral renal cell carcinomas. Translocations between chromosomes 3 and 8 and between 3 and 11 have been found in some cases of familial renal cancer and in a few sporadic cases. Hematuria is often the first symptom but often occurs late, after invasion of the renal vein or widespread metastases frequently to lung, bone, or brain. Renal cell carcinoma is predominantly of clear cell type with intracytoplasmic glycogen and lipid, but less often granular cells with numerous mitochondria or spindle cells occur. Diagnosis requires IVP, CT, and ultrasound to differentiate benign cysts, as well as percutaneous needle aspiration for cytology.

393. The answer is e. *(Cotran, 5/e, pp 462, 614.)* Wilms' tumor is the most common primary tumor of children, and its incidence is increased in several syndromes involving distinct chromosomal loci and congenital malformations. Patients with the WAGR syndrome, which is characterized by aniridia, genital abnormalities, and mental retardation, have a one-third chance of developing Wilms' tumor. The majority of patients with the Denys-Drash syndrome, characterized by gonadal dysgenesis (male pseudohermaphroditism) and nephropathy, develop Wilms' tumor. Both of these syndromes involve the Wilms' tumor-associated gene WT_1, located at band p13 on chromosome 11. A second Wilms' tumor gene, WT_2, located on chromosome 11 distal to WT_1, is associated with the Beckwith-Wiedemann syndrome, which is characterized by enlargement of body organs, hemihypertrophy, renal medullary cysts, and adrenal cytomegaly. These patients are also at an increased risk for developing Wilms' tumor. Hypoplasia of the radii, along with hypoplasia of the kidney and spleen, is associated with Fanconi's anemia, an autosomal recessive disorder of defective DNA repair.

394. The answer is e. *(Damjanov, 10/e, pp 887–888, 911–914, 1712.)* Cytomegalic inclusion disease is diagnosed in the immunosuppressed or AIDS patient by finding large intranuclear inclusions surrounded by a clear halo in enlarged cells in urinary sediment, in sputum or bronchial lavage, in spinal fluid specimens, or in liver biopsy. Small intracytoplasmic inclusions may be found. Cytomegalovirus (CMV) is a DNA member of the herpesvirus group that causes disseminated disease, including interstitial pneumonitis in the debilitated or immunosuppressed adult. Disseminated infection with CMV in AIDS is associated with pneumonitis, hepatitis, idiopathic ulcerative colitis, encephalitis, and retinitis. Rising antibody titers may not be detectable for up to 4 weeks after primary infection and early diagnosis may be achieved by finding typical inclusion bodies in cytologic or biopsy specimens. However, the shell vial technique has revolutionized detection of CMV in cell culture with detection of early antigen in 24 h instead of 1 to 3 weeks.

395. The answer is b. (*Cotran, 5/e, pp 997–1002.*) Approximately 90 percent of carcinomas of the bladder are of transitional cell type. They are more common in men. Known etiologic factors include cigarette smoking, persistent mucosal inflammation, exposure to certain chemicals (notably beta-naphthylamine), and administration of the immunosuppressive agent cyclophosphamide (Cytoxan). Infection by Schistosoma haematobium is associated with squamous cell cancer. All transitional cell cancers, regardless of grade, tend to recur; the frequency of recurrence increases with the tumor grade.

396. The answer is b. (*Damjanov, 10/e, pp 2179–2189.*) Most malignant germ cell tumors of the gonads, specifically the testis, typically occur in the younger man between the ages of 22 and 35. The seminoma has several types, most of which are found also in younger persons. The classic seminoma is populated by differentiated seminiferous tubule-type epithelium with intervening lymphocytes, while the anaplastic seminoma contains an increase in mitoses and a moderate degree of anaplasia. The spermatocytic seminoma, however, occurs in older patients, often between ages 55 and 65, and is a soft, yellowish, sometimes mucoid tumor that microscopically has several cell types: classic intermediate-sized germ cells; smaller, secondary spermatocytic-type cells; and large mononuclear and multinuclear giant cells. Polyembryoma and embryonal carcinoma are related, occur in the younger patient, and are less common than the seminomas. The most malignant germ cell tumor of the testis is the choriocarcinoma, which is characterized by large cytotrophoblastic and syncytiotrophoblastic cells. Teratocarcinomas are tumors of more than one histologic type that may contain seminomatous or embryonal components, or both.

397. The answer is b. *(Brawer, Hum Pathol 23:242–248, 1992. Cotran, 5/e, pp 1028–1029.)* Premalignant, intraepithelial abnormalities are found within several organ systems, including the endometrium, cervix, urothelium, respiratory tract, and prostate. Within the prostate these changes, which are referred to as prostatic intraepithelial neoplasia (PIN), consist of proliferation and dysplastic changes of the normal epithelial cells of the prostatic ducts and acini. Histologic features of PIN include cellular crowding and stratification, variation in cellular and nuclear size, hyperchromasia, and nucleoli. One of the major distinguishing features between PIN and carcinoma is that in PIN there remains the normal two distinct epithelial cell layers: the basal layer and the luminal layer. Prostatic carcinoma is characterized instead by a single layer of neoplastic, atypical epithelial cells, and stromal infiltration is present.

398. The answer is d. *(Cotran, 5/e, pp 1026–1031.)* Over 95 percent of prostatic cancers are adenocarcinomas. In nearly 75 percent of cases adenocarcinoma of the prostate arises in the posterior lobe, usually in a subcapsular location. The lateral lobes are the next, much less frequent site. Nodular hyperplasia occurs in the periurethral region. When prostatic cancer is extracapsular or metastatic (commonly osteoblastic metastases to pelvis and lumbar vertebrae), serum tumor markers such as prostatic acid phosphatase (PAP) or prostatic-specific antigen (PSA) are detectable by standard assays. Tumor growth may be inhibited by estrogen therapy; it is not estrogen-dependent. Invasion of capsule, blood vessels, and perineural spaces is useful in diagnosis of well-differentiated tumor. Diagnosis may include needle biopsy or fine needle aspiration (80 percent accuracy).

399. The answer is d. *(Cotran, 5/e, pp 1044–1045. Rubin, 2/e, pp 920–922.)* Neoplasms of the vagina are rare, but of these squamous cell carcinoma is the most common. Vaginal clear cell adenocarcinoma occurs occasionally (1 or less per 1000) in girls in their late teens whose mothers had received diethylstilbestrol during pregnancy. In about one-third of cases, such cancers arise in the cervix. More frequently, in about half of the population at risk, small glandular or microcystic lesions appear in the mucosa—vaginal adenosis. These benign lesions appear as red, velvety foci and are lined by mucus-secreting or ciliated columnar cells. From these areas the rarer clear cell adenocarcinoma arises. Sarcoma botryoides, which produces soft, polypoid, grapelike masses, is another rare primary vaginal cancer found usually in infants and children under age 5. It is a rhabdomyosarcoma that can also occur in the urinary bladder.

400. The answer is e. *(Fawcett, 12/e, pp 840–843. Damjanov, 10/e, pp 2262–2265. Cotran, 5/e, pp 1035–1037, 1053–1054.)* Histologic examination of the endometrium is important clinically to determine hormonal status, document ovulation, and evaluate the causes of dysfunctional uterine bleeding. After menses, under the influence of estrogen, the basal third of the endometrium proliferates rapidly (proliferative phase) to form straight, tubular glands lined by pseudostratified columnar cells. Characteristically, mitoses are numerous. Following ovulation the endometrium changes to a secretory-type endometrium, which is characterized by secretory vacuoles that form first in the basal parts of the cells, glandular secretions, stromal cell hypertrophy with abundant eosinophilic cytoplasm (predecidual change), and lack of glandular mitoses. Throughout the cycle lymphocytes may be found in the endometrium, but toward the end of the secretory phase there is a marked infiltrate of neutrophils. In contrast, the presence of any plasma cells within the endometrium is diagnostic of chronic endometritis.

401. The answer is d. *(Cotran, 5/e, pp 1057–1058.)* Cystic endometrial hyperplasia refers to the abnormal growth of endometrium associated with either an absolute or a relative estrogen excess. These are common findings at the time of menopause and in conditions causing an absolute excess of estrogen—e.g., Stein-Leventhal syndrome, functioning granulosa and thecal cell ovarian tumors, and the exogenous administration of estrogenic substances. The microscopic findings in an endometrial biopsy are dominated by the marked dilatation of the endometrial glands, which gives the tissue section the appearance of Swiss cheese. The glands are lined by benign columnar epithelium that is nonsecretory.

402. The answer is d. *(Damjanov, 10/e, pp 2269–2271.)* Endometrial carcinoma affects menopausal and postmenopausal women, with the peak incidence at 55 to 65 years of age. Although it was much less common than squamous cervical cancer several decades ago, it has not been controlled as effectively as cervical cancer by the Papanicolaou smear technique and therapy, so that it is now more common than invasive cervical cancer. However, the major symptom of endometrial carcinoma, postmenopausal bleeding, results in diagnosis while the tumor is still confined to the uterus (stage I or II), which permits cure by surgery or radiotherapy. The annual death rate in the U.S. from endometrial cancer is 3000, while more than 6000 deaths result from squamous cervical cancer. Risk factors for endometrial cancer include obesity and glucose intolerance or diabetes.

403. The answer is a. (*Cotran, 5/e, pp 1059–1060. Rubin, 2/e, p 945.*) The condition illustrated is a uterine leiomyoma (fibroid). This is an extremely common tumor occurring in up to 25 percent of women of reproductive age. The cause is unknown, but the growth is estrogen-dependent and for this reason the tumor may enlarge rapidly during pregnancy. If the tumor becomes very large, areas within it may undergo softening followed by liquefaction and cystic degeneration. Fibroids tend to regress in the postmenopausal period; with atrophy they become collagenous and calcification often occurs.

404–405. The answers are: 404-d, 405-e. (*Cotran, 5/e, pp 976–978.*) Benign nephrosclerosis (renal disease occurring in benign hypertension) is characterized by hyaline arteriolosclerosis with thickened hyalinized arteriolar walls and narrowed lumina. Fibroelastic hyperplasia occurs in the larger muscular arteries. Small kidneys with granular surfaces often result because of ischemic atrophy of nephrons. Renal arteriolar changes in malignant nephrosclerosis (malignant hypertension) include fibrinoid necrosis of arterioles (necrotizing arteriolitis), hyperplastic arteriolosclerosis (onion-skinning), necrotizing glomerulitis, and often a thrombotic microangiopathy. The clinical course is often downhill with only 50 percent of patients surviving 5 years; marked proteinuria, hematuria, cardiovascular problems, and finally renal failure contribute to death. The disease is often associated with accelerated preexisting benign essential hypertension, chronic renal disease (glomerulonephritis), or scleroderma.

406–407. The answers are: 406-c, 407-d. (*Cotran, 5/e, pp 875, 973–974, 1079–1081.*) Preeclampsia is characterized by hypertension, proteinuria, and edema that begins after 20 weeks of gestation but is obvious clinically after 32 weeks. Most common in the last trimester of a first pregnancy, it occurs in about 6 percent of all pregnancies. It may progress to eclampsia with convulsions and coma. Renal involvement involves the glomeruli with narrowing or obliteration of capillary lumina due to swelling of endothelial and mesangial cells (glomerular endotheliosis). Electron microscopy shows widening of the subendothelial region between basement membrane and endothelial cell by electron-lucent and dense material (fibrin); this change is similar to that in HUS. Pathogenesis includes placental ischemia with decreased production of vasodilator prostaglandins (PGI_2, PGE_2) and increased release of vasoconstrictors.

Analgesic abuse nephropathy (analgesic nephritis) occurs because of excessive intake of mixtures of aspirin and phenacetin. It requires the synergistic action of these drugs, and cases due to aspirin, or phenacetin, or acetaminophen alone are rare. Analgesic abuse nephropathy eventually results in papillary necrosis (necrotizing papillitis) with secondary chronic tubulointerstitial nephritis. Clinical findings include sterile pyuria, anemia, GI symptoms, urinary tract infections, and hypertension. Chronic renal failure may occur, but drug withdrawal often stabilizes kidney function. There is, however, an increased incidence of urothelial carcinoma of the renal pelvis.

408–409. The answers are: 408-i, 409-g. (*Cotran, 5/e, pp 994–995, 1007–1008. Damjanov, 10/e, pp 1710–1711, 2190–2191. Larsen, 1/e, pp 222–226.*) The cloaca is an embryonic structure that connects ventrally to the allantoic stalk and laterally to the mesonephric ducts. At about the eighth week of development a cloacal membrane forms within the cloaca and separates the cloaca into a dorsal rectum and a ventral urogenital sinus. The latter is the origin of the urachus, urinary bladder, and proximal urethra. Initially the urinary bladder is continuous with the allantois, which constricts and forms the thick, fibrous urachus. The urachus in turn becomes attenuated, but still remains attached to the bladder dome and forms the median umbilical ligament in the adult. Incomplete attenuation of the urachus (persistent urachus) can lead to formation of an urachal cyst, urachal sinus, or urachal fistula. The end attached to the bladder can remain and form a bladder diverticulum, while the central portion can remain and form an urachal cyst. Urachal sinuses and fistulas still connect the umbilicus to the urinary bladder, and therefore urine can leak at the site of the umbilicus.

Normally, mesodermal tissue grows onto the cloacal membrane to form the muscles of the lower abdominal wall. During this process the cloacal membrane is obliterated and disappears. In some embryos mesoderm does not grow onto the cloacal membrane..This leads to persistence of the cloacal membrane, which can become quite thin and rupture. This in turn causes the posterior bladder mucosa to evert through this defect in the anterior abdominal wall. This condition is called exstrophy and is associated with recurrent urinary infections and epispadias in males. There is also an increased incidence of neoplastic transformation, most commonly adenocarcinoma.

Meckel's diverticulum is a diverticulum found in the terminal ileum that is the result of persistence of the omphalomesenteric duct. It is usually about 2 inches long and is located less than 2 feet from the ileocecal valve. An omphalocele refers to protrusion of the intestines through an unclosed umbilical ring. This abnormality results from incomplete internalization of the intestines during fetal growth. A similar defect, gastroschisis, does not involve the umbilicus. Instead, viscera herniate through a defect in the anterior abdominal wall just lateral to the umbilicus.

Phimosis occurs when the orifice of the prepuce (foreskin) is too small to permit normal retraction. This may be due to inflammatory scarring or abnormal development of the prepuce. If a phimotic prepuce is forcibly retracted over the glans penis, a condition called paraphimosis may develop. This condition is extremely painful and may cause obstruction of the urinary tract or blood flow, which may lead to necrosis of the penis. Nonspecific infection of the glans and prepuce is called balanoposthitis. Genital malformations may cause an abnormal location of the urethral opening, either on the ventral surface of the penis (hypospadias) or the dorsal surface (epispadias). These abnormal developments may cause problems with infertility. Hypospadias is the result of failure of the urethral folds to close, while epispadias is the result of faulty positioning of the genital tubercle. The latter is also associated with exstrophy of the urinary bladder.

NERVOUS SYSTEM

Questions

30|4|01.

DIRECTIONS: Each question below contains five suggested responses. Select the **one best** response to each question.

410. The Arnold-Chiari malformation is characterized by

a. Hypoplasia of the cerebellar vermis
b. Herniation of the cerebellum and the fourth ventricle into the foramen magnum
c. Facial angiofibromata and tubers of the cerebral cortex
d. Hemangioblastomas of the retina and brain
e. Facial port-wine stains

411. Subdural hematomas occur most frequently in the

a. Supracerebellar region
b. Intracerebellar region
c. Cerebellopontine angle
d. Pituitary region
e. Cerebral hemisphere convexities

412. Which of the following conditions is the most frequent cause of intracerebral hemorrhage?

a. Ruptured aneurysm
b. Trauma
c. Blood dyscrasias
d. Angiomas
e. Hypertensive vascular disease

413. The majority of cases of subarachnoid hemorrhage result from

a. Transection of a branch of the middle meningeal artery
b. Bleeding from torn bridging veins
c. Rupture of a preexisting aneurysm
d. Rupture of an arteriovenous malformation
e. Cortical bleeding occurring opposite the point of a traumatic injury

414. Laminar necrosis and watershed infarcts are most suggestive of

a. Shock
b. Hypertension
c. Fat emboli
d. Vascular thrombosis
e. Venous sinus thrombosis

415. Hypertension is most closely related to the formation of which one of the following types of aneurysms?

a. Berry aneurysm
b. Atherosclerotic aneurysm
c. Mycotic aneurysm
d. Charcot-Bouchard aneurysm
e. Saccular aneurysm

416. Tabes dorsalis is characterized by

a. Hydrophobia
b. Increased neutrophils in the cerebrospinal fluid (CSF)
c. Involvement of the motor neurons of the spinal cord
d. Degeneration of posterior columns of the spinal cord
e. Infection of oligodendrocytes

417. Select the disorder below that has the most clinicopathologic features in common with postvaccinal encephalomyelitis.

a. Metachromatic leukodystrophy
b. Multifocal leukoencephalopathy
c. Guillain-Barré syndrome
d. Hypoxic encephalopathy
e. Hypertensive encephalopathy

418. An elevated IgG level in cerebrospinal fluid and an abnormal band on agar gel electrophoresis of cerebrospinal fluid are findings consistent with the diagnosis of

a. Secondary stage of syphilis
b. muscular dystrophy
c. Tumor involvement of the spinal cord
d. Meningeal involvement by leukemia
e. Multiple sclerosis

419. A 45-year-old man presents with weakness and cramping that involves both of his hands. Physical examination reveals atrophy of the muscles of both hands, hyperactive reflexes and muscle fasciculations involving his arms and legs, and a positive Babinski reflex. Sensation appears normal in his arms and legs. The most likely diagnosis for this individual is

a. Metachromatic leukodystrophy
b. Amyotrophic lateral sclerosis
c. Guillain-Barré syndrome
d. Huntington disease
e. Wilson disease

420. A 41-year-old male presents with involuntary rapid jerky movements and progressive dementia. He soon dies and gross examination of his brain reveals marked degeneration of the caudate nucleus. This individual's symptoms were caused by

a. Decreased functioning of GABA neurons
b. Increased functioning of dopamine neurons
c. Relative increased functioning of acetylcholine neurons
d. Relative decreased functioning of acetylcholine neurons
e. Decreased functioning of serotonin neurons

421. Which of the following tumors is characterized by pseudopalisading, necrosis, endoneurial proliferation, hypercellularity, and atypical nuclei?

a. Schwannoma
b. Medulloblastoma
c. Oligodendroglioma
d. Glioblastoma multiforme
e. Ependymoma

422. The most frequent of all the following intracranial tumors in adults is

a. Ependymoma
b. Medulloblastoma
c. Meningioma
d. Glioma
e. Metastasis

423. In subacute combined degeneration (SCD) there is

a. Association with hemolytic anemia
b. Usually involvement of gray matter of the spinal cord
c. Usually no motor impairment
d. Failure of the enzyme methylmalonic CoA mutase
e. Dermatitis, enteritis, and dementia

424. A 3-month-old male infant is being evaluated for severe neurological defects involving both of his legs, his urinary bladder, and his rectum. Physical examination reveals a cystic structure in his sacrolumbar region. Further examination reveals that this cystic structure contains meninges and portions of the spinal cord. What is the best diagnosis?

a. Anencephaly
b. Infantile hemiplegia
c. Myeloschisis
d. Spina bifida with meningocele
e. Spina bifida with meningomyelocele

425. True statements regarding neuroglial cells include all the following EXCEPT

a. They include astrocytes
b. They include oligodendrocytes
c. They include ependymal cells and microglial cells
d. All function to shelter and maintain neurons
e. All function as macrophages, when activated

426. A known alcoholic is brought to the emergency room following an altercation in a local bar. The intern observes respiratory irregularity, coma, and papilledema. Emergency surgery is planned in order to prevent all the following EXCEPT

a. Brainstem herniation
b. Cerebellar herniation
c. Duret hemorrhages
d. Ruptured aneurysm
e. Death of the patient

427. Cerebral embolism occurs frequently in association with all the following conditions EXCEPT

a. Cardiac mural thrombi
b. Left-sided endocarditis
c. Right-sided endocarditis
d. Cardiac catheterization
e. Prosthetic cardiac valves

428. All the following have been commonly associated with pyogenic brain abscesses EXCEPT

a. Congenital heart disease
b. Sinusitis
c. Lung abscess
d. Liver abscess
e. Mastoiditis

429. Characteristics of AIDS-related neurologic abnormalities include all the following EXCEPT

a. Areas of demyelination
b. Preferential infection of cortical neurons
c. Multinucleated giant cells
d. Vacuolar myelopathy
e. Increased incidence of progressive multifocal leukoencephalopathy (PML)

430. Creutzfeldt-Jakob disease displays all the following characteristics EXCEPT

a. Spongiform encephalopathy
b. Rapidly progressive dementia
c. Worldwide incidence of 1 case per 100,000 population
d. Absence of an inflammatory infiltrate
e. Inactivation by hypochlorite solution

431. Diseases that are classified as slow viral infections or unconventional agent (spongiform) encephalopathies include all the following EXCEPT

a. Reye's syndrome
b. Subacute sclerosing panencephalitis
c. Creutzfeldt-Jakob disease
d. Progressive multifocal leukoencephalopathy
e. Kuru

432. Alzheimer's disease is characterized by all the following EXCEPT

a. Cerebral atrophy in superior temporal and frontal lobes
b. Neuritic or senile plaques
c. Amyloid β-protein deposits
d. Lewy bodies
e. Granulovacuolar degeneration

433. All the following statements apply to ependymomas EXCEPT that

a. They are the most common type of intraspinal glioma
b. They are most commonly located in the lateral ventricles
c. Patients may present with headache and papilledema
d. They may require differentiation from choroid plexus papilloma
e. Histologic sections display rosettes

434. True statements about meningiomas include all the following EXCEPT

a. They usually present clinically with headaches or seizures
b. They constitute about 20 percent of primary brain tumors
c. They usually display rapid growth
d. They arise from arachnoid cap cells
e. They may be multiple in neurofibromatosis type 2

435. Intracerebral calcification is associated with all the following EXCEPT

a. Glioblastoma multiforme
b. Tuberous sclerosis
c. Oligodendroglioma
d. Craniopharyngioma
e. Hypoparathyroidism

436. True statements about classic neurofibromatosis (von Recklinghausen's disease) include all the following EXCEPT

a. Malignant degeneration may occur
b. Hamartomas of the iris are very common
c. Hemangioblastomas of the brain are associated
d. Acoustic neuroma is associated
e. Pheochromocytomas and meningiomas are associated

437. Transection of a peripheral nerve will result in all the following EXCEPT

a. Dissolution of the Nissl substance in the nerve cell body
b. Degeneration of the nerve fiber distal to the cut
c. Proliferation of the Schwann sheath from the proximal nerve segment
d. Loss of the entire Schwann sheath proximal to the cut
e. Degeneration of the axons from 1 to 3 nodes of Ranvier proximal to the cut

438. Syringomyelia is characterized by all the following EXCEPT

a. Segmental loss of pain and temperature sensation
b. Segmental loss of touch sensation
c. Loss of tissue (cavitation) within the cervical spinal cord
d. Small muscle atrophy of the hands
e. Kyphoscoliosis

439. All the following tumors may be found arising within the pineal gland EXCEPT

a. Teratoma
b. Pineoblastoma
c. Embryonal carcinoma
d. Choriocarcinoma
e. Craniopharyngioma

DIRECTIONS: Each group of questions below consists of lettered headings followed by a set of numbered items. For each numbered item select the **one** lettered heading with which it is **most** closely associated. Each lettered heading may be used **once, more than once, or not at all**.

Questions 440–441

Match each of the following clinical scenarios with the most likely diagnosis from the following list.

a. Astrocytoma
b. Berry aneurysm
c. Brown tumor
d. Cerebral lymphoma
e. Medulloblastoma
f. Metastatic carcinoma
g. Oligodendroglioma
h. Pseudotumor cerebri

440. A 9-year-old boy who had been suffering from a gait disturbance for several weeks was found to have a posterior fossa mass on CT scan.

441. A 55-year-old woman is suspected of having a brain tumor because of the onset of seizure activity. Computerized tomograms (CT scans) and skull x-rays demonstrate a mass in the right cerebral hemisphere that is markedly calcific.

Questions 442–443

Match each of the following clinical scenarios with the most likely location within the nervous system of the lesion that produced the abnormality.

a. Anterior horn of the spinal cord
b. Anterior pituitary
c. Basal ganglia
d. Caudate nucleus
e. Cerebellopontine angle
f. Cerebellum
g. Hippocampus
h. Midbrain
i. Substantia nigra
j. Third ventricle

442. A 65-year-old male presents with bradykinesia, tremors at rest, and muscular rigidity. Physical examination reveals the patient to have a "mask-like" facies. In this patient where would intracytoplasmic eosinophilic inclusions most likely be found?

443. A 45-year-old female presents with unilateral tinnitus and unilateral hearing loss. Physical examination reveals facial weakness and loss of corneal reflex on the same side as the tinnitus and hearing loss. This patient's symptoms might be produced by a tumor located where?

NERVOUS SYSTEM

Answers

410. The answer is b. (*Cotran, 5/e, pp 509, 1302–1303, 1354. Rubin, 2/e, pp 1446–1447.*) Developmental abnormalities of the brain include the Arnold-Chiari malformation, the Dandy-Walker malformation, and the phakomatoses, which include tuberous sclerosis, neurofibromatosis, von Hippel-Lindau disease, and Sturge-Weber syndrome. The Arnold-Chiari malformation consists of herniation of the cerebellum and fourth ventricle into the foramen magnum, flattening of the base of the skull, hydrocephalus secondary to the cerebral aqueduct, and spina bifida with meningomyelocele. Severe hypoplasia or absence of the cerebellar vermis occurs in the Dandy-Walker malformation. There is cystic distention of the roof of the fourth ventricle, hydrocephalus, and possibly agenesis of the corpus callosum. Tuberous sclerosis may show characteristic firm, white nodules (tubers) in the cortex and subependymal nodules of gliosis protruding into the ventricles ("candle drippings"). Other signs of tuberous sclerosis include a triad of seizures, mental retardation, and congenital white spots or macules (leukoderma). Facial angiofibromata (adenoma sebaceum) also occur. In von Hippel-Lindau disease, multiple benign and malignant neoplasms occur including hemangioblastomas of the retina, cerebellum, and medulla oblongata, angiomas of the kidney and liver, and renal cell carcinoma. Patients with Sturge-Weber syndrome, a nonfamilial congenital disorder, have angiomas of the brain, leptomeninges, and ipsilateral face, which are called port-wine stains (nevus flammeus).

411. The answer is e. (*Damjanov, 10/e, pp 2733–2736.*) When blood enters the potential space between the arachnoid and dura, a subdural hematoma forms. Subdural hematomas are most commonly located over the cerebral hemisphere convexities. The traditional explanation for the formation of subdural hematomas has been tearing of the bridging veins that pass from the cortical surface to the superior sagittal sinus. Blood may also leak from lacerated cortical vessels or arachnoidal vessels ruptured by a meningeal tear.

412. The answer is e. (*Cotran, 5/e, pp 1311–1312.*) Hypertension is 10 to 20 times more frequent than all the other causes of intracerebral hemorrhage and is also the most common cause of death from cerebrovascular disease. Major sites of hemorrhage are the putamen (more than 50 percent); the cortex and subcortex (15 percent); and the thalamus, the pons, and the cerebellum (each approximately 10 percent). Hypertensive hemorrhage shows a predilection for the distribution of the lenticulostriate arteries with small (lacunar) hemorrhages, or large hemorrhages obliterating the corpus striatum, including the putamen and internal capsule. It is possible that development of microaneurysms (Charcot-Bouchard aneurysms) with subsequent rupture is a precipitating factor.

413. The answer is c. (*Cotran, 5/e, pp 1304–1308.*) Trauma may cause bleeding within the brain parenchyma, on the surface of the brain, or within spaces overlying the brain. Epidural hemorrhages result from the rupture of one of the meningeal arteries, usually the middle meningeal artery, which run between the dura and the skull. Subdural hemorrhages result from bleeding of torn bridging veins, which connect the venous system of the brain with the large venous sinuses within the dura. About two-thirds of the cases of subarachnoid hemorrhage are the result of rupture of a preexisting arterial aneurysm rather than trauma, while in about 10 percent of cases, an arteriovenous malformation (AVM) is found. AVM's more commonly bleed into both the subarachnoid space and the brain parenchyma. Traumatic head injury may produce contusions (bruises) at the point of impact ("coup"), or if the head is in motion, such as in a backward fall, contusions may occur on the surface of the brain opposite the point of impact ("contrecoup").

414. The answer is a. (*Cotran, 5/e, pp 1308–1309, 1311. Rubin, 2/e, pp 1397–1403.*) Decreased brain perfusion may be generalized (global) or localized. Global ischemia results from generalized decreased blood flow, such as with shock, cardiac arrest, or hypoxic episodes (e.g., near-drowning or carbon monoxide poisoning). Global hypoxia results in watershed (border-zone) infarcts, which typically occur at the border of areas supplied by the anterior and middle cerebral arteries, and laminar necrosis, which is related to the short, penetrating vessels originating from pial arteries. The Purkinje cells of the cerebellum and the pyramidal neurons of Sommer's sector in the hippocampus are particularly sensitive to hypoxic episodes. Atherosclerosis, which predisposes to vascular thrombi and emboli, is related to regional ischemia. Hypertension damages parenchymal arteries and arterioles, producing small ischemic lesions (lacunar infarcts). Fat emboli, related to trauma of long bones, lodge in small capillaries to form petechiae. Venous sinus thrombosis is related to systemic dehydration, phlebitis, and sickle cell disease.

415. The answer is d. (*Cotran, 5/e, pp 1311–1314. Rubin, 2/e, pp 1393–1399.*) Hypertension results in the deposition of lipid and hyaline material in the walls of cerebral arterioles, which is called lipohyalinosis. This weakens the wall and forms small Charcot-Bouchard aneurysms, which may eventually rupture. Berry aneurysms (small saccular aneurysms) are the result of congenital defects of the media of blood vessels and are located at the bifurcation of arteries. Atherosclerotic aneurysms are fusiform (spindle-shaped) aneurysms, usually located in the major cerebral vessels. They rarely rupture, but may become thrombosed. Mycotic (septic) aneurysms result from septic emboli, most commonly from subacute bacterial endocarditis.

416. The answer is d. (*Cotran, 5/e, pp 1317–1318, 1320, 1322–1323.*) Neurosyphilis, a tertiary stage of syphilis, includes syphilitic meningitis, paretic neurosyphilis, and tabes dorsalis. Syphilitic meningitis is characterized by perivascular infiltrates of lymphocytes and plasma cells that cause obliterative endarteritis and meningeal fibrosis. Tabes dorsalis is the result of degeneration of the posterior columns of the spinal cord. This is caused by compression atrophy of the posterior spinal sensory nerves, which produces impaired joint position sensation, ataxia, loss of pain sensation (leading to joint damage, Charcot joints), and Argyll Robertson pupils (pupils that react to accommodation but not to light). Rabies, caused by a single-stranded RNA rhabdovirus, is transmitted by the bite of a rabid animal, usually a dog. The virus is transmitted through peripheral nerves to the brain, where it forms characteristic inclusions within neurons (Negri bodies). Symptoms related to destruction of neurons in the brainstem include irritability, difficulty in swallowing and spasms of the throat (these two resulting in "hydrophobia"), seizures, and delirium. The illness is almost uniformly fatal. Poliomyelitis is caused by an enterovirus that produces a nonspecific gastroenteritis and then secondarily invades the anterior horn motor neurons of the spinal cord, where it causes muscular paralysis. Progressive multifocal leukoencephalopathy (PML) is a viral infection of oligodendrocytes that causes demyelination and symptoms of dementia and ataxia. The causative agents of

PML are two closely related papovaviruses, JC virus and SV40. The pathognomonic feature of PML is oligodendrocytes in areas of demyelination with a "ground-glass" appearance of their nuclei. PML typically occurs as a terminal complication in immunosuppressed patients.

417. The answer is c. (*Cotran, 5/e, p 1279. Rubin, 2/e, p 1425.*) Guillain-Barré (GB) syndrome (acute inflammatory polyradiculoneuropathy) is similar to postinfectious (or postvaccinal) encephalomyelitis in that both cause a process of demyelination and show perivascular infiltrates of lymphoid cells (in the brain and brainstem in encephalomyelitis and in the craniospinal nerve, roots, and ganglia in GB syndrome). In addition, the anterior horn cells in GB syndrome may be degenerative. GB syndrome manifests clinically as lower limb weakness and paralysis with varying sensory disturbances, such as hypesthesia of the lower limbs. The disease is characterized by an ascending paralysis, which may progress to involvement of the musculature of the upper body, including the muscles of respiration, which in turn can lead to respiratory arrest in the absence of mechanical ventilatory assistance. GB syndrome was identified in some persons who were vaccinated with influenza vaccines during the late 1970s.

418. The answer is e. (*Henry, 19/e, pp 463–464. Cotran, 5/e, p 1326.*) Elevations in cerebrospinal fluid globulins often occur in multiple sclerosis (MS) and other demyelinating diseases. Most patients with MS have oligoclonal bands, which are the result of B-cell proliferation in the central nervous system. Late tertiary syphilis may cause these findings, but they would not occur in the secondary stage. Tumor or meningeal leukemia can also produce elevated levels of globulin in cerebrospinal fluid, but the presence of tumor cells and absence of an electrophoretic band would lead to the proper diagnosis.

419. The answer is b. (*Cotran, 5/e, pp 1279, 1336–1338.*) Amyotrophic lateral sclerosis (ALS), Lou Gehrig disease, is a degenerative disorder of motor neurons, principally the anterior horn cells of the spinal cord, the motor nuclei of the brain stem, and the upper motor neurons of the cerebral cortex. Clinically, this disease is a combination of lower motor neuron (LMN) disease with weakness and fasciculations and upper motor neuron (UMN) disease with spasticity and hyperreflexia. Early symptoms include weakness and cramping, then muscle atrophy and fasciculations. Reflexes are hyperactive in upper and lower extremities, and a positive extensor plantar (Babinski) reflex develops because of the loss of upper motor neurons. The triad of atrophic weakness of hands and forearms, slight spasticity of the legs, and generalized hyperreflexia—in the absence of sensory changes—suggests the diagnosis. The clinical course is rapid, and death may result from respiratory complications. There is no effective treatment for ALS. Theories about the etiology of ALS include viral infections, immunologic causes, or oxidative stress. The latter is related to defect in zinc-copper binding superoxide dismutase (SOD) on chromosome 21. Decreased SOD activity leads to apoptosis of spinal motor neurons.

Metachromatic leukodystrophy is an autosomal recessive disorder of sphingomyelin metabolism that results from deficiency of cerebroside sulfatase (aryl-sulfatase A). Sulfatides accumulate in lysosomes and stain metachromatically with cresyl violet. Diagnostic measures include amniocentesis, enzyme analysis, and measuring decreased urinary aryl-sulfatase A. Demyelination is widespread in the cerebrum and peripheral nervous system. Acute inflammatory demyelinating polyradiculoneuropathy (Guillain-Barré syndrome) is a life-threatening disease of the peripheral nervous system. The disease usually follows recovery from an influenza-like upper respiratory tract infection and is characterized by a motor neuropathy that leads to an ascending paralysis which begins with weakness in the distal extremities and rapidly involves proximal muscles. Sensory changes are usually minimal. The disease is thought to result from immune-mediated segmental demyelination. Huntington's disease is characterized by choreiform movements and progressive dementia that appear after the age of 30. Wilson's disease (hepatolenticular degeneration) is an autosomal recessive disorder of copper metabolism in which the total circulating copper is decreased, but the free copper is increased. This leads to athetoid movements, cirrhosis of the liver, and copper deposits in the limbus of the cornea that produce the Kayser-Fleischer ring.

420. The answer is a. (*Cotran, 5/e, p 1334.*) Huntington's disease, an autosomal dominant disorder that results from an abnormal gene on chromosome 4, involves the extrapyramidal system and atrophy of the caudate nuclei and putamen. Choreiform movements and progressive dementia appear after the age of 30. There is degeneration of GABA neurons in the striatum, which leads to decreased function (decreased inhibition) and increased movement. Huntington's disease is one of four diseases that are characterized by long repeating sequences of three nucleotides (the other diseases being fragile X syndrome, myotonic dystrophy, and spinal and bulbar muscular atrophy). Therapy for excessive movement (hyperkinetic) disorders can be attempted with dopamine antagonists. Decreased dopamine in the striatum theoretically will cause a relative increase in acetylcholine and an increase in excitation in the striatum. This will cause increased GABA function, which leads to increased inhibition of movement. The same result could theoretically be achieved with inhibition of acetylcholine breakdown (cholinesterase inhibitors). Compare this to the same treatment of hypokinetic (Parkinson) disorders. Dopamine agonists will increase the inhibition in the striatum, which will lead to decreased GABA in the striatum and decreased inhibition of movement (increased movement). The same result could theoretically be achieved with anticholinergics.

421. The answer is d. (*Cotran, 5/e, pp 1342–1349.*) The features listed in the question are characteristic of a glioblastoma multiforme. Schwannomas generally appear as extremely cellular, spindle cell neoplasms, sometimes with metaplastic elements of bone, cartilage, and skeletal muscle. Medulloblastomas occur exclusively in the cerebellum and microscopically are highly cellular with uniform nuclei, scant cytoplasm, and, in about one-third of cases, rosette formation centered by neurofibrillary material. Oligodendrogliomas, which are marked by foci of calcification in 70 percent of cases, commonly show a pattern of uniform cellularity and are composed of round cells with small dark nuclei, clear cytoplasm, and a clearly defined cell membrane. Ependymomas are distinguished by ependymal rosettes, which are ductlike structures with a central lumen around which columnar tumor cells are arranged in a concentric fashion.

422. The answer is d. (*Cotran, 5/e, pp 1342–1349. Silverberg, 2/e, pp 2093–2102.*) Gliomas are the most frequent intracranial tumors of adults; they constitute 40 to 50 percent of such tumors, with glioblastoma multiforme making up 25 to 30 percent. Gliomas at the opposite end of the spectrum include ependymoma and oligodendroglioma, each constituting only 2 to 3 percent. Medulloblastoma also forms 2 to 3 percent of intracranial tumors in adults. Astrocytomas have an 8 to 12 percent and meningiomas a 12 to 15 percent intracranial incidence. Metastatic tumors have an intracranial incidence of 25 to 30 percent; metastatic carcinoma (lung, breast, kidney, GI) and melanoma are predominant. Metastases are often multiple and demarcated from surrounding brain tissue.

423. The answer is d. *(Cotran, 5/e, pp 605–608, 1339–1340.)* Chronic deficiency of cobalamin (vitamin B12) has two major effects: a macrocytic megaloblastic anemia and a spinal cord degeneration, which may precede the anemia by months. The posterior columns and lateral corticospinal tracts undergo myelin degeneration, but the gray matter is rarely affected. Motor weakness with spasticity is the characteristic result, preceded by persistent paresthesias of the feet and hands. SCD is due to failure of the cobalamin-dependent enzyme methylmalonic CoA mutase, which is essential for maintenance of myelinated fibers. The classic triad of dermatitis, diarrhea, and dementia occurs in pellagra, which is due to niacin/nicotinic acid (vitamin B5) deficiency.

424. The answer is e. *(Cotran, 5/e, pp 1300–1304.)* Neural tube developmental defects are caused by defective closure of the neural tube. These defects, which may occur anywhere along the extent of the neural tube, are associated with maternal obesity and decreased folate during pregnancy. Neural tube defects are associated with increased maternal serum levels of alpha fetoprotein (AFP), which is a glycoprotein synthesized by the yolk sac and the fetal liver. Increased serum levels are also associated with yolk sac tumors of the testes and liver cell carcinomas. Neural tube defects are classified based on their location into caudal or cranial defects. Failure of development of the cranial end of the neural tube results in anencephaly. This abnormality, which is not compatible with life, is characterized by the absence of the forebrain. Instead there is a mass of vascularized neural tissue in this area, which is called the cerebrovasculosa.

Spina bifida is a general term that refers to abnormal fusion of the vertebral arches of the lowest vertebral arches, usually the sacrolumbar region. There are several disorders in this group of developmental abnormalities that have varying degrees of severity. Spina bifida occulta is the mildest form and is characterized by failure of vertebral fusion only. The spinal cord and meninges are normal. In spina bifida occulta the defect in the closure of the neural tube is covered by skin and dermis, with only a pinpoint sinus or hair-covered depression marking the site. Bacterial meningitis, or meningomyelitis, is the major potential risk in these patients.

The remaining types of spina bifida are classified as spina bifida cystica. Spina bifida with a meningocele is characterized by protrusion of a meningeal sac filled with cerebrospinal fluid (CSF) through the vertebral defect. Because the cord is in its normal location, there are minimal neurologic deficits. Next in severity is spina bifida with a myelomeningocele, which is characterized by herniation of the cord and a meningeal sac through the vertebral defect. This abnormality is often associated with severe neurologic defects in the lower extremities, bladder, and rectum. The most severe form of spina bifida, spina bifida aperta or myeloschisis, results from complete failure of fusion of the caudal end of the neural plate, which lies open on the skin surface. This abnormality also results in severe neurologic defects in the legs, bladder, and rectum.

Cranium bifidum refers to ossification defects of the occipital bone. The abnormalities produced by these defects are somewhat analogous to spina bifida. There may be protrusion of meninges (cranial meningocele), meninges and brain (meningoencephalocele), or meninges, brain, and ventricles (meningohydroencephalocele). Meningoencephalocystocele (a herniation at the roof of the mouth) together with cranial meningocele and cranial meningoencephalocele, occurs less frequently than the herniations associated with spina bifida. Cerebral palsy refers to any nonheritable, nonprogressive neurologic motor deficit with onset during the perinatal period, regardless of the etiology. Two examples of cerebral palsy are spastic diplegia and infantile hemiplegia. Spastic diplegia is characterized by spastic weakness of all four extremities, while infantile hemiplegia, usually resulting from unilateral infection or thrombosis of cerebral vessels, is associated with mild mental retardation and convulsions.

425. The answer is e. (*Fawcett, 12/e, pp 354–357. Cotran, 5/e, pp 1296–1298.*) The neuroglial cells—astrocytes, oligodendrocytes, ependymal cells, and microglial cells—provide supportive and protective functions for neurons. However, only microglial cells are phagocytic and, in response to injury or destruction of the brain, become activated as macrophages (gitter cells, compound granular corpuscles). Astrocytes support neurons and react to CNS injury by formation of glial scars (gliosis). Oligodendrocytes produce and maintain CNS myelin, and diseases affecting them include multiple sclerosis and the leukodystrophies. The lining ependymal cells do not produce or absorb cerebrospinal fluid. Cell processes of astrocytes, or "glial" fibers, contain vimentin and glial fibrillary acidic protein (GFAP).

426. The answer is d. (*Cotran, 5/e, pp 1298–1300. Rubin, 2/e, p 1439.*) The clinical constellation of altered sensorium and papilledema should call to mind the presence of intracranial pressure, regardless of the cause, which can be due to cerebral edema, tumor mass, or, more commonly, intracranial bleeding with hematoma formation. If the pressure is severe enough, downward displacement of the cerebellar tonsils into the foramen magnum may occur, producing further compression on the brainstem with consequent hemorrhage into the pons and midbrain (Duret hemorrhages). This is nearly always associated with death, since the vital centers, including respiratory control, are located in these regions. Subdural as well as epidural hemorrhages are sufficient to cause critical downward displacement of the cerebellar tonsils. The situation can be remedied with appropriate neurosurgical intervention. In this situation, the downward displacement could be due to hemorrhage-hematoma formation into the posterior intracranial fossa, caused by either a direct (coup) or an indirect (contrecoup) blow to the occiput.

427. The answer is c. (*Cotran, 5/e, pp 111–112, 1309–1310. Rubin, 2/e, pp 539–540.*) Cerebral embolism is probably the most common cause of stroke and most cerebral emboli arise in the heart. Myocardial infarction with mural thrombi, atrial fibrillation thrombi, and left-sided bacterial endocarditis are frequent sources, but in right-sided bacterial endocarditis (drug addicts, patients with gonococcal endocarditis or ventricular septal defect) emboli to organs other than the lungs are very rare, except in paradoxical embolism of septal defect. Endocarditis must be excluded when cerebral embolism is suspected. Thromboembolism from prosthetic heart valves has not been unusual. Cardiac catheterization and other invasive procedures involving an atherosclerotic aorta or femoral or iliac arteries may cause atheroemboli (cholesterol emboli) with resultant small infarcts of brain, kidney, gut, skin, or other organs. At least 35 to 40 percent of all strokes are embolic, and emboli are the predominant cause of infarction in the area supplied by the middle cerebral artery.

428. The answer is d. (*Damjanov, 10/e, pp 2715–2718.*) Pyogenic brain abscesses may have a number of possible sources, but the origin can often be determined from the location and number of abscesses in the brain parenchyma. Isolated lesions in the frontal lobes often arise from extension of sinus infections. In the temporal lobe or cerebellum, an isolated lesion may have the middle ear or mastoid as the primary site. Multiple lesions, especially in the superior aspects of the cerebrum, are seen with hematogenous dissemination, often from lung infection or in association with the lesions of congenital heart disease.

429. The answer is b. (*Cotran, 5/e, pp 225–227. Rubin, 2/e, pp 1419–1420.*) The nervous system is frequently affected in patients with AIDS. Opportunistic infections, such as toxoplasmosis, CMV, and PML, are increased in incidence, but in most patients the encephalopathy is the result of direct action of the virus itself. HIV-1 preferentially infects macrophages and microglial cells in the CNS, resulting in multinucleated giant cells, microglial nodules, and secondary loss of neurons and areas of demyelination. About one-third of patients have a vacuolar myelopathy marked by vacuolation of the posterior and lateral columns of the spinal cord, which is similar to the changes produced by decreased vitamin B12. This abnormality causes ataxia and spastic paraparesis.

430. The answer is c. (*Cotran, 5/e, pp 1323–1324.*) In Creutzfeldt-Jakob disease there is a spongiform change in the cortical gray matter and, sometimes, the basal ganglia are affected. There is little, or no, gross atrophy of the brain and no inflammatory response in brain tissue. The disease is similar to kuru in humans and scrapie in sheep and goats. Rapidly progressive dementia occurs. Worldwide incidence is about one case per million population. The disease is caused by transmissible agents, or prions, which are proteinaceous infective particles, resistant to formalin and ionizing radiation, but inactivated by autoclaving, hypochlorite solutions (bleach), and alcoholic iodine.

431. The answer is a. (*Adams, 5/e, pp 656–657. Cotran, 5/e, pp 865–866, 1322–1324.*) Subacute sclerosing panencephalitis (SSPE) is caused by the measles virus following infection early in life. There is a long latent period, protracted course, and high mortality. Histopathologic and electron-microscopic changes include perivascular mononuclear cell infiltrates, extensive neuronal loss, and intranuclear inclusions containing paramyxovirus particles in oligodendrocytes and neurons. The CSF contains oligoclonal immunoglobulins against viral components.

Progressive multifocal leukoencephalopathy (PML) is a viral infection of myelin-producing oligodendrocytes and causes primary demyelination. Oligodendroglial nuclei are enlarged and contain inclusion bodies, and bizarre giant astrocytes and foamy macrophages with myelin debris are seen in lesions. Electron microscopy reveals papovavirus particles in oligodendrocyte nuclei. Reye's syndrome occurs within 3 to 5 days of viral infection (influenza, chickenpox) treated with aspirin and is associated with severe or fatal brain edema. Creutzfeldt-Jakob disease, a spongiform encephalopathy, and kuru are probably transmitted by unconventional agents, or prions, that do not appear to be conventional viruses.

432. The answer is d. (*Cotran, 5/e, pp 1329–1331.*) Alzheimer's disease (AD) is characterized by numerous neurofibrillary tangles and senile plaques with a central core of amyloid β-protein. Both tangles and plaques are found to a lesser extent in other conditions, e.g., neurofibrillary tangles in Down's syndrome. Silver stains demonstrate tangles and plaques and Congo red shows amyloid deposition in plaques and vascular walls (amyloid angiopathy). In AD there are also numerous Hirano bodies, and granulovacuolar degeneration is found in more than 10 percent of the neurons of the hippocampus. AD often begins insidiously with impairment of memory and progresses to dementia. Grossly, brain atrophy (narrowed gyri and widened sulci) is predominant in frontal and superior temporal lobes. Lewy bodies are found in idiopathic parkinsonism and in diffuse Lewy body disease.

433. The answer is b. (*Cotran, 5/e, pp 1345–1346. Rubin, 2/e, pp 1438, 1441–1442.*) Ependymomas often occur in childhood and adolescence but have been noted at all ages. They form more than 60 percent of intraspinal gliomas, but only about 5 percent of intracranial gliomas. They are most commonly found in the fourth ventricle, not the lateral ventricles, which have a larger ependymal surface. Hydrocephalus can be a complication of intraventricular ependymoma. The papillary intraventricular ependymoma is similar grossly to the choroid plexus papilloma. Microscopically, the diagnostic rosette and pseudorosette formations are seen in the ependymoma, with tumor cells arranged around a central space (rosette) or around a blood vessel (pseudorosette). Blepharoplasts, the basal bodies of cilia, are pathognomonic if present.

434. The answer is c. (*Cotran, 5/e, p 1349. Rubin, 2/e, pp 1442–1443.*) Meningiomas arise from arachnoid villi of brain or spinal cord and have a female:male ratio of 3:2. Although they are usually tumors of middle or later life, a small number occur in persons 20 to 40 years of age. They commonly arise along the venous sinuses (parasagittal, sphenoid wings, and olfactory groove). Although benign and usually slow-growing, some meningiomas have progesterone receptors and rapid growth in pregnancy occurs occasionally. The rare malignant meningioma may invade or even metastasize. The typical case, however, does not invade the brain, but displaces it, causing headaches and seizures. Histologically, syncytial, transitional, and fibroblastic forms occur; psammoma bodies are found, particularly in the transitional pattern. The cut surface often has a whorled appearance. Meningioma is usually solitary, but multiple meningiomas occur, especially in neurofibromatosis type 2. Orbital meningiomas (female:male ratio of 5:1) may cause unilateral exophthalmos and often occur in patients under 20 years of age.

435. The answer is a. (*Cotran, 5/e, pp 1120–1121, 1147–1148, 1342–1345, 1354.*) Glioblastoma multiforme is a rapidly growing cerebral tumor in which calcification does not develop, but in which necrosis and hemorrhage are frequent. Both oligodendroglioma and craniopharyngioma show fairly frequent calcification; oligodendroglioma is often located in the frontal lobe, whereas craniopharyngioma occurs in the third ventricle. CT scan and particularly MRI are essential in diagnosis. Patchy intracerebral calcification may develop in tuberous sclerosis, an autosomal dominant disease characterized by the triad of epilepsy, mental retardation, and facial skin lesions (multiple angiofibromas). In addition, subependymal gliosis, cardiac rhabdomyoma, renal angiomyolipoma, and periungual fibroma occur. Calcification of the basal ganglia occurs in about 20 percent of patients with chronic hypoparathyroidism, which sometimes leads to a parkinsonian syndrome.

436. The answer is c. (*Cotran, 5/e, pp 148–149, 1354. Rubin, 2/e, pp 228–230.*) In von Hippel-Lindau disease, a rare autosomal dominant disorder, multiple benign and malignant neoplasms occur. These include hemangioblastomas of retina and brain (cerebellum and medulla oblongata), angiomas of kidney and liver, and renal cell carcinoma in 25 to 50 percent of cases. Classic neurofibromatosis (NF-1) is characterized by café-au-lait skin macules, axillary freckling, multiple neurofibromas, plexiform neurofibromas, and Lisch nodules (pigmented iris hamartomas). Lisch nodules are found in 95 percent of patients after age 6. Hamartomas of the iris are not present in central or acoustic neurofibromatosis (NF-2), though both types of neurofibromatosis have café-au-lait macules and neurofibromas. Only the central, or acoustic, form has bilateral acoustic neuromas; the classic form may have unilateral acoustic neuroma. There is increased risk of developing meningiomas or even pheochromocytoma. A major complication of NF-1 is the malignant transformation of a neurofibroma to a neurofibrosarcoma. The gene for the classic form (NF-1) is located on chromosome 17. It encodes for a protein, neurofibromin, which regulates the function of p21 ras oncoprotein.

437. The answer is d. (*Cotran, 5/e, pp 1277–1278.*) The axonal reaction that occurs when a peripheral nerve is cut includes a number of striking changes. In the cell body, swelling and dissolution of the Nissl substance are apparent within 24 to 48 h after transection. The axon and covering myelin or Schwann sheath distal to the lesion first degenerate and undergo resorption. In addition, the axis cylinder and Schwann sheath degenerate proximal to the cut over the distance of a few nodal segments. Regeneration occurs when the Schwann cells proliferate from the proximal portion to form a hollow myelin sheath through which the axons grow again.

438. The answer is b. (*Cotran, 5/e, p 1303. Rubin, 2/e, p 1382.*) Syringomyelia is a chronic myelopathy. There is cavitation involving the central gray matter of the spinal cord where pain fibers cross to join the contralateral spinothalamic tract. Interruption of the lateral spinothalamic tracts results in segmental sensory dissociation, with loss of pain and temperature sense, but preservation of the sense of touch and pressure, or vibration, usually over the neck, shoulders, and arms. Characteristic features also include wasting of the small intrinsic hand muscles (clawhand) and thoracic scoliosis. The cause of syringomyelia is unknown, although one type is associated with a Chiari malformation with obstruction at the foramen magnum.

439. The answer is e. (*Cotran, 5/e, pp 1168–1169. Rubin, 2/e, pp 1146–1147.*) Primary tumors of the pineal gland are very uncommon but are of interest, especially in view of the mysterious and relatively unknown functions of the pineal gland itself. The gland secretes neurotransmitter substances such as serotonin and dopamine, with the major product being melatonin. Tumors of the pineal gland include germ cell tumors of all types including embryonal carcinoma, choriocarcinoma, teratoma, and various combinations of germinomas. Germ cell tumors may arise extragonadal within the retroperitoneal space and the pineal gland, with the only commonality being that these structures are in the midline. Primary tumors of the pineal gland occur in two forms: the pineoblastoma and the pineocytoma. Pineoblastomas occur in young patients and consist of small tumors having areas of hemorrhage and necrosis with pleomorphic nuclei and frequent mitoses. Pineocytomas occur in older adults and are slow-growing; they are better differentiated and have large rosettes. Craniopharyngiomas occur not in the pineal gland but above the pituitary gland in the hypothalamus and are thought to arise from structures related to Rathke's pouch.

440–441. The answers are: 440-e,441-g. *(Cotran, 5/e, pp 1343–1345, 1347. Rubin, 2/e, pp 1440–1441.)* Astrocytomas are not at all uncommon in the younger age group, but when a child presents with clinical symptoms pointing to the intracranial posterior fossa, a cerebellar medulloblastoma should be suspected, especially if the child has no prior history of leukemia or neuroblastoma. Medulloblastomas occur predominantly in childhood and usually arise in the midline of the cerebellum (the vermis). They do occur (less commonly) in adults, in whom they are more apt to arise in the cerebellar hemispheres in a lateral position. They grow by local invasive growth and may block cerebrospinal fluid circulation (CSF block) by compression of the fourth ventricle. Recent aggressive treatment with the combined modalities of excision, radiotherapy, and chemotherapy have improved survival.

Although several lesions within the brain may be associated with dystrophic or metaplastic calcification, the presence of a calcified tumorlike mass lesion in the cerebral hemispheres should arouse suspicion of oligodendroglioma. Oligodendrogliomas are often slowly growing gliomas composed of round cells with clear cytoplasm ("fried-egg" appearance); they generally occur in the fourth and fifth decades of life. However, some oligodendrogliomas do proliferate in a rapid and aggressive fashion and may be associated with a malignant astrocytoma component. The brown tumor associated with hypercalcemia of hyperparathyroidism is associated with osteitis fibrosa cystica of bone. Some metastatic carcinomas may show microcalcifications in the form of psammoma bodies, as do some meningiomas. Papillary carcinomas of the thyroid and ovary are the best examples of such lesions, but the calcifications found in papillary carcinomas are rarely of the degree and magnitude of those found in some oligodendrogliomas.

442–443. The answers are: 442-i, 443-e. (Cotran, 5/e, pp 1332–1334, 1351–1352.) The degenerative diseases of the CNS are diseases that affect the gray matter and are characterized by the progressive loss of neurons in specific areas of the brain. In Parkinson's disease, characterized by mask-like facial expression, coarse tremors, slowness of voluntary movements, and muscular rigidity, there is degeneration and loss of pigmented cells in the substantia nigra, resulting in a decrease in dopamine synthesis. Lewy bodies (eosinophilic intracytoplasmic inclusions) are found in the remaining neurons of the substantia nigra. The decreased synthesis of dopamine by neurons originating in the substantia nigra leads to decreased amounts and functioning of dopamine in the striatum. This results in decreased dopamine inhibition and a relative increase in acetylcholine function, which is excitatory in the striatum. This excitation, however, is to increase the functioning of GABA neurons, which are inhibitory. The final effect, therefore, is increased inhibition or decreased movement. The severity of the motor syndrome correlates with the degree of dopamine deficiency. Therapy may be with dopamine agonists or anticholinergics. Similar degenerative changes that are seen with idiopathic Parkinson disease can be seen in other disorders. Von Economo's encephalitis was a transient infectious disorder that occurred from 1915–1918 concurrent with influenza pandemic, and was associated with a postencephalitic parkinsonism. Shy-Drager syndrome is associated with Parkinson-like signs along with autonomic dysfunction, postural (orthostatic) hypotension, and urinary incontinence. Other causes of Parkinson disease include trauma (especially boxers), certain drugs and toxins (MPTP, a meperidine analog found in illicit drugs), and copper (Wilson disease).

Schwannomas (neurilemomas) are single, encapsulated tumors of nerve sheaths, usually benign, occurring on peripheral, spinal, or cranial nerves. The acoustic neuroma is an example of a schwannoma that arises from the vestibulocochlear nerve (CN VIII). These tumors are typically located at the cerebellopontine angle or in the internal acoustic meatus. Initially when they are small, these tumors produce symptoms by compressing CN VIII and CN VII (facial). CN VIII symptoms include unilateral tinnitus (ringing in the ear), unilateral hearing loss, and vertigo (dizziness). Involvement of the facial nerve produces facial weakness and loss of corneal reflex. Histologically an acoustic neuroma consists of cellular areas (Antoni A) and loose edematous areas (Antoni B). Verocay bodies (foci of palisaded nuclei) may be found in the more cellular areas.

MUSCULOSKELETAL SYSTEM

Questions

DIRECTIONS: Each question below contains five suggested responses. Select the **one best** response to each question.

444. Characteristics of normal striated muscle include

a. Hypercontraction bands
b. Central location of majority of nuclei
c. Angulated fibers
d. Ring fibers
e. "Checkerboard" ATPase staining pattern

445. A pathognomonic feature of denervation followed by reinnervation is the histologic finding of

a. Atrophic fibers
b. Angular fibers
c. Type-specific grouping of fibers
d. Eosinophilic infiltrates
e. Lymphohistiocytic infiltrates

446. A 5-year-old boy presents with clumsiness, a waddling gait, and difficulty climbing steps. Physical examination reveals that this boy uses his arms and shoulder muscles to rise from the floor or the chair. Additionally, his calves appear to be somewhat larger than normal. This boy's physical findings are most consistent with a diagnosis of

a. Inclusion body myositis
b. Werdnig-Hoffman disease
c. Dermatomyositis
d. Duchenne's muscular dystrophy
e. Myotonic dystrophy

447. A 59-year-old woman presents with difficulty swallowing, ptosis, and diplopia. Which of the following is most consistent with these symptoms?

a. Antibodies to the acetylcholine receptor
b. Antibodies to the microvasculature of skeletal muscle
c. Lack of lactate production during ischemic exercise
d. Rhabdomyolysis
e. Corticosteroid therapy

448. Osteogenesis imperfecta type I is characterized by

a. A hereditary defect in osteoclastic function
b. Defective synthesis of type II collagen
c. Defective synthesis of osteoid matrix
d. Early death
e. Bone marrow aplasia

449. A 71-year-old female presents with the sudden onset of severe lower back pain. Physical examination reveals severe kyphosis, while an X-ray of her back reveals a compression fracture of a vertebral body in the lumbar area along with marked thinning of the bones. Serum calcium, phosphorus, alkaline phosphatase, and parathyroid hormone levels are all within normal limits. Her bone changes are most likely due to

a. Osteopetrosis
b. Osteoporosis
c. Osteomalacia
d. Osteitis fibrosa cystica
e. Osteitis deformans

450. Osteomalacia may best be characterized as

a. Failure of bone remodeling
b. Failure of bone mineralization
c. Failure of osteoid formation
d. Reactive bone formation
e. Reduction in amount of normally mineralized bone

451. A section of bone shows prominent osteoid seams, very large osteoclasts with more than 12 hyperchromatic nuclei, and viral-type inclusion particles. This is most characteristic of

a. Paget's disease
b. Gaucher's disease
c. Fibrous dysplasia
d. Giant cell tumors of bone
e. Brown tumor of bone

452. Features of the normal process of fracture healing include

a. Pseudoarthrosis
b. A sequestrum
c. An involucrum
d. A cloaca
e. A cartilaginous callus

453. The part of a long bone initially involved in hematogenous osteomyelitis is the

a. Metaphyseal region
b. Diaphysis
c. Epiphysis
d. Area around the entrance of the nutrient artery
e. Medullary cavity

454. Bilateral segmental osteonecrosis or avascular necrosis (AVN) of the femoral head is most often associated with

a. Systemic steroid therapy
b. Irradiation therapy
c. Sickle cell disease
d. Alcoholism
e. Fracture of the femoral neck

455. The most common tumor that involves bone is

a. A metastatic tumor from an extraosseous site
b. Osteogenic sarcoma
c. Multiple myeloma
d. Chondrosarcoma
e. A giant cell tumor

456. Which of the following fibroosseous bone disorders is most likely to be associated with skin lesions?

a. Osteoid osteoma
b. Albright's syndrome
c. Nonossifying fibroma
d. Polyostotic fibrous dysplasia
e. Monostotic fibrous dysplasia

457. The lesion illustrated in the photomicrograph below is most likely

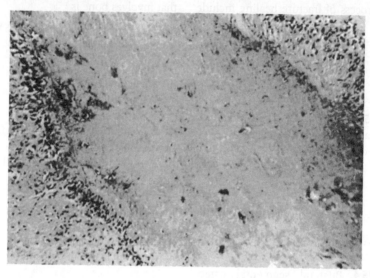

a. A rheumatoid nodule
b. Myositis ossificans
c. Necrotizing panniculitis
d. Polymyositis
e. Fat necrosis

458. A 54-year-old man presents with chronic knee pain. Resection of the patella reveals chalky white deposits on the surface of intraarticular structures. Histologic sections reveal long, needle-shaped, negatively birefringent crystals. The photomicrograph below was taken under polarized light. These findings are most consistent with a diagnosis of

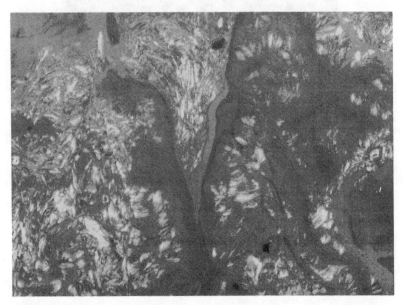

a. Osteoarthritis
b. Rheumatoid arthritis
c. Ochronosis
d. Gout
e. Pseudogout

459. A perivascular inflammatory infiltrate in skeletal muscle, as shown in the photomicrograph below, is likely to be seen in all the following EXCEPT

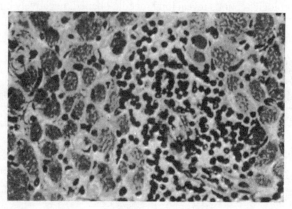

a. Hypersensitivity angiitis
b. Polymyositis
c. Polyarteritis nodosa
d. Cystic medial necrosis
e. Systemic sclerosis

460. The atypical rhabdomyoblasts illustrated in the photomicrograph below may be seen in all the following lesions EXCEPT

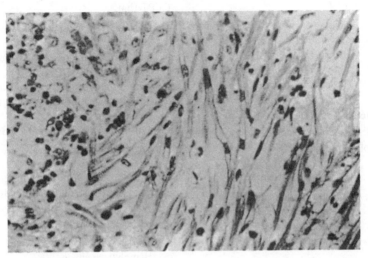

a. Sarcoma botryoides
b. Myositis ossificans
c. Mixed heterologous müllerian tumor of the uterus
d. Adult pleomorphic rhabdomyosarcoma
e. Embryonal rhabdomyosarcoma

461. Characteristics or components of normal bone in the adult skeleton include all the following EXCEPT

a. Osteoblasts
b. Osteoid
c. Type I collagen
d. Lamellar bone
e. Woven bone

462. Diseases affecting the epiphyseal plate include all the following EXCEPT

a. Cretinism
b. Achondroplasia
c. Osteopetrosis
d. Scurvy
e. Hurler's syndrome

463. Tuberculous spondylitis (Pott's disease) is characterized by all the following EXCEPT

a. Involvement of thoracic and lumbar vertebrae
b. Hematogenous spread
c. Proliferative synovitis with pannus
d. Destruction of intervertebral disks
e. Formation of psoas abscess

464. Osteosarcoma (osteogenic sarcoma) has an increased incidence in all the following conditions EXCEPT

a. Paget's disease
b. Retinoblastoma
c. Fibrous dysplasia
d. Plasmacytoma
e. Osteochondromatosis

465. All the following statements about chondrosarcoma are true EXCEPT that

a. It is most frequent in middle age or later
b. The peripheral type can arise from enchondroma
c. It is common in the pelvic bones
d. Histologic analysis is of prognostic significance
e. It is the second most common malignant bone tumor

466. Secondary gout may be seen in association with all the following EXCEPT

a. Polycythemia
b. Psoriasis
c. Hemolytic anemias
d. Myeloproliferative diseases
e. Chondrocalcinosis

DIRECTIONS: The group of questions below consists of lettered headings followed by a set of numbered items. For each numbered item select the **one** lettered heading with which it is **most** closely associated. Each lettered heading may be used **once, more than once, or not at all**.

Questions 467–468

For each bone lesion, select the lettered location and general configuration with which it is most likely to be associated in the diagram.

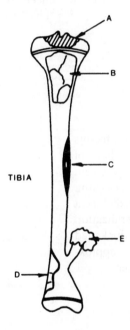

TIBIA

467. Giant cell tumor of bone (osteoclastoma)

468. Osteochondroma

Questions 469–470

Match each of the following clinical scenarios with the correct diagnosis from the following list.

a. Chondroblastoma
b. Chondroma
c. Chondromyxoid fibroma
d. Chondrosarcoma
e. Ewing's sarcoma
f. Fibrosarcoma
g. Fibrous dysplasia
h. Nonossifying fibroma
i. Osteoblastoma
j. Osteogenic sarcoma
k. Osteoid osteoma
l. Osteoma

469. A 17-year-old male presents with nocturnal pain in the bone of his left leg. He relates that the pain is quickly relieved by taking aspirin. X-rays reveal a round, radiolucent area with central mineralization that is surrounded by thickened bone. The lesion measures approximately 1.2 cm in diameter.

470. An 11-year-old boy presents with an enlarging, painful lesion that involves the medullary cavity of his left femur. X-rays reveal an irregular, destructive lesion that produces an "onion-skin" periosteal reaction. The lesion is resected surgically, and histologic sections reveal sheets of uniform small, round, "blue" cells.

MUSCULOSKELETAL SYSTEM

Answers

444. The answer is e. (*Cotran, 5/e, pp 1275–1277. Rubin, 2/e, pp 1350–1352.*) Two functional types of muscle fibers are determined by the lower motor neuron innervating the muscle fiber. "Slow-twitch" (type 1, red) fibers are high in myoglobin (a red pigment), oxidative enzymes, and mitochondria; "fast-switch" (type 2, white) fibers are high in glycolytic enzymes (Embden-Meyerhof pathway), glycogen, and phosphorylase. ATPase stains type 2 fibers darkly and type 1 fibers almost not at all. Since human skeletal muscle is normally composed of a random mixture of both type 1 and type 2 fibers, ATPase staining normally has a "checkerboard" pattern. Atrophic muscle fibers are smaller and have an angulated appearance on cross-section. In normal muscle, less than 5 percent of the fibers have central nuclei. An increase in the percentage of central nuclei is a nonspecific abnormal finding. Hypercontraction bands are particularly frequent in Duchenne's muscular dystrophy. Ring fibers, in which the peripheral myofilament runs abnormally in a circumferential pattern, are particularly characteristic of myotonic dystrophy.

445. The answer is c. (*Cotran, 5/e, pp 1277–1278. Rubin, 2/e, pp 1359–1361, 1365–1368.*) Histologic features of muscle biopsy specimens may suggest certain muscle disorders. Denervation causes atrophy of the fibers, which become angulated. Another change seen in denervated muscle is the presence of distinctive three-zoned fibers called target fibers. Reinnervation is characterized by type-specific grouping of fibers, which is in contrast to the mixed, "checkerboard" pattern of type 1 and type 2 fibers seen in normal skeletal muscle. Variation in size and shape along with degenerative changes and intrafascicular fibrosis are features of muscular dystrophy. Eosinophils within muscle are found in association with parasitic infections, the most common of which is trichinosis. Lymphocytes and macrophages within muscle are seen in polymyositis.

446. The answer is d. (*Cotran, 5/e, pp 213–214, 1285–1288.*) Duchenne muscular dystrophy (DMD) is a noninflammatory inherited myopathy that causes a progressive, severe weakness and degeneration of muscles, particularly the proximal muscles, such as the pelvic and shoulder girdles. The defective gene is located on the X chromosome and codes for dystrophin, a protein found on the inner surface on the sarcolemma. Histologically, the muscle fibers in patients with DMD show variations in size and shape, degenerative and regenerative changes in adjacent myocytes, necrotic fibers invaded by histiocytes, and progressive fibrosis. There are rounded, atrophic muscle fibers mixed with hypertrophied fibers. These muscle changes cause the creatine kinase levels in the serum to be elevated. The weak muscles are replaced by fibrofatty tissue, which results in pseudohypertrophy. In Duchenne's muscular dystrophy, symptoms begin before the age of 4, are progressive and lead to difficulty in walking, and are eventually followed by involvement of respiratory muscles, which causes death from respiratory failure before the age of 20. The classification of the muscular dystrophies is based on the mode of inheritance and clinical features. X-linked inheritance characterizes Duchenne's muscular dystrophy, autosomal dominant inheritance characterizes both myotonic dystrophy and fascioscapulohumeral type, while limb-girdle dystrophy is autosomal recessive. Sustained muscle contractions and rigidity (myotonia) are seen in myotonic dystrophy, the most common form of adult muscular dystrophy.

Dermatomyositis is an autoimmune disease that is one of a group of idiopathic inflammatory myopathies. The inflammatory myopathies are characterized by immune mediated inflammation and injury of skeletal muscle, and include polymyositis, dermatomyositis, and inclusion-body myositis. These diseases are associated with numerous types of autoantibodies, one of which is the anti-Jo-1 antibody. The capillaries are the principle target in patients with dermatomyositis. Damage is by complement-mediated cytotoxic antibodies against the microvasculature of skeletal muscle. In addition to proximal muscle weakness, patients typically develop a lilac discoloration around the eyelids with edema. Patients may also develop erythema over their knuckles (Gottron's sign). Histologically examination of muscles from patients with dermatomyositis reveal perivascular inflammation within the tissue around muscle fascicles This is in contrast to the other types of inflammatory myopathies, where the inflammation is within the muscle fascicles (endomysial inflammation). In particular, inclusion-body myositis is characterized by basophilic granular inclusions around vacuoles ("rimmed" vacuoles).

Werdnig-Hoffman disease is a severe lower motor neuron disease that presents in the neonatal period with severe proximal muscle weakness ("floppy infant").

447. The answer is a. *(Cotran, 5/e, pp 213–214, 1289–1291, 1292. Rubin, 2/e, pp 1359–1361, 1364–1365, 1370.)* Myasthenia gravis is an acquired autoimmune disease with circulating antibodies to the acetylcholine receptors at the myoneural junction. These antibodies cause abnormal muscle fatigability, which typically involves the extraocular muscles and leads to ptosis and diplopia. Other muscles may also be involved, and this may cause many different symptoms, such as problems with swallowing. Two-thirds of patients with myasthenia gravis have thymic abnormalities; the most common is thymic hyperplasia. A minority of patients have a thymoma. Lack of lactate production during ischemic exercise is seen in metabolic diseases of muscle caused by a deficiency of myophosphorylase. Dermatomyositis is an autoimmune disease produced by complement-mediated cytotoxic antibodies against the microvasculature of skeletal muscle. Rhabdomyolysis is destruction of skeletal muscle that releases myoglobin into the blood. This may cause myoglobinuria and acute renal failure. Rhabdomyolysis may follow an influenza infection, heat stroke, or malignant hyperthermia. Corticosteroid therapy may cause muscle weakness and selective type 2 atrophy.

448. The answer is c. *(Cotran, 5/e, pp 1218–1219.)* Osteogenesis imperfecta (OI), or brittle bone disease, constitutes a group of disorders often inherited as autosomal dominant traits and caused by genetic mutations involving the synthesis of type I collagen, which comprises about 90 percent of the osteoid, or bone matrix. Very early perinatal death and multiple fractures occur in OI type II, which is often autosomal recessive. The major variant of OI, type I, is compatible with survival; after the perinatal period fractures occur in addition to other signs of defective collagen synthesis such as thin, translucent, blue sclerae; laxity of joint ligaments; deafness from otosclerosis; and abnormal teeth. A hereditary defect in osteoclastic function with decreased bone resorption and bone overgrowth, which sometimes narrows or obliterates the marrow cavity, is characteristic of osteopetrosis, or marble bone disease.

449. The answer is b. *(Cotran, 5/e, pp 1219–1227. Chandrasoma, 3/e, pp 963–966.)* Osteopenia (reduction in the amount of bone) is seen in

osteoporosis, osteomalacia, and osteitis fibrosa. Osteoporosis is characterized by qualitatively normal bone that is decreased in amount. Histologic
bone sections reveal thin trabeculae that have normal calcification and
normal osteoblasts and osteoclasts. Osteoporosis predisposes patients to
fractures of weight-bearing bones, such as the femur and vertebral bodies.
Patients typically have normal serum levels of calcium, phosphorus, alkaline
phosphatase, and parathyroid hormone. Osteoporosis is classified as being
primary or secondary. Primary osteoporosis, the most common type of
osteoporosis, occurs most often in postmenopausal women and has been
related to decreased estrogen levels. Cigarette smoking is also associated with
an increased incidence of osteoporosis. Clinically significant osteoporosis is
related to the maximum amount of bone a person has (peak bone mass),
which is largely genetically determined. Secondary osteoporosis develops
secondary to many conditions such as corticosteroid administration, hyperthyroidism, and hypogonadism.

Osteopetrosis is a rare inherited disease having abnormal, decreased
functioning osteoclasts. This abnormality results in reduced bone resorption
and abnormally thickened bone. In these patients, multiple fractures are
frequent as the bones are structurally weak and abnormally brittle. Increased
fragility of bones is also present in osteomalacia (caused by abnormal
vitamin D metabolism in adults), and osteitis deformans (Paget's disease).
Osteitis fibrosa cystica (von Recklinghausan's disease of bone) is seen with
severe hyperparathyroidism and is characterized by increased bone cell
activity, peritrabecular fibrosis, and cystic bone lesions.

450. The answer is b. *(Cotran, 5/e, pp 1219–1223, 1225–1227. Rubin, 2/e,
pp 1300–1310.)* Osteomalacia (soft bones) is a disorder of adults characterized by inadequate mineralization of newly formed bone matrix and is most
often associated with abnormalities of vitamin D metabolism (such as dietary deficiency or intestinal malabsorption of vitamin D), hypoparathyroidism, or chronic renal diseases. Rickets is a similar condition that occurs
in children. Defective mineralization results in an increase in the thickness
of the osteoid seams, such as seen in vitamin C deficiency (scurvy), and not
in failure of osteoid formation. Osteopetrosis, marble bone, is a bone mod-
eling abnormality related to hypofunction of the osteoclasts. Osteoporosis
results from a reduction in the mass of bone, which still has the normal ratio
of mineral to matrix. Reactive bone formation occurs in bone or soft tissue
in response to such conditions as tumors, infections, or trauma.

451. The answer is a. (*Cotran, 5/e, pp 143–144, 1223–1227, 1242–1243, 1245.*) Paget's disease, osteitis deformans, is characterized by an uncoupling of osteoblastic and osteoclastic activity and is divided into three phases: an initial osteoclastic (osteolytic) resorptive stage, a mixed osteoblastic and osteoclastic activity stage, and a late sclerotic, burnt-out stage. Histologically, prominent osteoid seams separate irregular islands of bone into a mosaic ("jigsaw") pattern. The osteoclasts of Paget's disease are characteristically large with an increased number of hyperchromatic nuclei and viral inclusions. Because of the high bone turnover, the serum alkaline phosphatase level is markedly increased, and collagen breakdown products, such as hydroxyproline and hydroxylysine, are increased in amount in the serum and the urine. Gaucher's disease is characterized by the accumulation of glucocerebroside in macrophages, which then have an appearance described as "wrinkled tissue paper." These cells then accumulate in many organs, including the bone. Fibrous dysplasia histologically reveals a "Chinese-letters" effect of the bony trabeculae, which are surrounded by a cellular, fibrous stroma, with osteoblasts and osteoclasts decreased at the periphery of entrapped woven bone. Giant cell tumors of bone, usually occurring at the junction of the metaphysis and the epiphysis of a long bone, produce a multiloculated ("soap bubble") appearance on x-ray. They are composed of numerous osteoblastic giant cells found in a background of fibroblast-like neoplastic spindle cells. Brown tumors of bone are areas of fibrosis with hemosiderin-laden macrophages and many osteoclastic and foreign-body type giant cells. They occur in patients with primary hyperparathyroidism.

452. The answer is e. (*Cotran, 5/e, pp 1227–1231. Rubin, 2/e, pp 1288–1290, 1294–1296.*) Normal fracture healing is characterized initially by an inflammatory phase, which lasts a few days. This is followed by a reparative phase, which lasts a few weeks and is associated with the formation of a cartilaginous callus. Finally there is a remodeling phase, which lasts for months to years. Osteomyelitis is inflammation of bone caused by an infectious organism rather than fracture healing. Organisms may be introduced into the bone by direct penetration or hematogenous spread. The initial focus of infection of the bone in hematogenous osteomyelitis is the metaphyseal area. The area of infection, or abscess, may extend into the cortex, destroying perforating arteries and causing necrosis of the cortex. The necrotic bone within the inflammation and debris is the sequestrum, and it may be surrounded by periosteal new bone formation, the involucrum. The abscess may drain through the bone, forming a draining sinus called the cloaca. An area of infection may be walled off and contained but still a chronic nidus of infection. This is called a Brodie's abscess.

453. The answer is a. *(Rubin, 2/e, pp 1294–1296.)* Nutrient arteries to long bones divide to supply the metaphyses and diaphyses. In the metaphyses, the arteries become arterioles and finally form capillary loops adjacent to epiphyseal plates. This anatomic feature allows bacteria to settle in the region of the metaphysis and makes it the site initially involved in hematogenous osteomyelitis. As a consequence of vascular and osteoclastic resorption, the infected bone is replaced by fibrous connective tissue. Persistent chronic osteomyelitis is often associated with sequelae that include amyloidosis and the appearance of malignant tumors in old sinus tracts within the damaged bone.

454. The answer is a. *(Damjanov, 10/e, p 2624. Cotran, 5/e, pp 1229–1230.)* AVN of bone is a moderately frequent complication of high-dose systemic corticosteroid therapy—the usual cause of bilateral segmental infarction or AVN of the femoral head. Clinical features include sudden onset of severe pain and difficulty in walking. Within the femoral head a triangular yellow area of necrotic bone is found beneath the viable articular cartilage, and x-ray may show a crescent sign or space between cartilage and underlying infarct. Fracture of the subcapital femoral neck is frequently associated with unilateral AVN; the other conditions listed are much less frequently associated.

455. The answer is a. *(Damjanov, 10/e, pp 2531-2532, 2567. Cotran, 5/e, p 1246.)* Metastases account for the majority of bone tumors, followed in frequency by multiple myeloma and osteogenic sarcoma. Common carcinomas that metastasize to bone include lung, thyroid, breast, prostate, and renal cell carcinomas. Whereas most metastatic carcinomas to bone produce osteolytic radiologic lesions, prostate carcinoma tends to produce osteoblastic metastases. The serum calcium and alkaline phosphatase may be elevated in osseous metastases.

456. The answer is b. *(Cotran, 5/e, pp 1241–1244. Rubin, 2/e, p 1314.)* Fibroosseous lesions of bone classically include fibrous dysplasia (FD), nonossifying fibroma (fibrous cortical defect), and osteoid osteoma. Histologically, FD shows a characteristic "Chinese-lettering" effect of the bony trabeculae, which are surrounded by a cellular, fibrous stroma, with osteoblasts and osteoclasts conspicuously decreased at the periphery of the entrapped woven bone. Histologically, nonossifying fibroma shows characteristic foam cell histiocytes within the lesions of the metaphysis. Osteoid osteomas are found within the diaphysis of long bones and contain osteoid trabeculae in a cellular, fibrous matrix, but unlike FD, this disease demonstrates (singular) peripheral trabecular osteoblasts. FD produces radiolucent bone lesions involving long bones and thorax, skull, and facial bones. Monostotic FD refers to single-bone involvement, polyostotic FD refers to involvement of multiple lesions or bones, and Albright's syndrome refers to polyostotic bone lesions, endocrinopathy (hyperthyroidism, thyrotoxicosis, hyperpituitarism, Cushing's syndrome), precocious puberty in females, and café-au-lait spots on the skin. The pigmented, macular café-au-lait spots are usually more irregular ("coast of Maine") in outline than in the forms seen in neurofibromatosis. Monostotic FD is very rarely associated with the skin lesions.

457. The answer is a. (*Damjanov, 10/e, pp 2630–2634. Cotran, 5/e, pp 1249–1253.*) Rheumatoid arthritis frequently affects the small joints of the hands and feet. The larger joints are involved later. Subcutaneous nodules, with a necrotic focus surrounded by palisades of proliferating cells, are seen in some cases. In the joints, the synovial membrane is thickened by a granulation tissue pannus that is infiltrated by many inflammatory cells. Nodular collections of lymphocytes resembling follicles are characteristically seen. The thickened synovial membrane may develop villous projections, and the joint cartilage is attacked and destroyed.

458. The answer is d. (*Cotran, 5/e, pp 25–26, 1247–1253, 1255–1259.*) Gout is associated with increased serum levels of uric acid, even though less than 15 percent of all persons with elevated serum levels of uric acid develop symptoms of gout. Gout may be classified as primary or secondary. Secondary gout may result from increased production of uric acid or from decreased excretion of uric acid. Primary (idiopathic) gout usually results from impaired excretion of uric acid by the kidneys. Most patients present with pain and redness of the first metatarsophalangeal joint, the "great toe." Sodium urate crystals—needle-shaped, negatively birefringent crystals—

precipitate to form chalky white deposits. Urate crystals may precipitate in extracellular soft tissue, such as the helix of the ear, forming masses called tophi. Pseudogout is caused by deposition of calcium pyrophosphate dihydrate (CPPD) in synovial membranes, which also forms chalky white areas on cartilaginous surfaces. CPPD crystals are not needle-shaped like urate crystals, but are short, stubby, and rhomboid; they are also birefringent. The degenerative joint disease osteoarthritis is the single most common form of joint disease. It is a "wear and tear" disorder that destroys the articular cartilage, resulting in smooth (eburnated, "ivory-like") subchondral bone. Rheumatoid arthritis, a systemic disease frequently affecting the small joints of the hands and feet, is associated with rheumatoid factor. Rheumatoid factors are antibodies, usually IgM, which are directed against the Fc fragment of IgG. In the joints, the synovial membrane is thickened by a granulation tissue, a pannus, that consists of many inflammatory cells, mainly lymphocytes and plasma cells. Ochronosis, caused by a defect in homogentisic acid oxidase, is associated with deposition of dark pigment in the cartilage of joints and degeneration of the joints.

459. The answer is d. (*Cotran, 5/e, pp 210–214, 492–496, 502.*) Cystic medial necrosis is not inflammatory, but degenerative. Hypersensitivity angiitis primarily affects small vessels; polyarteritis nodosa affects small to medium-sized arteries. In addition to interstitial inflammation (often perivascular), patients with polymyositis have histologic evidence of muscle fiber death. Perivascular inflammation is one of the early skeletal muscle changes in scleroderma (systemic sclerosis).

460. The answer is b. (*Cotran, 5/e, pp 1264, 1267—1268.*) Myositis ossificans is a benign condition characterized by fibrous repair of a skeletal muscle or subcutaneous fat, hematoma with secondary cartilage formation, ossification, and calcification. The other lesions mentioned are malignant neoplasms that may contain a variety of mesodermal tissues. The rhabdomyoblasts, if elongated, are called "tadpole," or "strap," cells.

461. The answer is e. (*Cotran, 5/e, pp 1213–1216. Rubin, 2/e, pp 1276–1279.*) Bone is composed of cells, a mineralized matrix, and an organic matrix. The normal cellular component of bone includes osteoblasts (protein-synthesizing, alkaline phosphatase-containing cells arranged in a line along the bone surface), osteocytes (an osteoblast embedded in bone matrix that has lost the capacity for protein synthesis), and osteoclasts (large, multinucleate, bone-resorbing cells with numerous lysosomes, found on the surface of bones in Howship's lacunae). The mineralized matrix consists of hydroxyapatite, which is composed mainly of calcium and phosphate. The organic matrix consists mainly of type I collagen, which is secreted by osteoblasts. Bone may be organized into woven bone or lamellar bone, each of which may be mineralized or unmineralized. The unmineralized bone is called osteoid. Lamellar bone has a parallel arrangement of type I collagen and few osteocytes; it is formed slowly and its presence is normal in the adult skeleton. Woven bone has an irregular arrangement of type I collagen fibers and numerous osteocytes; it is formed rapidly and is always pathologic if found in the adult skeleton. It is found in newly formed bone, such as early in fracture repair or bone-forming tumors.

462. The answer is c. *(Cotran, 5/e, pp 1222–1223. Rubin, 2/e, pp 1282–1287.)* The epiphyseal plate (growth plate), a layer of modified cartilage lying between the diaphysis and the epiphysis, consists of the following zones: reserve (resting) zone, proliferating zone, zone of hypertrophy, zone of calcification, and zone of ossification. Many disorders affect the epiphyseal plate. Cretinism (congenital hypothyroidism) results in mental retardation and dwarfism. The skeletal abnormalities result in defects in cartilage maturation of the epiphyseal plate. In achondroplasia, the most common inherited form of dwarfism, the zone of proliferating cartilage is either absent or greatly thinned. This in turn causes the epiphyseal plate to be thin. Vitamin C is essential for the normal synthesis and structure of collagen. In scurvy (vitamin C deficiency) there is a lack of osteoblastic synthesis of collagen (causing excess growth of chondrocytes at the epiphyseal plate) and fragility of the basement membrane of capillaries (causing periosteal hemorrhage). Many of the mucopolysaccharidoses (MPS) involve skeletal deformities. Hurler's syndrome (MPS IH) is associated with increased tissue stores and excretion of dermatan sulfate and heparan sulfate. These mucopolysaccharides also accumulate in the chondrocytes of the growth plate, resulting in dwarfism. Gargoylism describes the characteristic clinical appearance of these patients. Osteopetrosis (marble bone disease) is a rare inherited disease that involves osteoclasts with decreased functioning and lack of the usual ruffled borders. This abnormality results in reduced bone resorption and bone overgrowth. Instead of affecting the epiphyseal plate, the long bones are widened in the metaphysis and diaphysis and have a characteristic "Erlenmeyer flask" appearance. Loss of the medullary cavity often results in anemia, and multiple fractures are frequent as the bones are structurally weak. The severe autosomal recessive form causes death in infancy, but the more common autosomal dominant adult form is relatively benign.

463. The answer is c. (*Cotran, 5/e, pp 1231–1232, 1249–1250.*) Pott's disease of the spine is caused by tuberculous infection of the lower thoracic and lumbar vertebrae. Destruction of the intervertebral disks and adjacent vertebral bodies causes them to collapse, and these compression fractures may result in angular kyphosis or scoliosis. Caseous material may extend from the vertebrae into paravertebral muscles and along the psoas muscle sheath to form a psoas abscess in the inguinal regions. Tuberculous osteomyelitis occurs most often in the long bones and spine and via hematogenous spread from a primary site elsewhere. Chronic proliferative synovitis with pannus formation is characteristic of rheumatoid arthritis and Lyme arthritis. In Lyme arthritis there is also hyperplastic "onion-skin" arteriolar thickening (similar to that in syphilis).

464. The answer is d. (*Cotran, 5/e, pp 1236–1244. Rubin, 2/e, pp 1318–1319.*) Osteosarcoma is the most common primary malignant bone tumor excluding multiple myeloma and lymphoma and is the most common bone cancer of children. In two-thirds of cases it is associated with mutations of the retinoblastoma (Rb) gene. Patients with retinoblastoma are at an increased risk for developing osteogenic sarcoma. In older patients, there is an association with multifocal Paget's disease of bone, radiation exposure (as in painters of radium watch dials), fibrous dysplasia, osteochondromatosis, and chondromatosis. Osteosarcomas usually arise in the metaphyses of long bones of the extremities, although they may involve any bone. They are composed of malignant osteoblasts and show marked variation histologically depending on the amount of type I collagen, osteoid, and spicules of woven bone produced. Osteosarcomas produce a characteristic sunburst x-ray pattern due to calcified perpendicular striae of reactive periosteum adjacent to the tumor. They may also show periosteal elevation at an acute angle (Codman's triangle) or penetrate cortical bone with extension into the adjacent soft tissue. These tumors metastasize hematogenously and usually spread to the lungs early in the course of the disease. With surgery, radiation, and chemotherapy the 5-year survival is now about 60 percent.

Plasmacytoma is not associated with an increased incidence of osteogenic sarcoma.

465. The answer is e. *(Cotran, 5/e, pp 1240–1241.)* Chondrosarcoma shows a peak incidence in the sixth and seventh decades. Most chondrosarcomas (85 percent) arise de novo, but the peripheral type, unlike the central type, may arise in benign tumors of cartilage, especially if they are multiple. Frequent sites of origin include pelvic bones (50 percent), humerus, femur, ribs, and spine. Although a fairly common form of bone cancer, chondrosarcoma is preceded in frequency by metastatic carcinoma, multiple myeloma, and osteosarcoma. Histologic grading is most important in prognosis since grade I and grade II lesions present very good 5-year survival rates following surgery, unlike grade III, poorly differentiated tumors, which invade quickly and metastasize to lungs.

466. The answer is e. *(Cotran, 5/e, pp 1255–1258.)* Diseases that lead to continued tissue synthesis and breakdown may produce hyperuricemia and clinical gout because of the resulting increase in nucleic acid turnover. This form of secondary gout may be seen in polycythemia vera, myeloid metaplasia, chronic leukemia, extensive psoriasis, and sarcoidosis. Cytotoxic drugs used in the chemotherapy of cancer may augment hyperuricemia. Decreased renal excretion of uric acid may also lead to secondary gout. Overproduction of uric acid may result from inborn errors of metabolism, as in the Lesch-Nyhan syndrome (deficiency of the enzyme hypoxanthine-guanine phosphoribosyltransferase (HGPRT). Chondrocalcinosis is pseudogout.

467–468. The answers are: 467-a, 468-e. *(Damjanov, 10/e, p 2532. Cotran, 5/e, pp 1237–1238, 1245–1246. Rubin, 2/e, pp 1315–1316.)* Osteoclastoma, the giant cell tumor of bone, usually produces a lytic lesion involving the epiphysis of long bones. The proximal tibia is a common site. There are many pitfalls involved in making a diagnosis of giant cell tumor of bone. The main problem involves the difficulty of distinguishing the bone destruction that is a true neoplasm from bone destruction that is the result of various types of osteoclastic-osteoblastic activity. Direct communication with the radiologist and, preferably, the orthopedic surgeon is, therefore, nearly mandatory for the pathologist when making a diagnosis.

Unicameral, or solitary, cysts are loculated, lytic lesions of bone that characteristically abut on the epiphyseal plate in older children and produce cortical irregularities. Regions involved in the benign lesion are prone to fracture.

Osteochondromas are cauliflower-like lesions that contain a core of cortical and medullary bone and a cartilage cap that decreases in width as age increases. They usually protrude from the metaphyses of long bones and may be multiple.

Nonossifying fibromas of bone—usually well-demarcated, eccentric, lytic metaphyseal lesions—most commonly occur in the tibia and femur. They are histologically identical to fibrous cortical defects and consist of a fibroblastic growth without concomitant bone formation.

469–470. The answers are: 469-k, 470-e. *(Cotran, 5/e, pp 814, 1233–1234, 1238–1239, 1244. Rubin, 2/e, p 1322.)* Many benign tumors of bone are capable of producing either bone or cartilage. Bone producing tumors include osteomas, osteoid osteomas, and osteoblastomas. Osteoid osteomas (OO) are bone tumors that are typically found in the cortex of the metaphysis. Osteoid osteoma occurs predominantly in children or young adults in the second and third decades of life as a benign osteoblastic (bone-forming) lesion of small size, which by definition is less than 3 cm. In osteoid osteoma malignant change does not occur, unlike the closely related but larger osteoblastoma, in which there is occasional malignant change. OO is often located in the diaphyseal cortex of tibia or femur, unlike osteoblastoma, which occurs in the spine (vertebral arch) or medulla of long bones. They are characteristically painful because of the excess production of prostaglandin E2. The pain occurs at night and is promptly relieved by aspirin. X-rays typically reveal a radiolucent area (the tumor itself) surrounded by thickened (reactive) bone. Histologic sections reveal a oval mass, the central nidus of which consists of interconnected trabeculae of woven bone having numerous osteoblasts and uncalcified osteoid. This central nidus is surrounded by a rim of sclerotic bone. Treatment is complete excision of the nidus to prevent recurrence.

A histologic picture which is identical to the central nidus of an osteoid osteoma is seen with the osteoblastoma. They are sometimes called giant osteoid osteomas. They differ from osteoid osteomas by their larger size (greater than 2 cm.) and lack of a decreased pain response to aspirin. These tumors also lack the surrounding sclerotic bone formation of osteoid osteomas and are found in the medulla of bone rather than the cortex. Osteomas are usually solitary and clinically silent. They may be multiple in patients with Gardener's syndrome (familial colonic adenomatous polyposis with mesenchymal lesions). Osteomas are composed of a circumscribed mass of dense sclerotic bone and are typically found in flat bones, such as the skull and facial bones. Chondromas usually occur at the diaphysis and may be found either within the medullary cavity (enchondromas) or on the surface of the bone. They are usually are solitary lesions, but may be multiple (Ollier's disease). X-rays reveal a characteristic "O-ring sign", which refers to radiolucent central cartilage surrounded by a thin layer of bone. Solitary enchondromas are not associated with malignant transformation, but there is an increased risk of chondrosarcoma in patients with Ollier's disease. Chondroblastomas, which usually occur at epiphyses, histologically reveal sheets of chondroblasts that are located within a background of "chicken-wire" mineralization and occasional non-neoplastic osteoclast-type giant cells. Ewing's sarcoma is an uncommon tumor primarily affecting patients younger than 20 years of age. It arises in the medullary cavity and is usually located in the diaphysis or metaphysis of the long bones, not the epiphysis. Most cases have a reciprocal translocation between chromosomes 11 and 22. In about half of the cases of

Ewing's sarcoma, reactive new bone formation may cause concentric "onion-skin" layering. Histologically the tumor is composed of small, uniform, round cells similar in appearance to lymphocytes. Occasionally the tumor cells form rosettes around central blood vessels (Homer-Wright pseudorosettes), indicating neural differentiation. PAS staining of glycogen-positive, diastase-sensitive cytoplasmic granules within the tumor cells of Ewing's sarcoma differentiates this lesion from lymphoma and neuroblastoma. With a combination of chemotherapy, radiation, and surgery, the 5-year survival is now 75 percent.

SKIN AND BREAST

Questions

DIRECTIONS: Each question below contains five suggested responses. Select the **one best** response to each question.

471. The clinical photograph below suggests that the patient

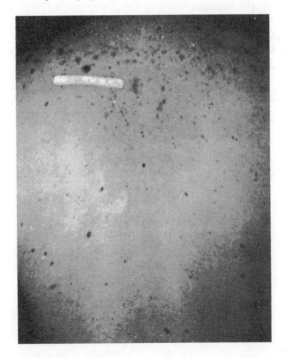

a. Has Leser-Trelat sign
b. Has multiple basal cell nevus syndrome
c. Is at risk for developing malignant melanoma
d. Has leopard syndrome
e. Has Torres's syndrome

472. A 68-year-old female presents with a single, uniformly brown round lesion that appears to be "stuck on" the right side of her face. Histologic sections from this lesion reveal hyperkeratosis with horn and pseudo-horn cyst formation. What is the correct diagnosis for this skin lesion?

a. Seborrheic keratosis
b. Squamous cell carcinoma
c. Verruca vulgaris
d. Keratoacanthoma
e. Actinic keratosis

473. Malignant or premalignant lesions of the skin include

a. Acrochordon
b. Senile (actinic) keratosis
c. Keratoacanthoma
d. Dermatofibroma
e. Dermoid cyst

474. Which of the following pairs of disorders would most appropriately be considered in the differential diagnosis for the lesion seen in the photomicrograph below?

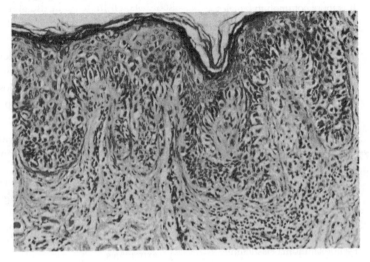

a. Superficial spreading malignant melanoma in situ and Paget's disease
b. Mycosis fungoides and metastatic carcinoma
c. Psoriasis and lichen planus
d. Lupus erythematosus and lupus vulgaris
e. Leukemia and lymphoma

475. The incidence of malignant melanoma of the skin appears to be increasing in the United States. Which of the following is most significant in predicting the clinical behavior following diagnosis?

a. The degree of pigmentation
b. The level and depth
c. The amount of inflammation
d. The degree of pleomorphism
e. The state of nutrition

476. Mycosis fungoides is correctly characterized by which of the following statements?

a. It is more common in females
b. It represents cutaneous spread of a primary nodal lymphoma
c. It is characterized histologically by microabscesses of Munro
d. It is a cutaneous lymphoma of CD4+ T-cell lineage
e. It is a cutaneous lymphoma of CD8+ T-cell lineage

477. Lobular panniculitis with vasculitis is seen in

a. Erythema nodosum
b. Erythema multiforme
c. Erythema induratum
d. Weber-Christian disease
e. Pseudoxanthoma elasticum

478. Histologic examination of a skin biopsy from an adult male reveals hyperkeratosis without parakeratosis, an increase in the granular cell layer, acanthosis, and a band-like lymphocytic infiltrate in the upper dermis involving the dermal-epidermal junction. Which one of the following describes the most likely clinical appearance of this patient's lesions?

a. Generalized skin eruptions with oval salmon-colored papules along flexure lines
b. Macules, papules, and vesicles on the trunk along with several target lesions
c. Pruritic purple papules and plaques on the flexor surfaces of his extremities
d. Red plaques covered by silver scales on the extensor surfaces of his elbows and knees
e. Soft yellow-orange plaques along the neck, axilla, and groin

479. A 34-year-old male presents with multiple large, sharply defined, silver-white scaly plaques on the extensor surfaces of his elbows, knees, and scalp. Physical examination reveals discoloration and pitting of his fingernails. Lifting of one of the scales on his elbows produces multiple, minute areas of bleeding (positive Auspitz sign). Histologic sections from one of the scaly plaques would most likely reveal

a. Subepithelial bullae
b. Regular elongation of the rete ridges
c. Liquefactive degeneration of the basal layer of the epidermis
d. Increased granular cell layer
e. Chronic inflammation below a zone of degenerated collagen

480. The photomicrograph below is from a small, papillary lesion found on the dorsal surface of the left hand of an 18-year-old woman. This lesion is most likely to be associated with human papillomavirus (HPV)

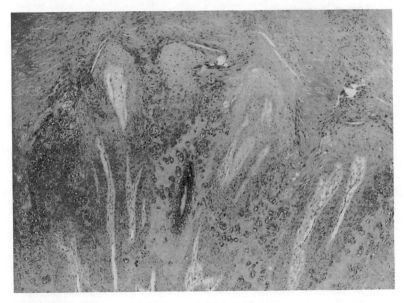

a. Types 1 or 3
b. Types 2 or 4
c. Types 5 or 8
d. Types 6 or 11
e. Types 16 or 18

481. During a routine breast self-examination, a 35-year-old female is concerned because her breasts feel "lumpy." She consults you as her primary care physician. After performing an examination, you reassure her that no masses are present, and that the "lumpiness" that she felt was due to fibrocystic changes. Considering this clinical opinion, a pathologic finding that is consistent with the nonproliferative form of fibrocystic change is

a. A blue-domed cyst
b. A radial scar
c. Atypical hyperplasia
d. Papillomatosis
e. Sclerosing adenosis

482. A 23-year-old woman presents with a rubbery, freely movable 2-cm mass in the upper outer quadrant of the left breast. A biopsy of this lesion would most likely histologically reveal

a. Large numbers of neutrophils
b. Large numbers of plasma cells
c. Duct ectasia with inspissation of breast secretions
d. Necrotic fat surrounded by lipid-laden macrophages
e. A mixture of fibrous tissue and ducts

483. A 16-year-old girl undergoes biopsy of a breast lump that shows the changes in the photomicrograph below. What is the most appropriate course of action?

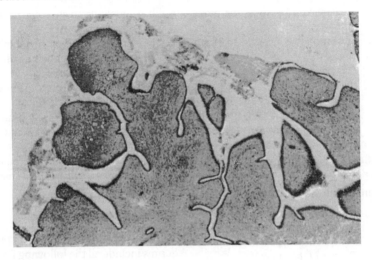

a. Radiotherapy
b. Local excision
c. Radical mastectomy
d. Modified radical mastectomy
e. No further therapy

484. A 37-year-old woman presents with a lump in the upper outer quadrant of the left breast, which shows a wide spectrum of benign breast disease on pathologic examination. Which of the following is considered to indicate the greatest risk for subsequent carcinoma of the breast?

a. Intraductal papillomatosis
b. Sclerosing adenosis
c. Focal papillomatosis
d. Marked apocrine metaplasia
e. Epithelial hyperplasia of the ducts

485. Which of the following statements most accurately describes inflammatory breast cancer?

a. Inflammation improves the prognosis
b. Inflammation is increased in Paget's disease
c. Acute inflammatory cells are present
d. Chronic inflammatory cells are present
e. Lymphatic permeation is present

486. The most important factor related to the prognosis of breast cancer is

a. The presence of activated oncogenes
b. The histologic type and grade
c. The size of the tumor
d. The status of axillary lymph nodes
e. The presence of estrogen receptors

487. All the following are the result of melanocytic hyperplasia EXCEPT

a. Freckle
b. Lentigo
c. Junctional nevus
d. Blue nevus
e. Spitz tumor

488. True statements concerning basal cell carcinoma of the skin include all the following EXCEPT

a. It is locally destructive but rarely metastasizes
b. Histologically it typically shows large cells with abundant, glassy, eosinophilic cytoplasm
c. Peripheral palisading is a common histologic feature
d. Clinical appearance is a pearly papule with raised margins and a central ulcer
e. Recognized variants include morphea-like, superficial, and pigmented

489. Diseases developing from cells found normally within the epidermis include all the following EXCEPT

a. Squamous cell carcinoma
b. Merkel cell carcinoma
c. Melanoma
d. Letterer-Siwe disease
e. Urticaria pigmentosa

490. The differential diagnosis of the lesion with dense lymphocytic infiltration depicted below could include all the following EXCEPT

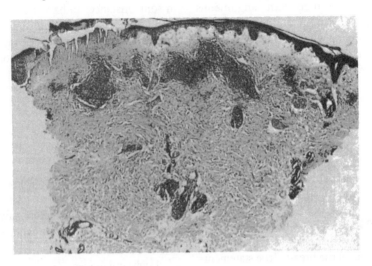

a. Lupus erythematosus
b. Urticaria pigmentosa
c. Polymorphous light eruption
d. Pseudolymphoma
e. Malignant lymphoma

491. An adult patient develops crops of bullae and vesicles in the mouth and later on the skin of the trunk. A skin biopsy is inconclusive but shows a suprabasal acantholysis of the overlying epidermis. Direct immunofluorescence of the skin can be used to identify all the following EXCEPT

a. Bullous pemphigoid
b. Pemphigus vulgaris
c. Dermatitis herpetiformis
d. Erythema multiforme
e. Discoid lupus erythematosus (DLE)

492. A papillary lesion is seen in a biopsy from a 32-year-old woman who presented with sanguineous discharge from the nipple. All the following would be useful in differentiating benign intraductal papilloma from papillary adenocarcinoma EXCEPT

a. A cribriform pattern
b. Knowledge of the presence or absence of cell uniformity
c. Fibrovascular cores
d. The age of the patient
e. Two cell types (epithelial and myoepithelial)

493. A menopausal woman is given a diagnosis of lobular carcinoma of the breast. True statements regarding this lesion include all the following EXCEPT

a. It represents about 10 percent of breast carcinomas
b. Epidermal infiltration is characteristic
c. Biopsies of the contralateral breast are indicated
d. It tends to be multifocal
e. A single file pattern of infiltration is characteristic

494. Clinical risk factors for development of carcinoma of the female breast include all the following EXCEPT

a. Early menopause
b. Nulliparity
c. History of endometrial cancer
d. Early menarche
e. Obesity

495. A number of malignant tumors of the breast have been known in some instances to have a deceptively bland histologic appearance and hence have at times been misdiagnosed as benign by the pathologist. These potentially deceptive tumors include all the following EXCEPT

a. Duct carcinoma
b. Tubular carcinoma
c. Angiosarcoma
d. Papillary carcinoma
e. Metastasizing mucinous carcinoma

496. All the following factors have shown an association with gynecomastia EXCEPT

a. Leydig cell tumors
b. Seminomas
c. Sertoli cell tumors
d. Alcoholic cirrhosis
e. Digitalis therapy

DIRECTIONS: Each group of questions below consists of lettered headings followed by a set of numbered items. For each numbered item select the **one** lettered heading with which it is **most** closely associated. Each lettered heading may be used **once, more than once, or not at all**.

Questions 497–498

Match each of the following clinical scenarios with the correct diagnosis from the following list.

a. Erythema migrans
b. Human papillomavirus
c. *Malassezia furfur*
d. Molluscum contagiosum
e. Pityriasis rosea
f. *Sarcoptes scabiei*
g. *Staphylococcus aureus*
h. h10Trichophyton rubrum

497. A 19-year-old male presents with a rash that involves a large, irregular portion of his trunk. Examination reveals several annular lesions having a raised papulovesicular border with central hypopigmentation. Examination of this area under a Wood's lamp reveals a yellow fluorescence. A scraping of this area viewed under the microscope after KOH is added reveals characteristic "spaghetti and meatball" forms.

498. A 45-year-old male presents with a 2mm pruritic lesion on his anterior chest. A biopsy from this lesion reveals homogeneous intracytoplasmic inclusions within the epidermal cells of the stratum granulosum.

Questions 499–500

Match each of the following clinical scenarios with the correct diagnosis from the following list.

a. Eczematous inflammation
b. Epidermoid carcinoma
c. Fat necrosis
d. Fibroadenoma
e. Mammary duct ectasia
f. Mammary fibromatosis
g. Paget's disease of the breast
h. Phylloides tumor, benign
i. Phylloides tumor, malignant

499. A 46-year-old woman presented with a 4 month history of a discharge from the nipple. An excisional biopsy of the nipple area revealed infiltration of the nipple by large cells with clear cytoplasm. These cells were found both singly and in small clusters in the epidermis and were PAS-positive diastase-resistant.

500. A 37-year-old female presents with a 4 cm mass in her left breast. The mass is excised and the microscopic examination reveals proliferation of fibrous tissue and ducts. The stroma appears densely cellular, but the ductal epithelial cells appear unremarkable. The stromal cells do not appear atypical. Mitoses are present, but they are rare.

SKIN AND BREAST

Answers

471. The answer is c. (*Cotran, 5/e, pp 1177–1178, 1181–1182. Rubin, 2/e, pp 1219–1220.*) The clinical photograph depicts the presence of the dysplastic nevus syndrome, first described by Dr. Wallace Clark and his coworkers Drs. Mark Greene, David Elder, and E. Bondi in Philadelphia during the mid 1970s. This valuable finding elucidated the presence of abnormal nevi that are at least a marker for the development of malignant melanoma. These nevi, while not malignant, have atypical features compared with those of normal nevi, such as irregular borders, a pink base, and irregular pigmentation. The Leser-Trelat sign refers to the development of multiple seborrheic keratoses over a short period of time in older patients who have visceral malignancy, while the basal cell nevus syndrome is dominantly inherited with the association of numerous basal cell carcinomas forming throughout life, bifid ribs, keratocysts of the mandible, unusual facies, and abnormalities of the central nervous system and reproductive system. A familial occurrence of dysplastic nevus syndrome with basal cell nevus syndrome was elucidated at the 1985 meeting of the International Academy of Pathologists by Elliot Foucar. The leopard syndrome refers to multiple flat lentigines that are not premalignant for melanoma, in addition to cardiac abnormalities and ocular hypertelorism. Recent studies have shown that the dysplastic nevus syndrome is not only familial, but may be sporadic in about 6 percent of the general population. The risk of developing melanoma in the dysplastic nevus familial situation is greatly increased over that in the general population. It has been stated that patients with dysplastic nevi belonging to a kindred with dysplastic nevus and familial malignant melanoma have a 100-fold risk of developing malignant melanoma over their entire lifetime.

472. The answer is a. (*Cotran, 5/e, pp 1181–1187.*) Keratosis refers to the proliferation of keratinocytes with excess keratin production. Seborrheic keratoses are benign, elevated ("stuck-on") lesions that usually occur in older individuals. Histologically these lesions reveal hyperkeratosis with horn and pseudo-horn cysts formation. The sudden development of large numbers of seborrheic keratoses (Leser-Trelat sign) may develop in association with another malignancy. This association with malignancies may also be seen with the malignant type of acanthosis nigricans, which consists of hyperpigmented areas of skin in the groin and axilla.

Keratoacanthomas (KA) are rapidly growing lesions that microscopically reveal a cup-shaped lesion with a central, keratin-filled crater surrounded by keratinocytes having eosinophilic ("glassy") cytoplasm. Atypia may be present, but these lesions are not considered to be malignant. The histologic appearance can make differentiating keratoacanthomas from squamous cell carcinomas on a histologic basis quite difficult. The clinical history of rapid development within several weeks is very helpful in making the correct diagnosis. Most cases of KA spontaneously resolve over several months. Human papillomavirus (HPV) causes several types of verrucae (warts), which are hyperkeratotic lesions. Verrucae vulgaris histologically reveal hyperkeratosis, papillomatosis, and koilocytosis. The latter term refers to large vacuolated cells with shrunken nuclei. Characteristically present are numerous, enlarged keratohyalin granules. Actinic (solar) keratoses, found on sun-damaged skin, microscopically shows hyperkeratosis, parakeratosis, atypia of the epidermal keratinocytes, and degeneration of the elastic fibers in the dermis. The latter finding is referred to as solar elastosis. Clinically actinic keratoses appear as irregular erythematous brown papules. When the atypia of the intraepidermal keratinocytes is extreme (full-thickness), the lesion is referred to as Bowen's disease. These lesions are in fat carcinomas in situ since there is no invasion into the underlying dermis. If invasion were present, the lesion would be diagnostic of a squamous cell carcinoma.

473. The answer is b. (*Cotran, 5/e, pp 1182–1186, 1188–1189.*) Fibrous histiocytoma (dermatofibroma, sclerosing hemangioma) is a benign dermal tumor of fibroblasts and histiocytes, proliferating in cartwheel or storiform pattern, in which small blood vessels may form a prominent component. Senile (actinic, solar) keratosis is a premalignant skin lesion with focal atypia of keratinocytes of the lower layers of the epidermis. There is often a history of chronic exposure to the sun, and there is a high incidence in the southern United States. Other precancerous skin lesions include erythroplasia of Queyrat and Bowen's disease. Keratoacanthoma, a benign tumor, may resemble squamous cell carcinoma both clinically and histologically, but penetration of the dermis never extends deeper than adjacent hair follicles. The lesion is cup-shaped with central keratin; biopsy or excision excludes squamous carcinoma. An acrochordon (skin tag) is a benign fibroepithelial polyp of the skin. The dermoid cyst is similar to the benign epidermal inclusion cyst except that it also has dermal appendage structures attached to the wall of the cyst.

474. The answer is a. (*Cotran, 5/e, pp 1105, 1179–1181, 1190–1192, 1197–1200.*) The photomicrograph was taken from a patient with superficial spreading malignant melanoma in situ; it shows individual cells resembling Paget's disease invading the upper regions of the epidermis. The basement membrane zone is intact and there are lymphocytes in the underlying dermis. Cells with clear cytoplasm and malignant-appearing nuclei such as shown here resemble those of Paget's disease, from which they must be distinguished. Some cells of mycosis fungoides will resemble this, but they occur in nest formations called Pautrier's abscesses. Metastatic carcinoma can produce lesions that resemble malignant melanoma, but these are problems relating to the dermis. Leukemia-lymphoma infiltrates mainly involve the dermis, although the epidermis may become ulcerated and atrophic. Lupus erythematosus and lichen planus produce subepidermal lymphocytic infiltrates with no involvement of the epidermis itself. Psoriasis produces parakeratosis and elongated rete ridges but no abnormal cells in the epidermis.

475. The answer is b. (*Cotran, 5/e, pp 1179–1181. Rubin, 2/e, pp 1218–1228.*) Although malignant melanoma of the skin is not as common as squamous and basal cell carcinoma, it is an exceedingly important and somewhat mysterious tumor owing to its often devastating clinical course and occasionally unpredictable behavior. There appear to be strong immune factors that presumably account for some well-documented remissions, lengthy survival after distant metastasis, and rapid growth in renal transplant patients. However, most patients with this form of cancer pursue a course characterized by eventual distant and visceral metastasis, especially if the histologic type is either nodular or superficial spreading. The subtype called lentigo maligna melanoma, found in the sun-exposed skin of elderly patients, generally has a much more favorable outlook. The most important predictors of outcome are the level of penetration into the subepidermis and reticular dermis (Clark levels I through V: I, in situ, V, invasion of subcutaneous fat) and the actual depth of invasion, measured in millimeters with an ocular micrometer (Breslow depth). The survival at 5 years is 90 percent if the tumor is Clark I or II and 0.76 mm or less in depth, but survival falls to 40 to 48 percent if the tumor is level III or IV and greater than 1.9 mm in depth. While some melanoma cells may show cytologic pleomorphism, many aggressive melanomas exhibit uniformity and blandness. Recent work has shown that melanomas arising in the region of the shoulder, upper trunk, and back in men behave in an aggressive fashion.

476. The answer is d. (*Cotran, 5/e, pp 1109–1192.*) Mycosis fungoides is part of the spectrum of malignant T-cell lymphomas, mostly of the CD4+ T-cell subset, with a predilection for the skin. It is more common in males and the incidence increases with age. It arises primarily in the skin but more than 70 percent of patients have extracutaneous spread with lymph nodes, spleen, liver, and lungs most often involved. Clinically it presents as cutaneous patches, plaques, or nodules and is often misdiagnosed as psoriasis or other dermatitides. Histologically there is a bandlike infiltrate in the upper dermis of atypical lymphocytes with markedly convoluted nuclei—the Sézary-Lutzner cells. These show epidermotropism and form characteristic intraepidermal clusters known as Pautrier's microabscesses. In some cases there is generalized erythroderma and Sézary-Lutzner cells in the peripheral blood. This is known as the Sézary syndrome.

477. The answer is c. (*Cotran, 5/e, pp 1195–1196. Rubin, 2/e, pp 1202–1204, 1213–1215.*) Inflammation of the subcutaneous adipose tissue, panniculitis, may affect the connective tissue septa (septal panniculitis) or the fat lobule (lobular panniculitis). Erythema nodosum is a self-limited disease triggered by several agents, including drugs and microorganisms. It consists of inflammation of the fibrous septa without vasculitis. Weber-Christian disease is characterized by recurring groups of tender nodules within the subcutaneous fat and inflammatory cells within the lobules with necrosis of adipocytes. There is no vasculitis. Erythema induratum is a chronic disease found primarily on the legs of women. It is associated with vasculitis and is considered to be a vascular hypersensitivity reaction. There is chronic inflammation in the subcutaneous lobules with tuberculoid granulomas and fat necrosis. Erythema multiforme is an acute, self-limited disorder that usually occurs as a reaction to a drug or infectious agent. Histologic examination reveals lymphocytic infiltration, with possible subepidermal bullae, and epidermal necrosis. Pseudoxanthoma elasticum is a hereditary disorder characterized by fragmented and thickened elastic fibers in the dermis and thickened, yellow-orange skin in the axillary folds and inguinal regions.

478. The answer is c. (*Cotran, 5/e, pp 1195–1199.*) Lichen planus is characterized by the formation of "pruritic, purple, polygonal papules" usually on flexor surfaces of the extremities, such as the wrists and elbows. These lesions may also have white dots or lines within them, which are called Wickham's striae. The basic defect in lichen planus is a decrease rate of keratinocyte proliferation, which is the exact opposite of the increased rate of keratinocyte proliferation in psoriasis. Histologically the skin reveals a characteristic band-like lymphocytic infiltrate in the superficial dermis, which destroys the basal cell layer of the epidermis and causes a "sawtooth" appearance of the rete ridges. Anucleate, necrotic basal epidermal cells may be found in the inflamed papillary dermis. These cells are called colloid bodies or Civatte bodies. Because of the decreased rate of keratinocyte proliferation there is an increase in the size of the granular cell layer, which is again the opposite of psoriasis.

Pityriasis rosea is a common idiopathic self-limited disease of the skin that is characterized by multiple oval salmon-pink papules that are covered by thin scales. The lesions typically follow flexure lines. Also present is a characteristic larger, sharply defined scaling plaque, which is called the "herald patch." Erythema multiforme (EM) is a hypersensitivity reaction to certain drugs and infections. Clinically patients develop lesions that are quite varied ("multiform") and include macules, papules, vesicles, and bullae. The characteristic lesion, however, is a target lesion that consists of a red macule or papule that has a pale center. Microscopic examination reveals epidermal spongiosis and necrosis with dermal vasculitis and edema. Psoriasis is a chronic skin disease having large, sharply defined silver-white scaly plaques. These skin lesions are usually found on the extensor surfaces of the elbows and knees, the scalp, and the lumbosacral areas. Pseudoxanthoma elasticum is a hereditary disorder characterized by fragmented and thickened elastic fibers in the dermis and thickened, yellow-orange skin in the axillary folds and inguinal regions.

479. The answer is b. (*Cotran, 5/e, pp 1195–1204.*) Psoriasis is a chronic skin disease having large, sharply defined silver-white scaly plaques. These skin lesions are usually found on the extensor surfaces of the elbows and knees, the scalp, and the lumbosacral areas, but additionally about one third of patients have nail changes including discoloration, pitting, and crumbling. The pathogenesis is not well understood, but about one third of patients have a familial history. The pathogenesis involves a faster turnover time of the epidermal keratinocytes. The normal turn-over time is about 28 days, but in patients with psoriasis this is decreased to about 3 days. Psoriasis is sometimes associated with other diseases, such as seronegative rheumatoid arthritis and AIDS. Clinically if the scale of psoriasis is lifted, it forms multiple, minute areas of bleeding. This is referred to as an Auspitz sign, and is due to increased, dilated vessels within the papillary dermis. The formation of new lesions at sites of trauma is referred to as the Koebner phenomenon, and this sign is also present. In patients with psoriasis, trauma may cause thickening of the epidermis (acanthosis), downward regular elongation of the rete ridges, hyperkeratosis, and parakeratosis. These changes may be related to faulty β-adrenergic receptors and decreased activity of adenyl cyclase in the lower epidermis. Since the keratinocyte turn-over time is faster, there is no granular cell layer. Characteristically, neutrophils infiltrate the epidermis and form Munro's microabscesses in the stratum corneum or Kogoj spongiform pustules in the subcorneal region. These areas within the epidermis are slightly spongiotic, but no bullae are formed. Lymphocytes below a zone of degenerated collagen in the superficial dermis is found in lichen sclerosis, and not psoriasis.

Two bullous diseases that can develop subepidermal bullae are bullous pemphigoid and dermatitis herpetiformis. Bullous pemphigoid is an autoimmune disease that is caused by IgG antibodies to a glycoprotein in the lamina lucida of the basement membrane zone. It is characterized by subepidermal blisters and linear deposits of IgG and C3 in the lamina lucida. Dermatitis herpetiformis is related to gluten sensitivity (celiac disease) and HLA haplotypes B8 and DRw3. Granular deposits of IgA, fibrin, and neutrophils accumulate at the dermal-epidermal junction at the tips of papillae. These changes result in subepidermal vesicles. In patients with systemic lupus erythematosus, patients typically have a malar "butterfly" rash. Histologic examination reveals liquefactive degeneration of the basal layers of the epidermis. Immunoglobulin (IgG) and complement are also deposited at the dermal-epidermal junction in a granular pattern.

480. The answer is b. (*Silverberg, 2/e, p 195. Cotran, 5/e, pp 1205–1206. Rubin, 2/e, pp 1228–1229.*) Verrucae (warts) are cutaneous lesions caused by human papillomaviruses (HPV) that belong to the DNA-containing papovavirus group. Verrucae are classified according to their location and morphology. Verruca vulgaris, the most common type of wart, may occur anywhere on the body, but most commonly, it is located on the dorsal surface of the hands. The photomicrograph reveals characteristic features of verrucae vulgaris including hyperkeratosis, papillary hyperplasia of the epidermis, and numerous, large, keratohyaline granules within the epidermal cells. Verrucae vulgaris have been associated with several types of HPV, including types 2 and 4. Plantar warts, hyperkeratotic lesions on the soles similar to a callus, are associated with HPV type 1, while verruca plana, typically found on the face, is associated with HPV type 3. Venereal warts, also called condyloma acuminata, are associated with HPV types 6 and 11. Carcinoma may develop in condyloma acuminata, in which case HPV types 16 and 18 are more frequently identified. Bowenoid papulosis, multiple hyperpigmented papules on the genitalia, are associated with HPV types 16 and 18. Epidermodysplasia verruciformis is an autosomal recessive disease associated with impaired cell-mediated immunity and the widespread development of multiple flat warts. These lesions have been associated with HPV types 5 or 8. Some of these lesions may develop into squamous cell carcinomas.

481. The answer is a. (*Cotran, 5/e, pp 1093–1097.*) Fibrocystic change of the breast is one of the most common features seen in the female breast. It is most likely associated with an endocrine imbalance that causes an abnormality of the normal monthly cyclic events within the breast. These fibrocystic changes are subdivided into nonproliferative and proliferative changes. Nonproliferative changes include fibrosis of the stroma and cystic dilatation of the terminal ducts, which when large may form blue-domed cysts. A common feature of the ducts in nonproliferative changes is apocrine metaplasia, which refers to epithelial cells with abundant eosinophilic cytoplasm with apical snouts. Proliferative changes include epithelial hyperplasia of the ducts. This hyperplastic epithelium may form papillary structures (papillomatosis when pronounced), or may be quite abnormal (atypical hyperplasia). Two benign, but clinically important, forms of proliferative fibrocystic change include sclerosing adenosis and radial scar. Both of these may be mistaken histologically for infiltrating ductal carcinoma, but the presence of my-oepithelial cells is a helpful sign that points to the benign nature of the proliferation. Sclerosing adenosis is a disease of the terminal lobules that is typically seen in patients 35 to 45 years old. It produces a firm mass, most often located in the upper outer quadrant. Microscopically there is florid proliferation of small ductal structures in a fibrous stroma, which on low power is stellate in appearance and somewhat maintains the normal lobular architecture. A radial scar refers to ductal proliferation around a central fibrotic area.

482. The answer is e. *(Cotran, 5/e, pp 1091–1093, 1097–1098. Rubin, 2/e, pp 978, 982.)* The most common benign neoplasm of the breast is the fibroadenoma. It typically occurs in the upper outer quadrant of the breast in women between the ages of 20 and 35. These lesions originate from the terminal duct lobular unit and histologically reveal a mixture of fibrous connective tissue and ducts. Clinically, fibroadenomas are rubbery, freely movable, oval nodules that usually measure 2 to 4 cm in diameter. Numerous neutrophils are seen in acute bacterial infection of the breast (acute mastitis), which is usually seen in the postpartum lactating or involuting breast. Dilatation of the breast ducts (ectasia) with inspissation of breast secretions is characteristic of mammary duct ectasia. It is common in elderly women. If large numbers of plasma cells are also present, the lesion is called plasma cell mastitis. Fat necrosis of the breast, associated with traumatic injury, is characterized by necrotic fat surrounded by lipid-laden macrophages and a neutrophilic infiltration.

483. The answer is b. *(Damjanov, 10/e, pp 2205–2206, 2363–2364. Cotran, 5/e, pp 1098–1099.)* The lesion depicted in the photomicrograph is that of a cellular fibroadenoma, a basically benign neoplasm of the breast. Mueller initially described cystosarcoma phylloides in 1838 and named it for the resemblance of the lesion to leaves. In older women if the stroma is hypercellular with mitoses and peripheral infiltrative borders, it has the capacity to metastasize. In the adolescent female, cellular stroma of spindle cells with occasional mitoses, such as in this example, may not behave in a malignant fashion as in older women. Because most lesions like these behave in a benign fashion, conservative but total excision with a small rim of normal tissue surrounding the lesion is all that is necessary in the adolescent.

484. The answer is e. (*Cotran, 5/e, pp 1093–1097.*) The spectrum of benign breast disease includes fibrocystic disease, which is probably a misnomer; adenosis, both sclerosing and microglandular; intraductal papillomas and papillomatosis; apocrine metaplasia; fibrous stromal hyperplasia; and hyperplasia of the epithelial cells lining the ducts and ductules of the breasts. At one time or another each of the above was considered to be a forerunner of carcinoma; however, with extensive studies in the literature, none of these has been shown to necessarily correlate with a greater risk of developing carcinoma with the exception of epithelial hyperplasia, particularly when atypical. With any of the features, but especially epithelial hyperplasia, adding a positive family history of breast cancer in a sibling, mother, or maternal aunt markedly increases the risk for developing carcinoma of the breast in the given patient. Owing to the advances and technology of xeromammography, there has been an increased interest in calcifications, which are markers for carcinoma of the breast. These calcifications, however, do not necessarily occur within the cancerous ducts themselves and can be found frequently in either adenosis adjacent to the carcinoma or even in normal breast lobules in the region. Stipple calcification as seen by xeromammography is regarded by some workers as an indication for a biopsy of the region.

485. The answer is e. (*Cotran, 5/e, p 1106.*) Inflammatory breast carcinoma is often misunderstood because of the qualifying adjective "inflammatory." The term does not refer to the presence of inflammatory cells, abscess, or any special histologic type of breast carcinoma; rather, it refers to more of a clinical phenomenon, in that the breast is swollen, erythematous, and indurated and demonstrates a marked increase in warmth. These changes are caused by widespread lymphatic and vascular permeation within the breast itself and in the deep dermis of the overlying skin by breast carcinoma cells. The clinical induration and erythema are presumably related to lymphatic-vascular blockage by tumor cells; if present, these findings mean a worse prognosis for the patient.

486. The answer is d. (*Cotran, 5/e, pp 1099, 1107–1108.*) Carcinoma of the breast still causes about 20 percent of female cancer deaths and is the leading cause of death worldwide in women over 40 years of age. It is difficult to predict survival rate, but the status of the axillary nodes is of major importance since negative nodes suggest 70 to 80 percent 10-year survival.

There is a significant decrease in 5-year survival if one to three nodes are positive (only 50 percent), and four or more positive nodes at the time of diagnosis usually mean about 20 percent disease-free survival. Obviously, a large size of involved nodes, invasion of the capsule, and fixation to adjacent tissue adversely affect survival. The histologic type and grade of tumor and its size are important also, but nodal involvement (number and size) is the outstanding factor in prognosis. Unfortunately, more than 20 percent of patients with negative lymph nodes do have recurrences and die within 10 years. Although they are of lesser prognostic importance in breast cancers, high levels of estrogen receptors have a better prognosis than lower levels or none, although the best response to endocrine (antiestrogen) ablation therapy is noted with tumors containing both estrogen and progesterone receptors. Amplified or activated tumor oncogenes, particularly c-erb B2, may be associated with an aggressive tumor and poor prognosis.

487. The answer is a. (*Cotran, 5/e, pp 1176–1181. Rubin, 2/e, pp 1218–1228.*) Melanocytic hyperplasia, which causes hyperpigmentation of the skin, can be classified into several types of lesions. A lentigo consists of melanocytic hyperplasia in the basal layers of the epidermis along with elongation and thinning of the rete ridges. Two types of lentigines are lentigo simplex and lentigo senilis ("liver spots"). Increased numbers of melanocytes may form clusters located either at the tips of the rete ridges in the epidermis (junctional nevus), within the dermis (intradermal nevus), or both at the tips of the rete ridges and within the dermis (compound nevus). A blue nevus is composed of highly dendritic melanocytes that penetrate more deeply into the dermis. This deep location gives the lesion its characteristic blue color. The Spitz tumor (epithelioid cell nevus) is a benign lesion composed of groups of epithelioid and spindle melanocytes found in children and young adults. It may be mistaken histologically for a malignant melanoma. A freckle (ephelis) is a pigmented lesion caused by increased melanin pigmentation within keratinocytes of the basal layer of the epidermis. There is no increase in the number of melanocytes. These lesions fade with the lack of sun exposure.

488. The answer is b. (*Cotran, 5/e, p 1187. Rubin, 2/e, pp 1230–1232.*) Basal cell carcinoma, arising from the pluripotential cells in the basal layer of the epidermis, is the most common tumor in patients with pale skin. This carcinoma is locally invasive and may be quite destructive. Metastasis, however, is quite rare. The classic clinical appearance is a pearly papule with raised margins and a central ulcer. Variants, which are not infrequent, include the superficial type (which may be multifocal), the morphea-like type (which has marked fibrosis and is difficult to eradicate locally), and the pigmented type (which may be mistaken clinically for malignant melanoma). Histologically the cells are deeply basophilic with palisading at the periphery of groups of tumor cells and peritumoral clefting. Abundant eosinophilic cytoplasm may be seen in squamous cell carcinomas, not basal cell carcinoma.

489. The answer is e. *(Cotran, 5/e, pp 1173, 1186–1188. Rubin, 2/e, pp 1179–1181, 1185.)* The skin is made up of the epidermis and the dermis. The epidermis is composed of stratified keratinocytes, which produce keratin, tonofibrils, and keratohyaline bodies. The epidermal keratinocytes may give rise to squamous cell carcinomas. Several cell types normally immigrate into the epidermis. Melanocytes are dendritic cells that originate in the neural crest, migrate into the basal layer of the epidermis, and contain melanosomes. They may give rise to malignant melanomas. Langerhans cells are dendritic cells that process antigens, contain distinctive organelles (the racket-shaped Birbeck granules), and may give rise to one of the forms of Langerhans cell histiocytosis (histiocytosis X), such as Letterer-Siwe disease. Merkel cells, attached to keratinocytes by desmosomes, have distinctive membrane-bound, dense-core granules and may give rise to Merkel cell carcinoma. Mast cells are normally found about venules within the dermis, not the epidermis. They may proliferate, causing the disease urticaria pigmentosa.

490. The answer is b. *(Damjanov, 10/e, pp 2409–2410, 2443–2445, 2449, 2457. Lever, 7/e, p 497.)* Dense lymphocytic infiltration of the skin carries with it a differential diagnosis that includes the five L's: lupus, light, lymphoma, pseudolymphoma, and lymphotic infiltration of the skin (Jessner). All are characterized by lymphoid hyperplasia of the dermis. Leukemic lymphomas are diagnosed by atypical sheets of lymphoblastic cells with mitoses; lupus erythematosus is characterized by lymphoid infiltration around the follicles and vessels of the dermis. Light eruptions are characterized by a lymphocytic perivascular inflammation of the skin of the face. A difficult differential diagnosis includes lymphocytic infiltration of the skin (Jessner), which often has an increase in dermal mucopolysaccharides that can be demonstrated by alcian blue stains. In urticaria pigmentosa, a localized cutaneous form of mastocytosis that affects mainly children, there is infiltration of mast cells in the upper and middle dermis.

491. The answer is d. (*Cotran, 5/e, pp 1199–1205. Rubin, 2/e, pp 1190–1205.*) Patients of either sex in the fourth to sixth decade who develop oral vesicles followed by disseminated bullae are likely to have pemphigus vulgaris, one of the blistering (bullous) dermatoses. The differential diagnosis in this setting is widespread and can include various forms of erythema multiforme (or Stevens-Johnson syndrome in the young) and bullous pemphigoid, as well as pemphigus vulgaris. Common to most bullous dermatoses is the presence of epidermal cell separation, which produces spaces and clefts (acantholysis) that are visible in ordinary tissue sections and specific to location within the epidermis. The bullae may be subcorneal, intraepidermal, suprabasal, or subepidermal, and multiple diseases can be grouped according to acantholysis location. To categorize the type of disease further, direct immunofluorescence testing can be done on a fresh skin lesion, using antibodies to immunoglobulins, fibrin, and complement. Pemphigus vulgaris shows a characteristic "basket-weave" pattern in the epidermis to IgG, IgA is found at the tips of the dermal papillae in dermatitis herpetiformis, and linear bands of IgG and complement are found in the subepidermal zones in bullous pemphigoid, whereas erythema multiforme has no immunofluorescent pattern. In DLE, direct immunofluorescence shows a granular band of immunoglobulin and complement at the dermoepidermal junction (lupus band test), and this may be present in "normal" skin in patients with systemic lupus erythematosus.

492. The answer is d. (*Damjanov, 10/e, pp 2365, 2375–2376.*) The histologic distinction between benign, cystic intraductal papillomas of the breast and papillary adenocarcinomas is based on multiple criteria. The age of the patient is not of immense importance, since papillomas occur in both younger and older women. Benign papillomas are structured with a complex arrangement of papillary fronds of fibrovascular stalks, covered by one or (usually) two types of cells (epithelial and myoepithelial). Papillary carcinomas are usually of one monotonous cell type and have either no fibrovascular stalks or only a few of them. Papillary carcinomas show a uniform growth of cells with similar appearance with enclosed tubular spaces; the whole arrangement bridges across the entire lumen at times or simply lines the outer rim of the duct (cribriforming). Peripheral invasion of the stroma, if present at all, makes the diagnosis of carcinoma rather certain. There are lesions in which the differentiation is exceedingly difficult, even in the hands of renowned surgical pathologists. Many competent pathologists understandably prefer to defer the diagnosis on all papillary lesions of the breast on frozen section until well-fixed and optimally prepared permanent sections are available.

493. The answer is b. (*Cotran, 5/e, pp 1105–1106.*) Lobular carcinoma composes up to 10 percent of all histologic types of breast cancer, with duct carcinoma being the most common (70 to 75 percent of the total). It presumably arises from the terminal duct epithelium of the lobule, and it carries a high propensity to multifocality and bilateral breast involvement. There is evidence that this form of breast cancer gives rise to multiple, separate primaries within both breasts. For this reason, breast therapists currently advocate biopsies of the contralateral breast when the tumor is diagnosed. The lobular architectural spectrum begins with lobular hyperplasia and may then progress to lobular neoplasia, atypical lobular neoplasia (lobular carcinoma in situ), and, finally, infiltrating lobular carcinoma. Histologically, the tumor cells infiltrate in a characteristic single file pattern. Invasion of the epidermis by malignant cells is characteristic of Paget's disease.

494. The answer is a. (*Cotran, 5/e, pp 1100–1101. Rubin, 2/e, pp 982–984.*) Long and continuous exposure to endogenous estrogens increases the risk of developing breast carcinoma. Therefore, late menopause (after age 50), early menarche (especially before age 13), and nulliparity are all risk factors. Endometrial adenocarcinoma and occasional ovarian cancers are also associated with continuous estrogen stimulation with a resultant higher risk of the development of breast cancer in the same patient. Other factors include obesity—estrogen metabolism is altered in obese women and synthesis of estrone increased. Family history is significant, especially if mother and sister had premenopausal breast cancer, in which case there is an increased risk of 50 times that of controls. A past history of breast cancer, especially of lobular type, means greater risk of contralateral breast carcinoma. Hormonal and genetic factors and obesity are probably the major risk factors.

495. The answer is a. (*Damjanov, 10/e, pp 2370–2376.*) The most notorious malignant tumor of the breast, presenting a deceptively innocuous histologic and cytologic appearance, is angiosarcoma, with its almost unrecognizable anastomosing clear channels lined by flattened and barely visible endothelial cells. If this combination is seen within unequivocal breast lobules and ducts, the pathologist must suspect angiosarcoma. Well-differentiated adenocarcinoma of the breast (tubular carcinoma) demonstrates a tumor that is rather benign in appearance, with small ducts lined by single and innocuous-appearing epithelial cells. Whereas the primary site of mucinous carcinoma of the breasts (colloid carcinoma), with its "cysts" filled with extracellular mucin and signet-ring cells, presents no problem in diagnosis, biopsies of metastatic lesions will not infrequently show sheets of bland granular cells with pinpoint nuclei resembling granular cell tumor of the skin, a benign lesion. Early intraductal papillary carcinomas have been misdiagnosed at times as benign intraductal papillomas, and the reverse error has also occurred. Infiltrating duct (scirrhous) carcinoma presents no diagnostic problem in either frozen or permanent section analysis for the pathologist.

496. The answer is b. *(Cotran, 5/e, pp 1109–1110.)* Gynecomastia is enlargement of the male breast with marked hyperplasia of duct epithelium and proliferation of periductal connective tissue. No lobular or acinar tissue exists. Gynecomastia often occurs in response to hyperestrinism and may be found with functioning testicular tumors such as Leydig (interstitial) cell or, rarely, Sertoli cell tumors. The major cause of hyperestrinism in the male is cirrhosis because of deficient breakdown of estrogenic substances by the damaged liver. Digitalis therapy occasionally causes gynecomastia, and Klinefelter's syndrome frequently does so because very reduced circulating androgen results in relative hyperestrinism.

497–498. The answers are: 497-c, 498-d. *(Cotran, 5/e, pp 1206–1209.)* Fungal infections of the skin can be classified into superficial mycoses, cutaneous mycoses, and subcutaneous mycoses. The superficial mycoses are characterized by infection of the superficial layers of the skin. The most common type is pityriasis versicolor (tinea versicolor), an infection of the upper trunk which is caused by *Malassezia furfur* (*Pityrosporum orbiculare*). Clinically, there are multiple groups of macules (discolorations) with a fine peripheral scale. These macules are hyperpigmented (dark) in white-skinned races, while they are hypopigmented (light) in dark-skinned races. These areas will fluoresce yellow under a Wood's lamp. Potassium hydroxide (KOH) is used to identify fungal infections from scrapings of the skin. The KOH dissolves the keratin, and then the mycelial fungi can be seen. With tinea versicolor, KOH examination reveals a characteristic "spaghetti and meatball" appearance. The fragments of hyphae are the "spaghetti," while the round yeast cells are the "meatballs." Different types of tinea include tinea capitis, tinea corporis, tinea pedis (athlete's foot), and tinea versicolor.

Intracytoplasmic inclusions are characteristic of viral diseases. Molluscum contagiosum is a poxvirus that has a characteristic brick-shape appearance with a dumbbell-shaped DNA core. Molluscum is a self-limited pruritic disease of the skin that typically occurs on the trunk or the anogenital region. Impetigo is a common bacterial infection of the skin caused by either coagulase-positive staphylococci or group A beta-hemolytic streptococci. Erythema migrans describes a characteristic expanding erythematous lesion that may be caused by either the bite of the brown recluse spider or by *Ixodes dammini*, the vector for the spirochete that causes Lyme disease. Pediculosis is a pruritic infection that may be caused by the head louse, the crab louse, or the body louse.

499–500. The answers are: 499-g, 500-h. (*Cotran, 5/e, pp 1097–1099, 1105. Rubin, 2/e, pp 986–987.*) Infiltration of the nipple by large cells with clear cytoplasm is diagnostic of Paget's disease. These cells are usually found both singly and in small clusters in the epidermis. Paget's disease is always associated with (in fact begins with) an underlying intraductal carcinoma that extends to infiltrate the skin of nipple and areola. Paget cells may resemble the cells of superficial spreading melanoma, but they are PAS-positive diastase-resistant (mucopolysaccharide- or mucin-positive), unlike melanoma cells. Eczematous dermatitis of the nipples is a major differential diagnosis but is usually bilateral and responds rapidly to topical steroids. Paget's disease should be suspected if "eczema" persists more than 3 weeks with topical therapy. Paget's disease occurs mainly in middle-aged women but is unusual. In Paget's disease of the vulvar-anal-perineal region, there is very rarely underlying carcinoma. Mammary fibromatosis is a rare, benign, spindle cell lesion affecting women in the third decade. Clinically, it may mimic cancer with retraction or dimpling of skin. It should be treated by local excision with wide margins since there is risk of local recurrence.

Neoplasms of the breast may arise from ductal elements or stromal elements. Neoplastic proliferations of the stroma of the breast may lead to the formation of either fibroadenomas or phylloides tumors. Fibroadenomas are characterized histologically by a mixture of fibrous tissue and ducts, with no increase in cellularity or mitoses. Only the stromal cells, not the glandular cells, are clonal proliferations. Another neoplastic tumor that arises from the stromal cells is the phyllodes tumor. It is distinguished from the fibroadenoma by a more cellular stroma and the presence of stromal mitoses. The phyllodes tumor, which has been called a cystosarcoma phyllodes, may either be benign or malignant. A benign phylloides tumor is characterized by increased stromal cells with few mitoses, while a malignant phylloides tumor has increased stromal cells that are atypical and numerous mitoses are present.

Mammary duct ectasia is characterized by dilatation of ducts with inspissation of secretions, while fat necrosis is characterized histologically by necrotic fat which is surrounded by lipid-filled macrophages. Neither of these latter two lesions is neoplastic.

HIGH-YIELD FACTS
FOR PATHOLOGY

I. Cell injury

REVERSIBLE CELL INJURY

- swelling of cell organelles and entire cell
- ribosomes dissociate from endoplasmic reticulum
- decreased energy production by mitochondria
- increased glycolysis → decreased pH → nuclear chromatin clumping

IRREVERSIBLE CELL INJURY

- dense bodies within mitochondria (flocculent densities in heart)
- release of cellular enzymes (e.g. SGOT, LDH, and CPK after MI)
- nuclear degeneration (pyknosis, karyolysis, karyorrhexis)
- cell death

2. Fatty change of the liver

MECHANISMS

1. Increased free fatty acid delivery to liver

   - starvation
   - corticosteroids
   - diabetes mellitus

2. Increased formation of triglyceride

   - alcohol (note: NADH > NAD)

3. Decreased formation of apoprotein

   - carbon tetrachloride
   - protein malnutrition (kwashiorkor)

3. Cell death

APOPTOSIS

- single cells (not large groups of cells)
- cells shrink → form apoptotic bodies
- gene activation → forms endonucleases
- condensation of chromatin
- no inflammatory response

Examples of apoptosis:

1. physiologic

   - involution of the thymus
   - cell death within germinal centers of lymph nodes

- fragmentation of endometrium during menses
- lactating breast during weaning

2. pathologic

- viral hepatitis
- cytotoxic T cell mediated immune destruction (type IV hypersensitivity)

NECROSIS

- many cells or clusters of cells
- cells swell
- cause → hypoxia or toxins (irreversible injury)
- inflammation present

Examples of necrosis:

- coagulative necrosis → ischemia (except the brain)
- liquefactive necrosis → bacterial infection (and brain infarction)
- fat necrosis → pancreatitis and trauma to the breast
- caseous necrosis → tuberculosis
- fibrinoid necrosis → autoimmune disease (type III hypersensitivity reaction)
- gangrene → ischemia to extremities → dry (mainly coagulative necrosis) or wet (mainly liquefactive necrosis due to bacterial infection)

4. Terms

ADAPTATION

- hypertrophy → increase in the size of cells
- hyperplasia → increase in the number of cells
- atrophy → decrease size of an organ
- aplasia → failure of cell production
- hypoplasia → decrease in the number of cells
- metaplasia → replacement of one cell type by another
- dysplasia → abnormal cell growth

ABNORMAL ORGAN DEVELOPMENT

- anlage → primitive mass of cells
- aplasia → complete failure of an organ to develop (anlage present)
- agenesis → complete failure of an organ to develop (no anlage present)
- hypoplasia → reduction in the size of an organ due to a decrease in the number of cells
- atrophy → decrease in size of an organ due to a decrease in the number of preexisting cells

5. Cardinal signs of inflammation

- rubor → red
- calor → hot

- tumor → swollen
- dolor → pain

6. Complement cascade

PRODUCTS

- C3b → opsonin
- C5a → chemotaxis and leukocyte activation
- C3a, C4a, C5a → anaphylatoxins
- C5—9 → membrane attack complex

DEFICIENCIES

- deficiency of C3 and C5 → recurrent pyogenic bacterial infections
- deficiency of C6, C7, and C8 → recurrent infections with Neisseria species
- deficiency of C1 esterase inhibitor → hereditary angioedema
- deficiency of decay accelerating factor → paroxysmal nocturnal hemoglobinuria

7. Thromboxane vs prostacyclin

THROMBOXANE

- produced by platelets
- vasoconstriction
- stimulates platelet aggregation

PROSTACYCLIN

- produced by endothelial cells
- vasodilation
- inhibits platelet aggregation

8. Granulomatous inflammation

CASEATING GRANULOMAS

- aggregates of activated macrophages (epithelioid cells)
- tuberculosis

NON-CASEATING GRANULOMAS

- sarcoidosis
- fungal infections
- foreign-body reaction

9. Collagen types

FIBRILLAR COLLAGENS

- type I → skin, bones, tendons, mature scars
- type II → cartilage
- type III → embryonic tissue, blood vessels, pliable organs, immature scars

AMORPHOUS COLLAGENS
- type IV → basement membranes
- type VI → connective tissue

10. Edema

EXUDATES

1. Composition
   - increased protein
   - increased cells
   - specific gravity greater than 1.020

2. Cause
   - inflammation
   - increased blood vessel permeability

TRANSUDATES

1. Composition
   - no increased protein
   - no increased cells
   - specific gravity less than 1.012

2. Cause → abnormality of Starling forces

   a. increased hydrostatic (venous) pressure
      - congestive heart failure
      - portal hypertension

   b. decreased oncotic pressure → due to decreased albumin
      - liver disease
      - renal disease (nephrotic syndrome)

   c. lymphatic obstruction
      - tumors or surgery
      - filaria

11. Carcinomas

SQUAMOUS CELL CARCINOMA
- skin cancer
- lung cancer
- esophageal cancer
- cervical cancer

ADENOCARCINOMA
- lung cancer
- colon cancer
- stomach cancer
- prostate cancer
- endometrial cancer

TRANSITIONAL CELL CARCINOMA

- urinary bladder cancer
- renal cancer (renal pelvis)

CLEAR CELL CARCINOMA

- renal cancer (renal cortex)
- vaginal cancer

12. Neoplasms

BENIGN

- slow growth
- remain localized
- may have well-developed fibrous capsule
- do not metastasize
- well-differentiated histologically

MALIGNANT

- rapid growth
- locally invasive
- irregular growth with no capsule
- capable of metastasis
- variable degrees of differentiation (well-differentiated, moderately differentiated, poorly-differentiated)

13. Oncogene expression

GROWTH FACTORS

1. *c-sis*
   - beta chain of platelet derived growth factor
   - astrocytomas and osteogenic sarcomas

GROWTH FACTOR RECEPTORS

1. *c-erb B1*
   - receptor for epidermal growth factor
   - breast cancer and squamous cell carcinoma of the lung

2. *c-neu*
   - receptor for epidermal growth factor
   - breast cancer

3. *c-fms*
   - receptor for colony stimulating factor (CSF)
   - leukemia

ABNORMAL MEMBRANE PROTEIN KINASE

1. *c-abl*
   - membrane tyrosine kinase
   - chronic myelocytic leukemia (CML)

GTP-BINDING PROTEINS

1. *ras*
   - p21 (protein)
   - adenocarcinomas

NUCLEAR REGULATORY PROTEINS

1. *c-myc* → Burkitt's lymphoma
2. *N-myc* → neuroblastoma
3. *L-myc* → small cell carcinoma of the lung
4. *c-jun*
5. *c-fos*

14. Chromosomes and cancer

POINT MUTATIONS
   - *c-ras* → adenocarcinomas

TRANSLOCATIONS
   - *c-abl* on chromosome 9 → CML
   - *c-myc* on chromosome 8 → Burkitt's lymphoma
   - *bcl-2* on chromosome 18 → nodular lymphoma

GENE AMPLIFICATION
   - *N-myc* → neuroblastoma
   - *c-neu* → breast cancer
   - *c-erb B2* → breast cancer

15. Anti-oncogenes

TUMOR SUPPRESSOR GENES
   - Rb → retinoblastoma and osteogenic sarcoma
   - p53 → many tumors and the Li-Fraumeni syndrome
   - WT-1 → Wilms' tumor and aniridia
   - NF-1 → neurofibromatosis type 1

16. Chemical carcinogens

INITIATORS
   - tobacco smoke → many tumors
   - benzene → leukemias
   - vinyl chloride → angiosarcomas of the liver
   - beta-naphthylamine → cancer of the urinary bladder
   - azo dyes → tumors of the liver
   - aflatoxin → hepatoma
   - asbestos → mesotheliomas and lung tumors
   - arsenic → skin cancer

PROMOTERS
- saccharin → bladder cancer in rats
- hormones (estrogen)

17. Viruses and cancer

RNA VIRUSES
- acute transforming viruses
- slow transforming viruses
- HTLV-1 → adult T cell leukemia/lymphoma

DNA VIRUSES

1. HPV (different subtypes)
   - cervical neoplasia
   - condyloma
   - verruca vulgaris

2. EBV
   - African Burkitt's lymphoma
   - carcinoma of the nasopharynx
   - B cell immunoblastic lymphoma

3. hepatitis B and hepatitis C
   - liver cancer

18. Paraneoplastic syndromes

- Cushing's syndrome (increased cortisol) → lung cancer
- Carcinoid syndrome (increased serotonin) → lung cancer or carcinoid tumor of the small intestine
- SIADH (syndrome of inappropriate ADH secretion) → lung cancer and intracranial neoplasms
- hypercalcemia → lung cancer or multiple myeloma
- hypocalcemia → medullary carcinoma of the thyroid (procalcitonin)
- hypoglycemia → liver cancer and tumors of the mesothelium (mesotheliomas)
- polycythemia (erythropoietin) → kidney tumors, liver tumors, and cerebellar vascular tumors

19. Tumor markers

β-HCG (HUMAN CHORIONIC GONADOTROPIN)
- gestational trophoblastic disease (e.g. choriocarcinoma, hydatidiform mole)
- dysgerminoma
- seminoma (10% of cases)

AFP (α-FETOPROTEIN)
- liver cancer
- germ cell tumors (e.g. yolk sac tumors, embryonal carcinoma, NOT seminoma)

PSA (PROSTATE SPECIFIC ANTIGEN)
PAP (PROSTATIC ACID PHOSPHATASE)
- adenocarcinoma of prostate

CEA (CARCINOEMBRYONIC ANTIGEN)
- adenocarcinomas of colon, pancreas, stomach, and breast (nonspecific marker)

CA-125
- ovarian cancer

S-100
- melanoma
- neural tumors

20. Protein-energy malnutrition (PEM)

KWASHIORKOR
- dietary protein deficiency
- anasarca (generalized edema)
- fatty liver (due to decreased apoproteins and decreased VLDL synthesis)
- abnormal skin and hair
- defective enzyme formation → malabsorption (hard to treat)

MARASMUS
- dietary calorie deficiency
- generalized wasting ("skin and bones")

21. Nutritional deficiencies

VITAMIN A
- night blindness
- dry eyes and dry skin
- recurrent infections

VITAMIN D
- decreased calcium
- bone → decreased calcification, increased osteoid
- children → rickets
- adults → osteomalacia

VITAMIN E
- degeneration of posterior columns of spinal cord

VITAMIN K

- decreased vitamin K-dependent factors → II, VII, IX, X, and proteins C and S
- increased bleeding
- increased PT and PTT

VITAMIN B1 (THIAMINE)

- beri-beri → wet (cardiac) or dry (neurologic)
- Wernicke-Korsakoff syndrome (lesions of mamillary bodies)

VITAMIN B3 (NIACIN)

- pellagra → dermatitis, dementia, diarrhea (and death)

VITAMIN B12 (COBALAMIN)

- megaloblastic (macrocytic) anemia
- hypersegmented neutrophils (more than 5 lobes)
- subacute combined degeneration of the spinal cord

VITAMIN C (ASCORBIC ACID)

- scurvy
- defective collagen formation → poor wound healing (wounds reopen)
- bone → decreased osteoid
- perifollicular hemorrhages ("cork-screw" hair)
- bleeding gums and loose teeth

FOLATE

- megaloblastic (macrocytic) anemia
- hypersegmented neutrophils
- associated with neural tube defects in utero

IRON

- microcytic hypochromic anemia (with increased TIBC)

22. Inheritance patterns

AUTOSOMAL DOMINANT (AD)

- disease produce in heterozygous state
- no skipped generations → parents affected (unless new mutation or reduced penetrance)
- father to son transmission possible
- males and females affected equally
- recurrence risk is 50%

AUTOSOMAL RECESSIVE (AR)

- disease produce in homozygous state
- heterozygous individuals are carriers
- skipped generations
- father to son transmission possible

- males and females affected equally
- recurrence risk is 25%

X-LINKED DOMINANT (XD)

- no skipped generations
- no male to male transmission
- females affected twice as often as males

X-LINED RECESSIVE (XR)

- skipped generations
- no male to male transmissions
- affected males more frequent than affected females

Y INHERITANCE

- only males affected
- only male to male transmission
- all males affected

MITOCHONDRIAL

- males and females affected
- only females transmit the disease

23. Examples of XR

HEMATOLOGY DISEASES

- glucose-6-phosphate dehydrogenase deficiency
- hemophilia A (deficiency of factor VIII)
- hemophilia B (deficiency of factor IX)

IMMUNODEFICIENCY DISEASES

- Bruton's agammaglobulinemia
- chronic granulomatous disease
- Wiskott-Aldrich syndrome

STORAGE DISEASES

- Fabry disease
- Hunter's syndrome

MUSCLE DISEASES

1. Duchenne muscular dystrophy

   - defective dystrophin gene (muscle breakdown)
   - pseudohypertrophy of calf muscles
   - Gower maneuver (using hands to rise from floor)

2. Becker's muscular dystrophy

METABOLIC DISEASES

- diabetes insipidus
- Lesch-Nyhan syndrome

OTHER DISEASES
- red-green color blindness
- Fragile X syndrome

24. Chromosomes

TERMS
- haploid → number of chromosomes in germ cells (23)
- diploid → number of chromosomes found in non-germ cells (46)
- euploid → any exact multiple of the haploid number
- aneuploid → any non-multiple of the haploid number
- triploid → three times the haploid number (69)
- tetraploid → four times the haploid number (92)
- trisomy → three copies of same chromosome

25. Autosomal trisomies

TRISOMY 13 (PATAU SYNDROME)
- mental retardation
- microcephaly and microphthalmia
- holoprosencephaly (fused forebrain)
- fused central face ("cyclops")
- cleft lip and palate
- heart defects

TRISOMY 18 (EDWARD'S SYNDROME)
- mental retardation
- micrognathia
- heart defects
- rocker-bottom feet
- clenched fist with overlapping fingers

TRISOMY 21 (DOWN'S SYNDROME)
- most cases due to maternal nondisjunction during meiosis I
- associated with increased maternal age
- minority of cases due to Robertsonian (balanced) translocation
- mental retardation (most common familial cause)
- oblique palpebral fissures with epicanthal folds
- horizontal palmar crease
- heart defects (endocardial cushion defect is most common)
- acute lymphoblastic leukemia (first 2 years of life)
- Alzheimer's disease (almost 100% incidence after age 35)
- duodenal atresia (double-bubble sign on X-ray)

26. Chromosomal deletions

5p- (CRI DU CHAT)
- high pitched cry

- mental retardation
- heart defects and microcephaly

11p-

- Wilms tumor
- absence of iris

13q-

- retinoblastoma

15q-

1. Maternal deletion → Angelman syndrome
   - stiff ataxic gait with jerky movements
   - inappropriate laughter ("happy puppets")
   - may be due to two copies of paternal 15 chromosome (paternal uniparental disomy)

2. paternal deletion → Prader-Willi syndrome
   - mental retardation
   - short and obese
   - small hands and feet
   - hypogonadism
   - may be due to two copies of maternal 15 chromosome (paternal uniparental disomy)

27. Hypogonadism

KLINEFELTER'S SYNDROME

- most common genotype is 47XXY
- male hypogonadism
- testicular dysgenesis → small firm atrophic testes
- decreased testosterone
- increased FSH, LH, estradiol
- decreased secondary male characteristics
- tall, gynecomastia, and female distribution of hair
- infertility

TURNER'S SYNDROME

- most common genotype is 45XO
- female hypogonadism
- ovarian dysgenesis → streak ovaries
- decreased estrogen
- increased LH, FSH
- primary amenorrhea
- decreased secondary female characteristics
- skeletal abnormalities → short stature
- web neck (cystic hygroma)

28. Ambiguous sexual development

TRUE HERMAPHRODITE

- ovaries and testes both present

FEMALE PSEUDOHERMAPHRODITE (XX)

- ovaries
- male or ambiguous external genitalia
- due to excess androgens (e.g. congenital adrenal hyperplasia)

MALE PSEUDOHERMAPHRODITE (XY)

- testes
- female external genitalia
- due to decreased androgen effects (most common → testicular feminization)

ANDROGEN INSENSITIVITY SYNDROME (XY INDIVIDUAL)

- testicular feminization
- Müllerian duct regresses (due to MIF)
- Wolffian duct regresses (due to lack of testosterone receptors)
- phenotypic female (due to lack of receptors for DHT)

DECREASED 5 α REDUCTASE (XY INDIVIDUAL)

- testes form (due to presence of Y chromosome)
- Müllerian duct regresses (due to MIF)
- Wolffian duct develops (due to testosterone)
- decreased DHT (due to lack of 5 α reductase)
- variable external genitalia (due to decreased DHT)

TURNER'S SYNDROME (XO INDIVIDUAL)

- streak gonads (due to lack of two X chromosomes)
- Müllerian duct develops (due to lack of MIF)
- Wolffian duct regresses (due to lack of testosterone)
- external female (due to lack of DHT)
- decreased secondary female characteristics (due to decreased estrogen)

CONGENITAL ADRENAL HYPERPLASIA (XX INDIVIDUAL)

- ovaries develop (due to two X chromosomes)
- Müllerian duct develops (due to lack of MIF)
- Wolffian duct regresses (due to lack of local testosterone production)
- external male (due to excess systemic formation of DHT)

29. Disorders of trinucleotide repeats

1. Fragile X syndrome → CGG repeats
   - mental retardation (second most common familial cause)
   - long face with large ears

- large testes (macro-orchidism)
- trinucleotide sequence expanded in females, not males

2. Huntington's syndrome → CAG repeats
3. Myotonic dystrophy → GCT repeats
4. Spinal-bulbar muscular atrophy → CAG repeats

30. Lymphocytes

B CELLS

- form plasma cells which secrete immunoglobulin
- surface antigen receptor composed of immunoglobulin
- rearrange immunoglobulin genes from germ-line configuration
- CD19 → pan-B cell marker
- CD20 → pan-B cell marker, also called L26
- CD21 → pan-B cell marker, receptor for EBV
- CD22 → pan-B cell marker

T CELLS

- secrete lymphokines
- surface antigen receptor (TCR) is attached to CD3
- rearrange genes for T cell receptor
- CD2 → receptor for sheep erythrocyte (E rosette)
- CD3 → attached to T cell receptor
- CD4 → helper T cells, binds with MHC class II antigens
- CD5 → pan-T cell marker
- CD7 → pan-T cell marker
- CD8 → cytotoxic T cells, binds with MHC class I antigens

NATURAL KILLER CELLS

- large granular lymphocytes
- do not need previous sensitization
- CD16 → receptor for Fc portion of IgG

31. Immunoglobulins

IgM

- large molecule (pentamer)
- secreted early in immune response (primary response)
- can not cross the placenta
- can activate complement
- contains a J chain

IgG

- most abundant immunoglobulin in serum
- secreted during second antigen exposure (secondary or amnestic response)
- can cross the placenta

- can activate complement
- can function as opsonin

IgE

- allergies, asthma, parasitic infection
- found attached to the surface of basophils and mast cells
- participates in type I hypersensitivity reactions

IgA

- usually a dimer with a J chain and a secretory component
- found along GI tract and respiratory tract
- secretory immunoglobulin
- can activate alternate complement pathway

IgD

- receptor for B cells
- found on the surface of mature B cells

32. T lymphocytes

CD4+ CELLS

- helper T lymphocytes
- respond to MHC class II antigens

subtypes

1. T-helper-1 cells (T_H1)
   - secrete → IL-2, IL-3, GM-CSF, γ-interferon, and lymphotoxin (β TNF)
   - stimulate cell-mediate immune reactions → fight intracellular organisms
2. T-helper-2 cells (T_H2)
   - secrete → IL-3, IL-4, IL-5, IL-6, IL-10, and GM-CSF
   - stimulate antibody production → fight extracellular organisms

CD8+ CELLS

- cytotoxic T lymphocytes
- respond to MHC class I antigens

33. Major histocompatibility complex (MHC)

CLASS I ANTIGENS

- found on all nucleated cells
- transmembrane alpha glycoprotein chain with beta2 microglobulin
- react with antibodies and CD8-positive lymphocytes
- fight virus infected cells and transplants

CLASS II ANTIGENS

- found on antigen-presenting cells, B cells, and T cells
- transmembrane alpha chain and beta chain

- react with CD4-positive lymphocytes
- fight exogenous antigens which have been processed by antigen-presenting cells

34. Diseases associated with HLA types

- ankylosing spondylitis → HLA-B27
- primary hemochromatosis → HLA-A3
- 21-hydroxylase deficiency → HLA-BW47
- rheumatoid arthritis → HLA-DR4
- insulin-dependent (type I) diabetes mellitus → HLA-DR3/DR4
- systemic lupus erythematosus → HLA-DR2/DR3

35. Hypersensitivity reactions

TYPE I

- binding of antigen to previously formed IgE bound to mast cells and basophils
- release of histamine and leukotrienes C4 and D4
- urticaria (hives)
- anaphylaxis

TYPE II

- antibody (IgG or IgM) binds to antigens insitu
- cells destroyed by complement or cytotoxic cells (antibody-dependent cell-mediated cytotoxicity)
- linear immunofluorescence (IF)
- transfusion reactions

TYPE III

- antibody (IgG or IgM) binds to antigens forming immune complexes
- granular IF
- systemic → serum sickness
- local reaction → Arthus reaction

TYPE IV

1. delayed-type hypersensitivity
   - CD4 lymphocytes
   - extrinsic antigen associated with class II MHC
   - formation of activated macrophages (epithelioid cells) → granulomas
   - PPD skin test
   - contact dermatitis (poison ivy, poison oak)
2. cell-mediated immunity
   - CD8 lymphocytes
   - intrinsic antigen associated with class I MHC
   - viral infections and transplant rejection

36. Autoantibodies

NUCLEAR

- diffuse (homogenous) → DNA (many diseases), histones (drug-induced SLE)
- rim (peripheral) → double-stranded DNA (SLE)
- speckled (non-DNA extractable nuclear proteins) → Smith (SLE), SS-A and SS-B (Sjögren's syndrome), Scl-70 (progressive systemic sclerosis)
- nucleolar (RNA) → many (e.g. progressive systemic sclerosis)
- centromere → CREST syndrome

CYTOPLASMIC

- mitochondria → primary biliary cirrhosis

CELLS

- smooth muscle → lupoid hepatitis (autoimmune chronic active hepatitis)
- neutrophils → Wegener's granulomatosis and microscopic polyarteritis
- parietal cell and intrinsic factor → pernicious anemia
- microvasculature of muscle → dermatomyositis

PROTEINS

- immunoglobulin → rheumatoid arthritis
- thyroglobulin → Hashimoto's thyroiditis

STRUCTURAL ANTIGENS

- lung and glomerular basement membranes → Goodpasture's disease
- intercellular space of epidermis → pemphigus vulgaris
- epidermal basement membrane → bullous pemphigoid

RECEPTORS

- acetylcholine receptor → myasthenia gravis
- thyroid hormone receptor → Graves' disease
- insulin receptor → diabetes mellitus

37. Antineutrophil cytoplasmic antibodies (ANCA)

1. c-ANCA (cytoplasmic)
   - proteinase 3 → Wegener's granulomatosis
2. p-ANCA (perinuclear)
   - myeloperoxidase → microscopic polyarteritis

38. Amyloidosis

AMYLOID

- any protein having β-pleated sheet tertiary configuration
- apple-green birefringence with Congo red stain

SYSTEMIC DEPOSITION

- multiple myeloma → deposits of amyloid light protein
- chronic inflammatory diseases → deposits of amyloid associated protein
- hemodialysis → deposits of beta2-microglobulin

LOCALIZED DEPOSITION

- senile cardiac disease → deposits of amyloid transthyretin
- Alzheimer's disease → deposits of beta2 amyloid protein
- medullary carcinoma of thyroid → deposits of procalcitonin
- non-insulin dependent diabetes mellitus (type II) → amyloid deposits in islets of Langerhans of pancreas

39. Defects in inflammation or immunity

CHEDIAK-HIGASHI SYNDROME

- autosomal recessive
- defective polymerization of microtubules
- giant lysosomes in leukocytes
- recurrent infections
- albinism (abnormal formation of melanin)

CHRONIC GRANULOMATOUS DISEASE

- defective NADPH oxidase (enzyme on membrane of lysosomes)
- recurrent infections with catalase positive organisms
- abnormal nitroblue tetrazolium dye test

SEVERE COMBINED IMMUNODEFICIENCY (SCID)

1. X-linked form

   - defect in IL-2 receptor

2. autosomal recessive form (Swiss type)

   - lack of adenosine deaminase
   - prenatal diagnosis and gene therapy possible

X-LINKED AGAMMAGLOBULINEMIA OF BRUTON

- defective maturation of B lymphocytes past the pre-B stage
- absence of germinal centers and plasma cells
- bacterial infections begin at the age of nine months (loss of maternal antibody)
- therapy with immunoglobulin injections

COMMON VARIABLE IMMUNODEFICIENCY

- variable clinical presentation
- recurrent infections → especially bacteria and Giardia
- hyperplastic B cell areas
- therapy with immunoglobulin injections

ISOLATED DEFICIENCY OF IgA

- most patients are asymptomatic
- may develop anti-IgA antibodies
- risk of anaphylaxis with transfusion

DiGEORGE'S SYNDROME

- defective development of pharyngeal pouches 3 and 4
- deletion of chromosome 22
- lack of thymus → no T cells (recurrent viral and fungal infections)
- lack of parathyroid glands → (hypocalcemia and tetany)
- congenital heart defects

ACQUIRED IMMUNODEFICIENCY SYNDROME (AIDS)

- cause → HIV
- infection of CD4+ T lymphocytes
- inversion of CD4:CD8 ratio (normal is 2:1)
- decreased humoral and cell-mediated immunity → recurrent infections
- increased incidence of malignancy (Kaposi sarcoma and immunoblastic lymphoma)

40. Viral changes

GIANT CELLS

- herpes simplex virus (HSV)
- cytomegalic virus (CMV)
- measles (Warthin-Finkeldey giant cells)
- respiratory syncytial virus

INCLUSIONS

- herpes simplex virus (Cowdry A bodies)
- smallpox virus (Guarnieri bodies)
- rabies virus (Negri bodies)
- molluscum contagiosum (molluscum bodies)

GROUND GLASS CHANGE

- nucleus = herpes simplex virus
- cytoplasm (of hepatocytes) = hepatitis B

ATYPICAL CELLS

- atypical lymphocytes → Ebstein-Barr virus
- smudge cells → adenovirus (respiratory epithelial cells)
- koilocytosis → human papillomavirus (HPV)

41. Systemic mycoses

CANDIDIASIS

- *Candida albicans*
- pseudohyphae
- white plaques (thrush)

HISTOPLASMOSIS
- *Histoplasma capsulatum*
- found within the cytoplasm of macrophages
- bird droppings
- Ohio and Mississippi valleys

ASPERGILLOSIS
- aspergillus species
- septate hyphae with acute-angle branching
- fruiting bodies (when exposed to air → fungus ball in lung cavity)

BLASTOMYCOSIS
- *Blastomyces dermatitidis*
- broad-based budding

COCCIDIOMYOCOSIS
- *coccidioides immitis*
- large spherules filled with many small endospores
- Southwest United States (San Joaquin Valley)

CRYPTOCOCCOSIS
- *cryptococcus neoformans*
- CNS infection in immunosuppressed patients
- mucicarmine-positive capsule
- India ink stain of CSF

MUCORMYCOSIS
- nasal infection in diabetic patients
- broad, non-septate hyphae with right angle branching

42. Familial hyperlipidemia

TYPE I HYPERLIPOPROTEINEMIA
- familial hyperchylomicronemia
- mutation in lipoprotein lipase gene
- increased serum chylomicrons

TYPE II HYPERLIPOPROTEINEMIA
- familial hypercholesterolemia
- mutation involving LDL receptor
- increased serum LDL
- increased serum cholesterol

TYPE III HYPERLIPIDEMIA
- floating or broad β disease
- mutation in apolipoprotein E
- increased chylomicron remnants and IDL
- increased serum triglyceride and cholesterol

TYPE IV HYPERLIPIDEMIA
- familial hypertriglyceridemia
- unknown mutation
- increased serum VLDL
- increased serum triglyceride and cholesterol

TYPE V HYPERLIPIDEMIA
- mutation in apolipoprotein CII
- increased serum chylomicrons and VLDL
- increased serum triglyceride and cholesterol

43. Aneurysms

ATHEROSCLEROTIC ANEURYSMS
- cause → atherosclerosis
- location → abdominal aorta (between renal arteries and bifurcation of the aorta)
- pulsatile mass
- may rupture → sudden, severe abdominal pain in male older than 55

LUETIC ANEURYSMS
- cause → syphilis (treponema) infection
- obliterative endarteritis (plasma cells around small blood vessels)
- location → ascending (thoracic) aorta
- may produce aortic regurgitation or rupture

DISSECTING ANEURYSMS
1. due to cystic medial necrosis of aorta
   - hypertension
   - Marfan syndrome → due to defect in fibrillin gene
2. "double-barrel" aorta on X-ray

BERRY ANEURYSMS
- location → bifurcation of arteries in circle of Willis
- most commonly bifurcation of anterior communicating artery
- subarachnoid hemorrhage
- associated with polycystic renal disease

44. Cardiac hypertrophy

CONCENTRIC HYPERTROPHY
- response to pressure overload (e.g. hypertension or aortic stenosis)
- sarcomeres proliferate in parallel
- increased ventricular thickness
- no change in size of ventricular cavity

ECCENTRIC HYPERTROPHY

- response to volume overload
- sarcomeres proliferate in series
- no increase in ventricle thickness
- increase in size of ventricular cavity

45. Congenital heart defects

LEFT-TO-RIGHT SHUNTS

1. ventricular septal defects (VSD) → most common congenital cardiac anomaly
2. atrial septal defects (ASD)
3. patent ductus arteriosus (PDA)
   - "machine-like" heart murmur
   - indomethacin closes PDA

RIGHT-TO-LEFT SHUNTS

1. Tetralogy of Fallot (TOF) → most common cause of congenital cyanotic heart disease
   - pulmonary stenosis
   - ventricular septal defect
   - dextroposition (over-riding) aorta
   - right ventricular hypertrophy

NO SHUNTS

1. coarctation of the aorta
   - infantile type (preductal)
   - adult type (postductal) → rib notching, increased BP in upper extremities, decreased BP in lower extremities
2. transposition of the great vessels
   - need shunt to be present to survive (e.g. PDA)
   - PGE keeps ductus open

46. Atrophy of the stomach

TYPE A → AUTOIMMUNE GASTRITIS

- autoantibodies to parietal cells and intrinsic factor → pernicious anemia
- decreased vitamin B12 → megaloblastic anemia
- increased serum gastrin levels
- histologic changes found in fundus of stomach

TYPE B → ENVIRONMENTAL

- no autoantibodies present

- associated with *Helicobacter pylori* (urease positive)
- decreased serum gastrin levels
- histologic changes found in antrum of stomach

47. Inflammatory bowel disease (IBD)

ULCERATIVE COLITIS

- crypt abscesses (microabscesses) and crypt distortion
- disease begins in rectum and extends proximally (no skip lesions)
- does not involve small intestines
- superficial mucosal involvement (not transmural)
- increased risk of colon cancer and toxic megacolon

CROHN'S DISEASE

- granulomas
- segmental involvement (skip lesions)
- may involve small intestines (regional enteritis or ileitis)
- transmural involvement → fissures, fistulas, and obstruction

48. Gallstones

CHOLESTEROL STONES

- yellow stones
- risk factors → fat, female, fertile, forty
- increased incidence in Native Americans

BILIRUBIN (PIGMENT) STONES

- black stones
- risk factors → chronic hemolysis and infections of biliary tract
- increased incidence in Asians

49. Congenital adrenal hyperplasia (CAH)

21-HYDROXYLASE DEFICIENCY

- decreased cortisol → increased ACTH
- decreased aldosterone
- sodium loss in the urine → salt-wasting form of CAH
- hyperkalemic acidosis
- virilism in females

11-HYDROXYLASE DEFICIENCY

- decreased cortisol → increased ACTH
- decreased aldosterone
- increased DOC and 11-deoxycortisol → increased mineralocorticoid effects
- sodium retention → hypertensive form of CAH
- hypokalemic alkalosis
- virilism in females

17-HYDROXYLASE DEFICIENCY

- decreased cortisol → increased ACTH
- no decreased aldosterone
- decreased sex hormones
- females → primary amenorrhea
- males → pseudohermaphrodites

50. Multiple endocrine neoplasia

TYPE I (WERMER'S SYNDROME)

- parathyroid
- pituitary
- pancreas

TYPE II (SIPPLE'S SYNDROME)

- parathyroid
- medullary carcinoma of thyroid
- pheochromocytoma

TYPE III (MEN IIb)

- medullary carcinoma of thyroid
- pheochromocytoma
- mucosal neuromas

51. Renal (glomerular) syndromes

NEPHROTIC SYNDROME

- marked proteinuria → hypoalbuminemia and edema
- increased cholesterol → oval fat bodies in the urine

examples (non-proliferative glomerular disease)

1. minimal change disease (lipoid nephrosis)

   - normal light microscopy
   - EM reveals fusion of foot processes of podocytes

2. focal segmental glomerulosclerosis (FSGS)

3. membranous glomerulonephropathy (MGN)

   - thickening of basement membrane ("spikes and domes")
   - uniform subepithelial deposits

4. diabetes mellitus

NEPHRITIC SYNDROME

- hematuria (red blood cells and red blood cell casts in urine)
- variable proteinuria and oliguria
- retention of salt and water (hypertension and edema)

examples (proliferative glomerular disease)
1. focal segmental glomerulonephritis (FSGN)
   - mesangial deposits of IgA
   - Berger's disease
2. acute (diffuse) proliferative glomerulonephritis (DPGN)
   - post-streptococcal glomerulonephritis
   - large, irregular subepithelial deposits
3. membranoproliferative glomerulonephritis (MPGN)
   - subendothelial deposits → type I MPGN
   - intramembranous deposits → type II MPGN (dense deposit disease)
   - splitting of basement membrane by mesangium → "tram-track" appearance
4. rapidly progressive glomerulonephritis (RPGN)

52. Glomerular deposits

SUBEPITHELIAL
   - Diffuse Proliferative Glomerulonephritis (DPGN) → irregular and large
   - Membranous Glomerulopathy (MGN) → uniform and small

INTRAMEMBRANOUS (BASEMENT MEMBRANE)
   - Membranoproliferative Glomerulonephritis (MPGN), type II

SUBENDOTHELIAL
   - Membranoproliferative Glomerulonephritis, type I
   - SLE

MESANGIAL
   - Focal Segmental Glomerulonephritis (FSGN)
   - Henoch-Schonlein purpura

53. Rapidly progressive glomerulonephritis (RPGN)

LINEAR IMMUNOFLUORESCENCE
   - anti-membrane antibody
   - Goodpasture's disease

GRANULAR IMMUNOFLUORESCENCE
   - immune complexes
   - other glomerular or systemic disease

MINIMAL OR NEGATIVE IMMUNOFLUORESCENCE
   - pauci-immune disease
   - Wegener's granulomatosis
   - microscopic polyarteritis nodosa

54. Cerebral hemorrhage

EPIDURAL HEMATOMA

- severe trauma
- arterial bleeding (middle meningeal artery)
- symptoms occur rapidly

SUBDURAL HEMATOMA

- minimal trauma in elderly
- venous bleeding (bridging veins)
- symptoms occur slowly

SUBARACHNOID HEMORRHAGE

- rupture of berry aneurysm
- "worst headache ever"
- bloody or xanthochromic spinal tap

55. Infections of the meninges

BACTERIAL INFECTIONS

- increased neutrophils and protein in CSF
- decreased glucose in CSF
- life-threatening

Age	Organism
neonates	*Escherichia coli*
6 months to 6 years	*Streptococcus pneumoniae*
6 years to 16 years	*Neisseria meningitidis* (meningococcus)
older than 16 years	*Streptococcus pneumoniae*
epidemics	*Neisseria meningitidis*

VIRAL INFECTIONS

- increased lymphocytes in CSF
- normal glucose in CSF
- mild and self-limited

56. Atrophy of the nervous system

ALZHEIMER'S DISEASE

- diffuse atrophy of cerebral cortex
- dementia (most common cause in elderly)
- senile plaques (with β-amyloid core)
- neurofibrillary tangles (with abnormal tau protein)

PICK'S DISEASE

- unilateral frontal or temporal lobe atrophy

HUNTINGTON'S DISEASE

- atrophy of caudate and putamen → decreased GABA and acetylcholine

- progressive dementia
- choreiform movements

PARKINSON'S DISEASE

- substantia nigra (depigmentation)
- decreased dopamine in corpus striatum
- cogwheel rigidity and akinesia
- tremor
- treatment → dopamine agonists

57. Joints

RHEUMATOID ARTHRITIS

- rheumatoid factor (IgM antibody against antibody)
- pannus formation in synovium (hyperplastic synovium with lymphocytes and plasma cells)
- ulnar deviation of fingers
- subcutaneous rheumatoid nodules (at pressure points)
- pain worse in morning

OSTEOARTHRITIS

- degenerative joint disease ("wear and tear")
- loss of articular cartilage → smooth subchondral bone (eburnation)
- osteophyte formation (DIP → Heberden's nodes, PIP → Bouchard's nodes)
- pain worse in evening

GOUT

- hyperuricemia → precipitation of monosodium urate crystals (needle-shaped negatively birefringent crystals)
- first MTP joint (big toe)
- tophus formation
- increased production of uric acid → Lesch-Nyhan syndrome
- increased turnover of nucleic acid → leukemias and lymphomas
- decreased excretion of uric acid → chronic renal disease, ethanol intake, diabetes

58. Stains

ROUTINE (H&E)

1. Hematoxylin
   - blue and basic
   - stains negatively charged structures → DNA and RNA
2. Eosin
   - pink and acidophilic
   - stains positively charged structures → mitochondria

SPECIAL STAINS
- fats → oil red O
- glycogen → PAS positive, diastase sensitive
- iron → Prussian blue
- hemosiderin → Prussian blue
- amyloid → Congo red
- alpha-1-antitrypsin → PAS positive, diastase resistant
- calcium → von Kossa

59. Enzymes

AMINOTRANSFERASES (AST, ALT)
- myocardial infarction (AST)
- alcoholic hepatitis (AST > ALT)
- viral hepatitis (ALT > AST)

CREATINE KINASE (CK OR CPK)
- myocardial infarction (CPK-MB)
- muscle diseases (DMD)

LACTATE DEHYDROGENASE (LDH)
- myocardial infarction (LDH1 > LDH2)

AMYLASE OR LIPASE
- acute pancreatitis

60. Histologic "bodies"

1. psammoma bodies:
   - papillary carcinoma of the thyroid
   - papillary tumors of the ovary
   - meningioma
2. immunoglobulin
   - Russel body → cytoplasmic or extracellular
   - Dutcher body → nucleus (Waldenstroms)
3. Councilman body → viral hepatitis
4. Mallory body → alcoholic hyaline
5. Cowdry A body → herpes
6. Aschoff body → rheumatoid fever
7. ferruginous body → asbestos
8. Negri body → rabies
9. Lewy body → Parkinson's
10. Heinz bodies (denatured hemoglobin) → G6PD deficiency
11. Barr body → number of X chromosomes minus one

61. Healing of the myocardium after a myocardial infarction

	Gross	Light
0-12 hours	none	usually none (?wavy fibers)
12-24 hours	pallor	coagulative necrosis
1-3 days	hyperemic (red) border	above + neutrophils
4-7 days	pale-yellow	above + macrophages
7-14 days	red-purple border	above + granulation tissue
> 2 weeks	gray-white scar	fibrosis (scar)

62. Familial storage disorders

Storage disease	Enzyme deficiency	Substance accumulating
· Pompe Disease	α-1,4-glucosidase (acid maltase)	glycogen
· Hurler's Syndrome	α-L-iduronidase	heparan sulfate, dermatan sulfate
· Hunter's Syndrome	L-iduronosulfate sulfatase	heparan sulfate, dermatan sulfate
· Niemann-Pick Disease	sphingomyelinase	sphingomyelin
· Tay-Sachs Disease	hexosaminidase A	GM_2-ganglioside
· Sandhoff disease	hexosaminidase A and B	GM_2-ganglioside and globoside
· Gaucher Disease	glucocerebrosidase	glucocerebroside
· Fabry Disease	α-galactosidase A	ceramide trihexosidase

BIBLIOGRAPHY

Abenhaim L, Moride Y, Brenot F, et al: Appetite-suppressant drugs and the risk of primary pulmonary hypertension. *N Engl J Med* 335(9): 609–16, 1996.

Adams RD, Victor M: *Principles of Neurology*, 5/e. New York, McGraw-Hill, 1993.

Alberts B, et al: *Molecular Biology of the Cell*, 3/e. New York, Garland Publishing, 1994.

Brawer MK: Prostatic intraepithelial neoplasia: A premalignant lesion. *Hum Pathol* 23:242–248, 1992.

Chandrasoma P, Taylor CR: *Concise Pathology*, 3/e. Stamford, Appleton and Lange, 1998.

Connolly HM, Crary JL, et al: Valvular heart disease associated with fenfluramine-phentermine. *N Engl J Med* 337(9): 581–8, 1997.

Cotran RS, Kumar V, Robbins SL: *Pathologic Basis of Disease*, 5/e. Philadelphia, Saunders, 1994.

Damjanov I, Linder J (eds): *Anderson's Pathology*, 10/e. St. Louis, Mosby, 1996.

Duchin JS, et al: Hantavirus pulmonary syndrome: A clinical description of 17 patients with a newly recognized disease. *N Engl J Med* 330:949–955, 1994.

Fawcett DW: *A Textbook of Histology*, 12/e. New York, Chapman & Hall, 1994.

Flake AW, Roncarolo MG, et al: Brief report: Treatment of x-linked severe combined immunodeficiency by in utero transplantation of paternal bone marrow. *N Engl J Med* 335(24): 1806–10, 1996.

Ganong WF: *Review of Medical Physiology*, 17/e. Norwalk, CT, Appleton & Lange,1995.

Henry JB, et al (eds): *Clinical Diagnosis and Management by Laboratory Methods*, 19/e. Philadelphia, Saunders, 1996.

Isselbacher KJ, et al (eds): *Harrison's Principles of Internal Medicine*, 13/e. New York, McGraw-Hill, 1994.

Joklik WK, et al (eds): *Zinsser Microbiology*, 20/e. Norwalk, CT, Appleton & Lange, 1992.

Larsen WJ: *Human Embryology*, 1/e. New York, Churchill Livingstone, 1993.

Lee GR, et al (eds): *Wintrobe's Clinical Hematology*, 9/e. Philadelphia, Lea & Febiger, 1993.

Lever WF, Schaumberg-Lever G: *Histopathology of the Skin*, 7/e. Philadelphia, Lippincott, 1990.

Rubin E, Farber JL: *Pathology*, 2/e. Philadelphia, Lippincott, 1994.

Silverberg SG (ed): *Principles and Practice of Surgical Pathology*, 2/e. New York, Churchill Livingstone, 1990.